Consuming and Producing Research in Communication Sciences and Disorders

DEVELOPING POWER OF PROFESSOR

Consuming and Producing Research in Communication Sciences and Disorders

DEVELOPING POWER OF PROFESSOR

Robert Goldfarb, PhD

PLURAL PUBLISHING INC.

PLURAL PUBLISHING
INC.

5521 Ruffin Road
San Diego, CA 92123

e-mail: information@pluralpublishing.com
Website: http://www.pluralpublishing.com

Typeset in 10.5/13 Palatino by Flanagan's Publishing Services, Inc.
Printed in the United States of America by Integrated Books International

Library of Congress Cataloging-in-Publication Data

Names: Goldfarb, Robert (Robert M.), author.
Title: Consuming and producing research in communication sciences and disorders : developing power of professor / Robert Goldfarb.
Description: San Diego, CA : Plural Publishing, [2021] | Includes bibliographical references and index.
Identifiers: LCCN 2019015046 | ISBN 9781635500677 (alk. paper) | ISBN 1635500672 (alk. paper)
Subjects: | MESH: Communication Disorders | Research Design | Biomedical Research
Classification: LCC RC423 | NLM WL 340.2 | DDC 362.196/855--dc23
LC record available at https://lccn.loc.gov/2019015046

CONTENTS

PART III. DISSEMINATING RESEARCH IN CSD

INTRODUCTION

Power of attorney has been part of general business law since 1948 and includes durable and nondurable forms, with the former continuing in effect even if the individual who grants the power becomes disabled or incompetent. Nondurable general power of attorney gives a designated person powers to handle property, acting as an agent. These powers end if the person designating the power becomes disabled or incompetent. The powers permit the assigned individual to mortgage, sell, or dispose of any real or personal property without advance notice or approval. This power does not authorize anyone to make medical or other health care decisions, which require a health care proxy.

Just as the above powers are consistent with the duties of a licensed attorney-at-law, the power to conduct research is consistent with the duties of a professor. The job description of any university professor is likely to include references to the three areas of academic instruction; service to department, school, university, and professional organizations; and research, including publication in refereed, peer-reviewed journals. The proposal here is to begin a discussion of what constitutes power of professor and what obligations an individual, professor or not, has before being permitted to do research. This book represents some preliminary thoughts.

Unlike other texts on evaluating research in communication sciences and disorders (CSD), this book includes the "doing" of research, considering the welfare and confidentiality of patients and participants. Preparation for power of professor should also include an understanding of types of research, threats to reliability and validity, philosophy of science, and the relationships among theory, research, and therapy. The emphasis is NOT on professors, but on clinically oriented professionals who can perform the research associated with professors, much as individuals who are not attorneys can perform contractual work. The purpose of the book is to guide nonprofessors in attaining the competencies required to consume, produce, and disseminate research (and achieve power of professor).

Why have I chosen to write this book? I have spent my career as a practicing speech-language pathologist as well as a consumer and producer of research—as a professor teaching master's- and doctoral-level courses in Research Methods and as a research mentor to students and junior faculty. Further, for nearly 30 years, I have also been a senior administrator or program director in three university settings where research is a major focus.

Who is this book written for? It is a core textbook for undergraduate and first-year graduate students taking Research Methods courses in speech-language pathology and audiology. It is not for advanced graduate students, especially those in Research 1 universities where students are supported by senior faculty who have multiyear, renewable grants. Those privileged students will not need this book to develop power of professor because it is likely that they will earn doctorate (PhD) degrees and become professors. My hope is that students whose passions and goals are to provide best practices to individuals with communication disorders will realize that evidence-based practice is research-based practice. I hope these students, as well as their clinical supervisors and other practicing clinicians, will learn how much fun it is to do research, that is, to discover a small piece of truth about communication sciences and disorders. It is well worth the hard work involved in mastering research methodologies, because the payoffs are better treatment of the individuals we serve and a deeper understanding of communication disorders and clinical interventions.

There are many fine books on evaluating research in CSD, including some published by Plural, that tend to focus either on statistics or on the student as a consumer of research. The relevant chapter (Chapter 6) of the current text addresses only the statistics most essential to interpreting the Results section of a journal article. Part I also includes academic–clinical integration of research, as well as information required for consumption of research such as research ethics, the scientific method, types of research, and how to critique a journal article and a diagnostic test. The second part of the book should help guide the undergraduate student in producing a capstone project or senior thesis and the master's student in producing a graduate thesis or research project. Part II of the book also addresses mentoring, the Institutional Review Board, and conducting academic and clinical research. Part III addresses dissemination of research, from the traditional (presenting and publishing academic and clinical research) to the nontraditional (marketing, social media, and Web 2.0 technologies).

There is a shortage of people with PhDs in CSD. In fact, some university searches to replace faculty who retire from or leave their positions fail because of a lack of an adequate application pool. If we restrict clinical CSD research only to individuals who have a PhD, then it will be necessary to have scholars in other disciplines (e.g., psychology) answer our research questions for us. If that happens, our right to exist as an independent discipline will be in jeopardy. The quality of experimental research in CSD is not at risk; in fact, it gets more competitive (in terms of success in funding multiyear, renewable grants), sophisticated (in terms of use of technology and advanced instrumentation), and valid (in terms of adhering to the highest standards of research) with each passing year. In other words, evidence-based practice is in pretty good shape. Practice-based evidence, on the other hand, is not, nor is dissemination of research.

This book is meant to empower students who want to be clinicians to generate the clinical evidence that will go back to the laboratories for experimental researchers to generate new theories about communication disorders. It is meant to help translate new research findings not only from the lab to the clinic (called "bench-to-bedside" in the medical community) and back again, but also from clinic to community and back again, as well as to influence public health policies. My vision is to help create a cohort of students who are equipped with power of professor when they graduate. Individuals with power of professor will have the knowledge and skills provided in this book that are necessary and sufficient to conduct research, even if they do not have a PhD degree.

I take certain liberties in using the first person ("I," rather than "the author") when referring to some of my own clinical and research experiences and the second person ("you," rather than "the reader") when referring to some of the skills needed to develop power of professor. There is also some intentional redundancy when I find it useful to rephrase some important concepts in different contexts. Finally, although I have tried to include a wide variety of topics and authors, including some articles that have won awards from ASHA, I include many of my own studies, not to be self-serving (I hope), but because I have been intimately involved in the research.

The book is organized in three parts devoted to consuming, producing, and disseminating research.

PART I. CONSUMING RESEARCH IN CSD

It is important to become an educated consumer of research before attempting to produce or disseminate it. You need to know what typical researchers do before attempting it, just as your undergraduate CSD curriculum was structured to include typical language development and basic hearing and speech science before delving into communication disorders. Recall that your undergraduate CSD curriculum started with phonetics, anatomy and physiology of the speech and hearing mechanisms, speech and hearing science, and typical acquisition of language before you learned about language, speech, and hearing disorders. Chapters 1 through 8 focus on educating the consumer of research with a primary focus on clinical research, although laboratory and group studies are also addressed.

Chapter 1. Developing Power of Professor: The Nature of Research in CSD

Learning Objectives

After reading this chapter, the student will be able to

- explain why academic and clinical research is important;
- critically evaluate whether research is independent or self-serving; and
- outline the research review process.

The discussion in Chapter 1 includes reasons why students and professors do research, differences between research and development (R & D) and objective research, the need for skepticism, and the concept of power of professor. A clinical case study conducted by the author and a first-year graduate student in our university's speech and hearing center illustrates some of the concepts that are reviewed.

Chapter 2. Academic–Clinical Integration of Research

Learning Objectives

After reading this chapter, the student will be able to

- interpret how professors and clinical supervisors bridge the academic–

clinical practicum gap in educating CSD students;
- describe how evidence-based practice is research-based practice; and
- synthesize a large body of literature by studying systematic reviews and meta-analyses.

The discussion in Chapter 2 includes types of research evidence, including levels of evidence; the International Classification of Functioning, Disability, and Health (ICF); clinical trials; and systematic reviews and meta-analyses. The chapter highlights best practices and evidence-based practice. Finally, a model of therapy considers dosage of therapy, whether or not exercises and practice should be massed or distributed in the therapy session, a consideration of what constitutes an adequate stimulus, and the implications of noncompliance. Starting with this chapter and including all the following chapters, advanced study includes practice in the subject matter of the chapter that is needed for the student to earn power of professor.

Chapter 3. Ethics of Research

Learning Objectives

After reading this chapter, the student will be able to

- describe the rules of ethics;
- infuse the highest ethical standards in research and clinical practice;
- comply with standards for best practices; and
- prepare for the Praxis II examination in speech-language pathology and audiology.

The discussion in Chapter 3 includes seven rules of ethics; unintended consequences of research, both positive and negative; the NIH/CITI online training course on the protection of human research participants; the Belmont Report that guides the Institutional Review Board (IRB) as well as ethical decision making in research; and some examples of ethical blindness and society's responses, including an example from CSD. The chapter continues with a summary of the research portion of the code of ethics of both the American Academy of Audiology (AAA) and the American Speech-Language-Hearing Association (ASHA), and concludes with a discussion of the Health Insurance Portability and Accountability Act of 1996 (HIPAA).

Chapter 4. The Scientific Method

Learning Objectives

After reading this chapter, the student will be able to

- describe the scientific method;
- differentiate the rules of science from "common sense" and pseudoscience; and
- formulate experimental and clinical hypotheses.

The discussion in Chapter 4 addresses the rules of science and the scientific method. The rules of science include empirical verification, operational definition, controlled observation, statistical generalization, and empirical confirmation. In comparison to the scientific method, "common sense" (which is sometimes nonsense) includes psychological verification, verbal definition, uncontrolled observation, overgeneralization, and psychological confirmation. Differences between the scientific method and pseudoscience is that the latter may be untestable; unchanged in the light of new data; may lack confirming evidence, including only anecdotal or inadequate evidence; and may avoid peer review.

Chapter 5. Types of Research

Learning Objectives

After reading this chapter, the student will be able to

- evaluate different types of research;
- interpret clinical files and design evidence-based clinical research studies; and
- critically examine survey forms.

The discussion in Chapter 5 addresses experimental, quasiexperimental, and nonexperimental designs. Single-subject and case studies are addressed in terms of strengths and weaknesses, as are proof-of-concept and pilot studies. The chapter also shows strengths and weaknesses of group designs, including quantitative, qualitative, and mixed-methods designs; retrospective research; survey research; longitudinal studies; and translational research.

Chapter 6. Really Basic Statistics

Learning Objectives

After reading this chapter, the student will be able to

- reject innumeracy and feel confident about basic math skills;
- interpret the Results section of a journal article; and
- select appropriate measures of statistical analysis to answer some clinical or academic research questions.

Before you have a MEGO (my eyes glaze over) moment, remember that only ninth grade math skills (elementary algebra) are all you need. In fact, to paraphrase a song from the Beatles, all you need are sums of squares to calculate variance and standard deviation, as well as *t*-tests, one-way analyses of variance, and the correlation coefficient *r*. Descriptive statistics include measures of central tendency and dispersion that should be a review for most readers. The chapter also includes some statistical concepts including random sampling, with the potential of Type I and Type II errors, degrees of freedom, and the *P* value. One nonparametric test, the chi-square (χ^2) test of independence, is included because it is often used to analyze demographic data. There is an alphabetical list of definitions of terms in statistics that should help as a reference as well as a guide for exams. Finally, there are a few more advanced concepts such as Bayesian inference and repeated measure analysis at the end of the chapter.

Chapter 7. Journal Article Critique

Learning Objectives

After reading this chapter, the student will be able to

- identify the structure of a journal article;

- control threats to internal and external validity of experiments; and
- explain the peer-review process.

Empirical research published in a peer-reviewed journal typically adheres to a formal style that is described and explained in Chapter 7. The experimenter seeks to control threats to the internal and external validity of the study in order to maximize generalizability of the findings. The peer-review process leads to a recommendation to accept or reject a manuscript submitted to a journal, and I provide two sample ad hoc reviews.

Chapter 8. Diagnostic Test Critique

Learning Objectives

After reading this chapter, the student will be able to

- evaluate sensitivity and specificity of diagnostic tests;
- explain what motivates his or her decision to use a particular diagnostic test; and
- identify threats to validity and reliability in tests and measurements.

Before evaluating a diagnostic test or writing a critique of one, it is important to recognize some problems in diagnosis. These problems may relate to the limited knowledge we have about a disorder, our tendency to underdiagnose or overdiagnose depending on the whims of the profession, and shortcomings in our theories or working models. Chapter 8 also goes through the structure of a typical diagnostic test manual, addressing theory, development, administration, and scoring of the test.

PART II. PRODUCING RESEARCH IN CSD

Chapters 9 through 12 address the "doing" of research from the perspective of a student or a new researcher. Since 2000, all proposed research that uses human participants must be approved by an Institutional Review Board (IRB) and the applicant must have satisfactorily completed the review course on the protection of human research participants (NIH certification or CITI certification as of October 2018). New researchers need mentors, and the student beginning to produce research will likely be guided by faculty, clinical supervisors, and even peers. As our practice is built on an evidence base (evidence-based practice [EBP]), most undergraduate and virtually all graduate CSD programs require an EBP project. Finally, undergraduate students are usually required to produce a research project in their major, called a capstone project or senior thesis, and graduate students are required to produce a clinical research project, a master's thesis, or both.

Chapter 9. Mentoring

Learning Objectives

After reading this chapter, the student will be able to

- establish mentor–student relationships;

- establish peer mentoring relationships; and
- end or advance mentoring relationships.

The mentor–student relationship usually refers to a younger person (the student) receiving academic, clinical, and employment guidance from an older person (faculty member, clinical supervisor, and employer, respectively). Chapter 9 includes these relationships as well as others, such as peer mentoring and even mentoring of clinicians by clients. In addition, I raise ethical concerns of mentoring and discuss the ASHA S.T.E.P. model of mentoring, as well as e-mentoring and e-supervision.

Chapter 10. Institutional Review Board (IRB) Research Approval

Learning Objectives

After reading this chapter, the student will be able to

- describe the history and purpose of the IRB;
- earn the certificate of completion from the National Institutes of Health (NIH) or Collaborative Institutional Training Initiative (CITI) training course on protection of human research participants; and
- prepare a research proposal that will be approved by the local IRB.

Chapter 10 is constructed in two sections: an overview of the IRB that looks at breaches of ethics that motivated creation of IRBs, university policies of IRBs, and common mistakes that appear in an IRB proposal by a student; and the second section that guides the student in completing an IRB review form.

Chapter 11. Conducting Clinical Research

Learning Objectives

After reading this chapter, the student will be able to

- apply the scientific method to clinical practice;
- develop a capstone project in evidence-based practice; and
- set clinical goals.

Producing clinical research starts with developing a clinical hypothesis that is based on critical thinking about relevant professional literature. You will also learn how to determine the appropriate experimental design for your study, how to set goals and take data, and how to disseminate the results of your work. A large part of this chapter is devoted to the operant conditioning paradigm that will guide you in goal setting and data collection.

Chapter 12. Conducting Academic Research

Learning Objectives

After reading this chapter, the student will be able to

- conduct research at basic and more advanced levels of education;
- decide which CSD programs in U.S. colleges and universities are the best fit; and

- explore options of funding for research.

Through spreadsheets and descriptions from university websites, Chapter 12 presents a selection of undergraduate and graduate requirements for CSD research. These include capstone projects and senior theses for undergraduates, master's theses and clinical evidence-based projects for master's students, and other, often archival, research projects for those who pursue the doctorate of audiology (AuD), clinical doctorate in SLP, or PhD degrees.

PART III. DISSEMINATING RESEARCH IN CSD

This last part of the book includes three chapters on dissemination of research. In the first two parts of this book you have learned how to be an educated consumer of research and a producer of clinical research. This third part addresses what to do with completed research. At one time, students and scholars depended on books for professional information. Books are fine (or I would not be writing this one), but are hardly cutting edge information. For example, I received a contract for the present book from Plural Publishing, Inc. in 2017. Most of the references in the book are from 2017 or earlier, representing work that was probably conducted 2 to 3 years before publication. After peer reviewers sent back corrections and recommendations, the completed manuscript was sent to Plural by June 1, 2019. In short, by the time the book gets to you, portions of it may be out of date.

If your goal is to learn the latest information on a professional subject, then, books are unlikely to be your best choice. As noted in Chapter 13, ad hoc peer reviewers for journals have access to the most current studies that are about to be published, so serving as an external peer reviewer should be a goal for someone who wants a future in academia. Chapter 14 addresses conference presentations as well as opportunities for continuing education that are required for maintenance of clinical certification and state licensure. Research that is being presented at scientific meetings is likely to be current and may even be still in progress. Chapter 15 that ends the book considers nonacademic dissemination of research. While every effort is made to present advocacy groups and social media that are currently relevant to CSD, these sources are most likely to change over time.

Chapter 13. Dissemination by Publication

Learning Objectives

After reading this chapter, the student will be able to

- identify aspects of peer review;
- identify the editorial process for acceptance or rejection of a manuscript; and
- identify how chapters are reviewed and edited differently from journal articles.

Research is traditionally disseminated in peer-reviewed journals. Chapter 13 begins by addressing advantages and disadvantages of peer review and continues with a discussion of the editorial process and how to respond to ad hoc peer reviewers. There is also a section on open-access and predatory journals. Peer review may be less clear when it comes to books and portions of books, and the rest of the chapter is devoted to determining whether or not a book has been peer reviewed, as well as publishing a contribution to a book and some tips on writing style.

Chapter 14. Oral Presentation of Research

Learning Objectives

After reading this chapter, the student will be able to

- write an abstract for a platform or poster presentation;
- prepare and rehearse the presentation;
- present the poster or platform information orally; and
- use educational technology to support the presentation.

Oral presentation of research often refers to conference presentations. The content in Chapter 14 moves from submitting an abstract to preparing and rehearsing the talk to delivering a poster or platform presentation. Practice-based networks are another less formal way of disseminating research. Whether the presentation is formal or informal, education technology offers a variety of ways to enhance your presentation. The chapter ends with some strategies to secure funding for travel.

Chapter 15. Nontraditional Dissemination of Research

Learning Objectives

After reading this chapter, the student will be able to

- describe a marketing strategy for a device, instrument, therapy, or test you have developed;
- describe differences between Web 1.0 and Web 2.0 technologies; and
- describe how to disseminate research through social media.

Nontraditional dissemination of research addresses some challenges to dissemination such as marketing, distribution, and making use of new Web technologies and social media. Some other areas of difficulty in dissemination are raised, including moving research findings from the clinic to the community and from the community to public health policies. An alphabetical list of some support groups in major areas of communication disorders offers contacts to the world outside the laboratory, clinic, and classroom. The last part of the chapter, and of the book, provides information on advocating for the professions and how to highlight your research in university and association news publications.

ACKNOWLEDGMENTS

In recognizing the many people who helped with this project, I want to begin with the peer-review process of Plural Publishing, Inc. Thank you to all reviewers for giving your time and expertise so freely. Plural Publishing continues to be very supportive to its authors, with Valerie Johns and Kalie Koscielak of most notable help in the present project.

Versions of the present book, even before I considered writing it, were shaped by the reactions of my students to information in Research Methods courses at Lehman College; The Graduate Center, CUNY; Adelphi University; and the National Pedagogical University, Bogotá, Colombia. I have also had the extraordinary good fortune of working with two superb master's-level research assistants, Emily Goldman and Yulia Kovalenko for two years. In addition, another graduate student, Monica Fernandes, helped me translate information on the scientific method into South American Spanish for use in Bogotá. The notion of good therapy being a parallel of an experiment where $n = 1$ was shaped by more than 30,000 therapy sessions with homebound adults with aphasia and dysarthria. Thank you for welcoming me into your homes and your lives.

Some very generous colleagues offered comments on various chapters in the book: Reem Khamis-Dawkar inspired the chapter on academic–clinical integration; Elizabeth V. Goldfarb provided information on informed consent for the chapter on ethics; Melissa Randazzo helped with the organization of the chapter on types of research; Fran Redstone clarified an early version of the chapter on statistics, Matthew D. Simon offered a tutorial on Bayesian statistics; Lawrence J. Raphael helped with the organization of the chapter on the IRB; and Wendy Papir Bernstein offered information about nontraditional forms of dissemination.

I offer heartfelt thanks to Chris Code, Audrey Holland, and Leonard L. LaPointe who served as professional and personal cheerleaders during my recent harrowing medical adventure. I will say that there are better ways to improve one's empathy for those who have had a stroke than by having one yourself.

To Shelley, my bride and muse for a half century, this book is dedicated to you. To our daughter, Elizabeth V. Goldfarb—a superb cognitive neuroscience researcher—and our son-in-law, Matthew D. Simon—a world-class molecular biochemist—we love you madly. You have both already had a significant impact on Yale University and the world. Finally, to our granddaughter, Tessera Rose Goldfarb Simon, you are still a baby, but the lives you touch are already enriched by knowing you.

REVIEWERS

Plural Publishing, Inc. and the author would like to thank the following reviewers for taking the time to provide their valuable feedback during the development process.

Mary Jo Santo Pietro, PhD, CCC-SLP, ASHA Fellow
Professor
School of Communication Disorders and Deafness
Kean University
Union, New Jersey

Alfred Valdez, PhD, CCC-SLP
Interim Academic Department Head
Department of Communication Disorders
New Mexico State University
Las Cruces, New Mexico

Anniversary Waltz (to Shelley)

Like a dog, circling before he sleeps,
I have burrowed my head in my pillow
in just the right place.
You choose this moment
to request a kiss.
I am thrilled to comply.

PART I

Consuming Research in CSD

1

Developing Power of Professor: The Nature of Research in CSD

INTRODUCTION

Consuming research in communication sciences and disorders (CSD) is not optional for students, clinicians, and academic faculty. Increasingly, all are also required to produce the products of their research, even if it does not result in a conference presentation or journal article. Students at all levels, from the BA or BS through the MA or MS and AuD or PhD degrees, are required to produce evidence of their research in the forms of term papers as well as a senior thesis or capstone project, master's thesis or evidence-based practice report, and doctoral dissertation, respectively (see Chapter 12 for details). Clinicians critically evaluate diagnostic and assessment materials and protocols, instrumentation and devices, and intervention techniques before using them in their clinical practices. Academic faculty members evaluate and synthesize the professional literature to create and update course syllabi. All are required to engage in continuing education throughout their professional careers.

Everyone does research, from comparison shopping, to finding a good plumber or accountant, to trying to understand current events. The standard that students, clinicians, and professors have for conducting research is much higher, and there are many rules to be learned and followed. This book is organized to guide the student through the process of becoming an educated consumer of research, to beginning the process of conducting research, and to understanding the options for disseminating research. The theme, as elaborated on at the end of this chapter, is to enable students and clinicians, as well as new faculty, to gain the knowledge and skills necessary to develop what I am calling "power of professor."

Learning Objectives

After reading this chapter, the student will be able to

- explain why academic and clinical research is important;
- critically evaluate whether research is independent or self-serving; and
- outline the research review process.

WHY PROFESSORS AND CLINICIANS DO RESEARCH

Not all professors and clinicians do publishable research. For example, some professors work in teaching institutions that do not require scholarly output in terms of peer-reviewed publications and presentations. The teaching load is usually much higher in institutions that focus mainly on teaching than in research-intensive, or research 1 universities (sometimes referred to as "R1: Doctoral Universities–highest research activity"), where external funding and peer-reviewed publications are required for retention, promotion, and tenure. Evidence of research is critical to college and university peer-review committees that evaluate faculty on three criteria: teaching; scholarship or creative work; and service to the university, community, and profession.

All professors do research to prepare for their courses, and all clinicians do research to prepare for clinical intervention in speech-language pathology (SLP) and audiology (A). At least they should. Many of us have sat through courses where it seemed that the instructor had not updated the curriculum in decades, or observed clinicians who implemented only the same therapies that they used for decades. As noted in Chapter 3, this may be legal, but it is not ethical. Good teaching as well as good therapy is hard work that requires continual updating through critical evaluation of current research, synthesis of professional literature, and continuing education. The student clinician is not finished with education upon graduation. Nearly all states in the United States require licensure for the professional practice of SLP and A, with continuing education hours needed to maintain the professional license.

Some institutions of higher education are known for conservatory programs where creative work (e.g., in art, dance, music, and theatre) is of paramount importance. Communication sciences and disorders (CSD) departments are not located in conservatory programs. The old expression, "publish or perish" applies to faculty in most CSD programs. The requirement for faculty to publish can be a boon to students who may be paid or receive tuition remission to work as a research assistant to a faculty member (see Chapter 9). However, just as all university clinicians and academics must do research for therapy and teaching, respectively, even if they do not publish, students must do research for courses and other institutional requirements even if they do not work as a research assistant to a faculty member. Most colleges and universities require some written or archival document that is based on research at every level of education. Undergraduate CSD students usually prepare what is known as a capstone project or senior thesis in their major; some master's-level students write a thesis, but nearly all will prepare an evidence-based (or research-based) therapy project for clinical practicum; and doctoral students often do preliminary (or "brown bag") research projects, run pilot studies, and write a dissertation. All will produce research-based written term papers for courses at every level.

Expanding the original question, what is involved when we, as students, professors, or clinicians do research, and why do we do it? The main outlets for the products of our research are peer-reviewed or refereed conference presentations (local, state, national, and international), journal articles, and books or portions of books. The peer-review process that involves evaluation of research by volunteer experts in the field will be discussed in detail in Chapter 7. As professors, we may work for years preparing a journal article to submit to a peer-reviewed publication, and if we are lucky, we get to give it away for free. Sometimes we even have to pay page charges. Your friends in business schools will no doubt find this surprising. We need to publish in order to be tenured and promoted, but there is a more basic motivation. Our business is the pursuit and dissemination of knowledge, and it is exhilarating to find a little piece of truth that had not been uncovered before. As clinicians, we are not required to publish, but the positive effect that our research has on a client's communicative behaviors is more than enough motivation to stay current with the literature. Finally, as students, you get to do both academic and clinical research, either to fulfill your university's scholastic requirements or to succeed in clinical practicum.

RESEARCH AND DEVELOPMENT (R & D) VERSUS OBJECTIVE RESEARCH

R & D

Think of the advertisement that claims a product is "clinically proven to be effective at . . . " (you fill in the sentence). This advertisement is an interpretation of research and development (R & D) that you should not believe. Hypotheses, theories, and therapies are never proven (we can falsify or reject them, but we can only support or strengthen them; see Chapter 5 for an expanded discussion of this topic). By its very existence as an advertisement, there is a potential conflict of interest in the claim of effectiveness; that is, the motivation to sell a product can be at odds with the desire to discover the truth (R & D is usually conducted in an ethical manner, but see Chapter 3 on Ethics of Research for more information).

Private support of research is crucial to the development of new knowledge, as governments cannot afford to pay for all the expenses that research entails. Even though R & D is driven by the profit motive, results of privately supported research can be enormously consequential and even publishable in the best journals if the authors include a disclosure statement. Most scientific convention presentations and journals require authors to state if they have a personal or financial interest in the outcome of the research. The following is part of a critique where the present author served as an ad hoc reviewer for an article submitted to a journal in our field. (The reviewer posed the question and the authors of the article provided the response.)

Response to reviewers:

Q. The purpose of the paper seems to be to support the use of ABaCo (presumably the assessment battery they developed) as a tool to assess the pragmatic language disorder in schizophrenia. If the authors have a financial interest in this tool, it should be stated as a disclosure.

R. We have modified the introduction in order to make clearer that the purpose of the paper was not to promote the use of ABaCo as much as to provide a wide-ranging picture of communicative abilities in patients with schizophrenia.

Following a resubmission with the requested revisions from two reviewers, the paper was accepted for publication in the journal, and a disclosure statement appeared on the first page of the article.

Objective Research

Errors may still appear in objective research, but there are several checks to prevent them. Assume that you are planning your first experiment to fulfill an academic requirement. The first check will be done by your academic adviser and possibly by other faculty members of your thesis or dissertation committee as well. The faculty will help you to write an experiment that you can complete in a reasonable amount of time and that will yield important information. For example, with the approval of the faculty, you plan to implement a protocol to assess expressive syntax in 5-year-old children with specific language impairment (SLI). Your research population is from a protected class (their status as children means that researchers must make extra efforts to protect them from any potential harm in an experiment; see Chapter 3), so you will not be able to get an expedited review from your university's Institutional Review Board (IRB; you will learn how to complete an application to the IRB in Chapter 10). The second check by the IRB will make sure that your research proposal ensures respect for persons, beneficence, and justice for the research participants, as delineated in the Belmont Report (National Commission for the Protection of Human Subjects of Biomedical and Behavioral Research, 1979; see Chapter 3 for an extended discussion of the Belmont Report), and will also provide a check on the experiment's purpose, methodology, and design. In most instances, the IRB will ask for clarification or additional information, and the proposal will have to be resubmitted for a final approval.

Now assume that you will need funding to complete your experiment. You can fund your study alone or with your adviser in many ways: through an internal or university-based grant, through a private agency, through a professional association (e.g., the American Speech-Language-Hearing Association [ASHA] or the American Academy of Audiology [AAA]), through a government agency, or as part of your adviser's funding for an existing grant. The application for funding must be thorough and competitive, as there are many more applications than available funds. The third check by the funding agency will result in useful feedback, whether or not your proposal is funded (some funding opportunities for students at different levels of education, as well as for junior and senior faculty, are described in Chapter 12).

The fourth check will result from a pilot study, where you and your adviser will determine if your protocol is working properly. If adjustments need to be made, and there probably will be some, then piloting, perhaps with neurotypical children, before running the experiment will allow for modifications. If you start running participants with SLI and there are problems with the protocol, then you may have to throw out the data you collected.

Finally, you have completed running the experiment. Your faculty committee must approve the document you wrote (a fifth check), and you may be required to defend it in front of the faculty or at a public event.

Congratulations! You have completed your research, you have earned the approval of your advisers, and you have defended what you have written. Now it is time to disseminate your research (see Chapters 13 through 15 for traditional and nontraditional dissemination opportunities). Together with your adviser and perhaps with other faculty as well, you submit a proposal for presentation at a professional meeting; for example, ASHA or AAA. Proposals for presentation at these conventions are peer reviewed (a sixth check where experts in SLI will evaluate the accuracy and relevance of your work, as well as suitability to the professional society hosting the meeting) to make sure that the content is appropriate for the target audience, is consistent with the theme of the convention, and has scholarly or professional merit. You and the faculty may also decide that the research qualifies for submission to a peer-reviewed journal (a seventh check where ad hoc reviewers with expertise in SLI will determine if the manuscript should be accepted, rejected, or accepted with major or minor revisions). This is a painstaking process that will probably involve responding to journal editors and ad hoc peer reviewers, as well as some rewriting.

These seven checks do not guarantee that everything you read in a refereed journal or elsewhere is of a high quality or even correct. Errors can elude even the most diligent reviewers, and new evidence can falsify old hypotheses. The Internet can sensationalize findings or generalize them incorrectly. Book authors, including this one, can make mistakes in synthesizing a large body of literature. On very rare occasions, researchers cheat. These cheaters may feel pressure to justify a grant, to get promoted or tenured, or to publish what they are sure is correct, even if the data indicates otherwise. The consequences of being caught at cheating are so severe that virtually all researchers are honest. It is likely that the cheating will be discovered, with resultant loss of job and reputation, and sometimes incarceration.

CLINICAL RESEARCH: A CASE STUDY

Danielle, a graduate student, and I sat on child-size chairs next to a child-size table at our university's Center for Communicative Disorders on a hot day in early June. We were waiting for our new client, a 4;5-year-old female with a diagnosis of cerebral palsy and profound hearing loss who was reportedly nonverbal. We had brought toys and other stimulus materials and planned to devote our first therapy session to establishing rapport and evaluating the current status of the client. CM, a thin, white middle-class female entered the therapy room wearing shorts and a tank top, her knees bent in from her wide stance as she walked shifting her weight from side to side. CM's mother, who stayed in the waiting room, was a homemaker, and her father owned a pizza restaurant. We greeted CM who threw herself on the floor and started screaming.

Danielle, astonished, asked what we should do. I said I didn't know, but suggested we get down on the floor with some of our toys and engage in parallel play. After a brief time, CM started to play with some of the toys, and we shifted our strategy to interactive play. As we were playing with plastic food, CM picked up an apple and said, "poo." I told Danielle that I thought CM might not be deaf as she spontaneously produced the second syllable of a word that had most of its acoustic power in the first syllable, a stressed vowel. CM then picked up a piece of plastic pizza and said, "Dada." I said to Danielle that CM might not be nonverbal either, as her father owned a pizzeria. We spent the rest of the session interacting with CM who seemed to have been misdiagnosed. As an aphasiologist, I suspected that CM's ambulation and language behavior might have resulted from an in utero stroke.

We obtained an MRI that was done when CM was 1 year, 11 months that revealed mild relative prominence of the lateral ventricles, without evidence for acute hydrocephalus. Our university's Faculty Center for Professional Excellence helped me to add ultraviolet digital enhancement to the image that revealed ventricular enlargement in the area of the primary auditory cortex (Figure 1–1).

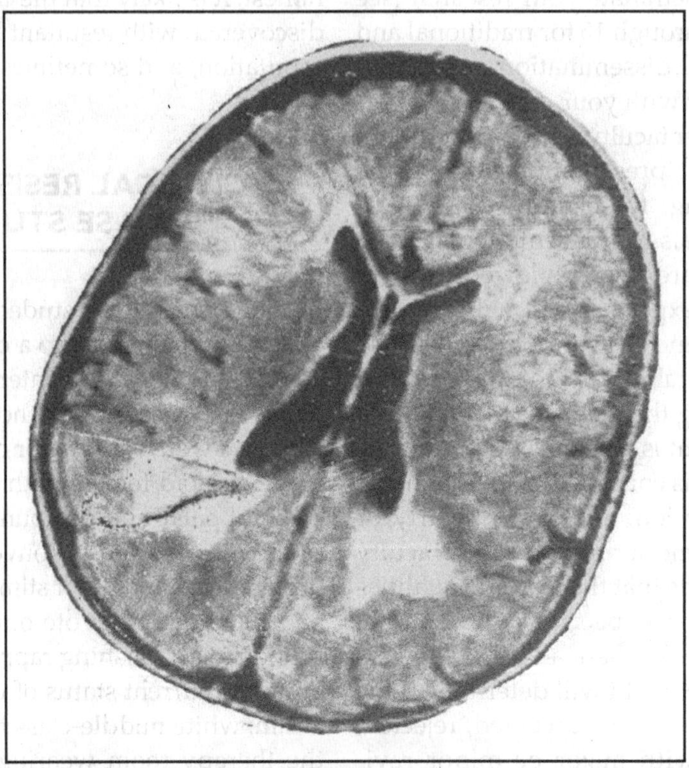

Figure 1–1. *MRI of CM's brain at 23 months of age*

One of our department's audiology faculty members, who became a coauthor on the subsequent ASHA presentation and journal article, needed five testing sessions with CM. The audiologist ultimately obtained sound-field warble tone thresholds that indicated a spondee reception threshold (SRT) of 15 dB HL in the left ear and an SRT of 25 dB HL in the right ear for octave frequencies from 500 to 4000 Hz, suggesting adequate hearing through the speech frequencies in the better ear. We concluded that part of the behavior that had been attributed to a profound hearing loss may have resulted from an auditory processing deficit secondary to in utero stroke, or CVA.

Treatment for CM focused on providing augmentative and alternative communication (AAC) interventions for 10 weeks, 2 times per week for 30-min durations. A faculty colleague who was a certified speech-language pathologist with extensive AAC experience provided recommendations for the introduction of AAC materials. CM's verbal language and communicative competence improved to the extent that she did not require special education placement. Follow-up contacts with the family revealed that CM had scored above average on standardized verbal skills testing.

We wrote the results of the clinical experience with CM as a case study and submitted it to ASHA—where Danielle won the AAC Institute Award for best student presentation--and published it in a peer-reviewed journal (Arroyo, Goldfarb, Cahill, & Schoepflin, 2010). We did not go into the first therapy session with CM expecting to publish a case study. However, our philosophy of seeing therapy as a way of testing clinical hypotheses (preparing for a therapy session with a clinical hypothesis rather than a lesson plan is described in Chapter 11) led us to reject the initial diagnosis that CM had cerebral palsy that resulted in her status of being nonverbal with a profound hearing loss.

When clinical intervention is seen as no different from a research study where hypotheses are tested on a population of 1, then the divide between experimental research and clinical practice narrows. Academic–clinical integration (the subject of Chapter 2) facilitates this process.

SKEPTICISM

Did you know that you can go to the dentist to get cavities? Think about it. You may have tooth decay that causes pain, so the dentist drills out the decay and fills the hole (cavity) he drilled with amalgam. In other words, the dentist created a cavity in your tooth by drilling. As another example, an SLP graduate student observes her supervisor demonstrate "diaphragmatic breathing" to a client with multiple sclerosis. This would be somewhat akin to a physical therapist demonstrating "leg walking" to the same client. The diaphragm is contracted and lowered for inspiration and relaxed and raised back up to its dome shape for expiration, even though you cannot localize the muscle in your body. There are muscles that move the rib cage up and out for inspiration, just as there are muscles in the hips and buttocks used for walking, but the diaphragm and the legs are the principal players for breathing and walking, respectively. (Yes, some acrobats are capable of walking on their hands, but let's not quibble.)

We understand that the dentist is using the term "cavity" in a way that is specific to the profession of dentistry, and the SLP is using the term "diaphragmatic breathing" as a metaphor (similar to the injunction to "breathe from the soles of your feet") to remind the client to engage the abdominal musculature more and the thoracic musculature less. The skeptical researcher insists on more precision in professional literature and uses what are called "operational definitions" (such as whether "articulation" refers to the production of speech sounds or to connective tissue where articulation of bones forms a joint; see Chapter 7) for clarity.

Just because something has been published does not mean that it was done well, or even correctly. As skeptical researchers, we ask if the hypothesis is falsifiable (it must be or the hypothesis is not interesting; see Chapter 4), if there are alternative explanations for the findings (the fewer the better; see Chapter 7), if threats to validity (truthfulness and generalizability) and reliability (consistency) have been controlled (see Chapter 7), and if the statistical analysis was rigorous and appropriate (see Chapter 6).

Here is an example. A 6-year-old girl with a cleft palate has been diagnosed with a phonological disorder because she says "treat" instead of "street" and "doe" instead of "go." The phonological processes involved are said to be cluster reduction and velar fronting. Indeed, there are journal articles that claim phonological disorders are responsible for articulation errors in the speech of children with cleft palate. The skeptical researcher asks, "Who needs phonology when you have phonetics?" Phonology is part of linguistic competence or the underlying set of rules that make articulation possible, whereas phonetics codes the features of place and manner of actual articulation. What have been called disorders of phonology in our hypothetical child may not be velar fronting but simplification of articulation caused by velopharyngeal insufficiency (making it easier to substitute the voiced alveolar plosive in "doe" for the voiced velar plosive in "go"). What was called cluster reduction may be the simplification of a three-consonant cluster that starts with a fricative (because of nasal emission from the cleft palate that results from attempts to say /s/) to a two-consonant cluster that starts with a plosive.

Similarly, our case study of CM would never have occurred if we were not skeptical about her diagnosis as a child who was nonverbal with a profound hearing loss. One major point of this book (see Chapter 2) is that clinical research and clinical practice depend on academic–clinical integration. Another major point is we do not currently disseminate new findings (see Part III on disseminating research) in ways that get to the practicing clinician expeditiously; we also need to do a better job of translating cutting-edge research from "bench to bedside" and from "bedside to community" (translational research and other kinds of research are described in Chapter 5).

POWER OF PROFESSOR

The term, "power of professor" is intended to evoke comparisons with power of attorney. You or a member of your family may obtain power of attorney to sell property, trade stocks and bonds, and transact banking on behalf of an aged or disabled relative, even though you are not a lawyer. Similarly, a person with power of professor would be authorized to conduct academic and clinical research, even if that individual does not have a PhD degree. However, there are proposed differences in the two powers. A speech-language pathologist (SLP) and audiologist (A) would be required to demonstrate competencies, as indicated in this textbook, before earning power of professor. The clinical researcher, SLP or A, will be equipped to treat therapeutic or diagnostic interactions as miniexperiments where hypotheses are being tested on a population of one person.

At the end of each of the following chapters is a section called, "Advanced Study." There is a template indicating that power of professor requires signatures from a mentor, faculty adviser, program director, or department chair when the student answers a series of questions related to the topics covered in the chapter.

We need SLPs and As to earn power of professor, because there simply are not enough practitioners with PhD degrees, nor are there likely to be anytime soon. The proposal here is to begin a discussion of what constitutes power of professor and what obligations an individual, professor or not, has before being permitted to do research. This book is designed to enable the reader not only to understand, but also to do research, considering the welfare and confidentiality of patients and participants. There is also the major issue of the need for theory where clinical researchers inform laboratory researchers who do group studies that provide information for new theories. Preparation for power of professor should also include an understanding of the relationships among theory, research, and therapy. Finally, those who have earned power of professor will know how to disseminate their research.

Granted power of professor, an individual with an MA, MS, or AuD might earn research privileges based on competencies. In hospitals and medical centers it is often the case that SLPs and As with general privileges can engage in diagnosis and treatment of patients; those with specialized privileges (e.g., with expertise in cochlear implants or augmentative and alternative communication devices) can treat patients with more complicated needs; and those with research privileges (the highest designation) can submit proposals to the IRB to conduct research with a clinical population (Goldfarb, 1989). ASHA might extend the Knowledge and Skills Assessment protocol to focus on research, or a Special Interest Division might be established to grant power of professor.

When I first proposed the concept of power of professor in a book I edited more than 10 years ago (Goldfarb, 2006), one of the contributors who had also been my teacher suggested that the topic was important enough to consider in book form. Professor Oliver Bloodstein is no longer with us, but I consider this book to be a promise kept to him.

REFERENCES

Arroyo, C., Goldfarb, R., Cahill, D., & Schoepflin, J. (2010). AAC interventions: Case study of in-utero stroke. *Journal of Speech-Language Pathology and Applied Behavior Analysis, 5*, 32–47.

Goldfarb, R. (1989). Organization of speech, language, and hearing programmes in United States hospitals. *The College of Speech Therapists Bulletin, 452*, 2–7.

Goldfarb, R. (Ed.). (2006). *Ethics: A case study from fluency*. San Diego, CA: Plural.

National Commission for the Protection of Human Subjects of Biomedical and Behavioral Research. (1979). *The Belmont Report: Ethical principles and guidelines for the protections of human subjects of research* (GPO Office 887-890). Washington, DC: Government Printing Office.

2

Academic–Clinical Integration of Research

INTRODUCTION

The university clinic and the classroom should be closely aligned, rather than being considered as separate entities. After all, students register for clinical practica at their *university* speech and hearing center, not their *hospital* speech and hearing center. Tenured or tenure-track faculty members often spend time supervising or demonstrating in the clinic, and clinical supervisors often serve as adjunct instructors. Integrating academic and clinical perspectives helps to make therapy sessions mini experiments and makes course information come alive for students. Collaborations among academic faculty, clinical supervisors, student observers, and student clinicians stimulate clinical research. We had a sign in a speech and hearing center where I worked that read, "All of us are smarter than any of us."

Power of professor to undertake clinical research comes with responsibilities to understand what clinical research is, how clinical research has been conducted in the past, how to differentiate among various kinds of clinical research, and what clinical questions have yet to be answered. This chapter addresses levels of research evidence and a research protocol, explains systematic reviews and meta-analyses, explores best practices and evidence-based practice, provides a model of therapy, and raises concerns about clinical research that follows academic–clinical integration.

Learning Objectives

After reading this chapter, the student will be able to

- interpret how professors and clinical supervisors bridge the academic–clinical practicum gap in educating CSD students;
- describe how evidence-based practice is research-based practice; and

- synthesize a large body of literature by studying systematic reviews and meta-analyses.

TYPES OF RESEARCH EVIDENCE

Levels of Research Evidence

Levels of evidence categorize studies based on methodological quality of their design, validity, and applicability to patient/client care. The highest level (Level I), by convention of the scientific community, has the greatest strength of recommendation (Ackley, Swan, Ladwig, & Tucker, 2008). This ranking of strength or grade of recommendation should not be considered absolute, because some research designs are better than others at answering certain clinical questions. For example, systematic reviews are ranked as Level I if they include meta-analyses of randomized controlled trials (RCT) and as Level V if they include meta-syntheses of descriptive and qualitative studies, according to Ackley et al. (2008). Systematic reviews may be the suggested research design for information on general or overall clinical questions because they provide summary knowledge in our field. Meta-analyses and review articles are similar to textbooks in that they condense many points of view, but they are more timely sources of information. Evidence from RCTs (Level I) results from studies with the most scientific rigor and is the least susceptible to experimental bias, whereas evidence derived from expert opinion (Level IV) represents the least rigor and is the most susceptible to bias.

What is bias? The Centre for Clinical Effectiveness in Melbourne, Australia (Harris & Turner, 2011, p. 18) defines bias as systematic errors in designing or conducting a study. Bias also means that errors in analysis distort the results of the study away from the truth. Bias may result in an over- or underestimation of an intervention, an exposure, or a relationship. Types of bias include:

- *selection bias*, where errors in participant selection or group allocation impact the results of the study; and
- *information bias*, where there are errors in measurement of the data about participants (inaccurate or incomplete), their exposure, or effects of intervention.

The "gold standard" of RCT (Level I) is recommended for an individual study of therapy, etiology, diagnosis, and prevention. In RCTs, there is masked outcome assessment. Masking or blinding refers to a design intended to withhold knowledge about treatment assignment. That is, the participants and sometimes the investigators do not know who is in the experimental or control group. In some medical experiments, knowledge is withheld about who is getting the active drug and who is getting the placebo. For RCT studies, masking is done to prevent bias in assessment of subjective outcomes, such as comfort of hearing aids, self-perception of stuttering, or food aversions. RCTs are also prospective studies. The design of a prospective study involves collecting data, whereas the design of a retrospective study involves analyzing data that has already been collected for another purpose, such as clinical use.

Evidence-based practice and research designs depend on information that is filtered or unfiltered. There are more studies with the weakest designs than there are with the strongest.

- *Unfiltered information:* The largest number of studies tend to be those providing background information and expert opinion (Level IV; Box 2–1). You can find this kind of information in textbooks, encyclopedias, and handbooks. Case controlled studies, also called case series or case reports (Level III), are less numerous than Level IV studies. There are usually two or more participants or two or more treatments for one participant, where one shows that a treatment leads to the outcome of interest and the other does not show the same outcome. If groups are the focus of the research design, then they are called cohort studies. RCTs (Level I or Level II, depending on the degree of control) include randomized placement of participants in either an experimental group or control group. The experimental group receives the treatment of interest and both groups are followed up for the outcomes or variables of interest.
- *Filtered information:* The largest number of studies that also have the lowest quality of evidence are article synopses or critical appraisal of individual articles. Authors who evaluate and synthesize many articles produce evidence synthesis or critical appraisal of topics; there are fewer of these. The fewest studies and the ones with the highest quality of evidence are systematic reviews and meta-analyses.

Another classification system for levels of evidence considers risks associated with clinical interventions (Box 2–2). Level I studies have the most scientific rigor and the least likelihood of experimenter bias, and Level IV studies are the least rigorous and the most susceptible to bias.

Box 2–1. Levels of Evidence

Level I studies

Prospective, randomized controlled clinical trials; masked outcome assessment; representative population with qualifiers

Level II studies

Prospective, matched group cohorts; masked outcome assessment; representative population; lacking one criterion for Class I evidence

Level III studies

All other controlled trials where outcome assessment is independent of patient treatment; representative population

Level IV studies

Evidence from uncontrolled studies, for example, case studies, expert opinion

Box 2–2. Evidence Regarding Interventions and Risk

Level I

Evidence obtained from a systematic review (or meta-analysis) of all relevant randomized controlled trials

Level II

Evidence obtained from at least one randomized controlled trial

Level III

1. Evidence obtained from pseudo-randomized controlled trials (alternate allocation or some other method)
2. Evidence obtained from comparative studies (including systematic reviews of such studies) with concurrent controls and allocation not randomized, cohort studies, case control studies, or interrupted time series with a control group
3. Evidence obtained from comparative studies with historical control, two or more single-arm studies, or interrupted time series without a parallel control group

Level IV

Evidence obtained from case series, either post-test or pretest/posttest

Source: Harris & Turner, 2001, p. 26. Reprinted with permission.

Systematic Reviews and Meta-Analyses

There has been an explosive increase in the number of research journals and journal articles. Critical evaluation of both print and online journals, as well as the structure of a journal article appear later in this book. There is no substitute for reading the article yourself and determining if it is important and useful; otherwise, you trust someone else (like this author) to synthesize and explain the article. However, the reality is that in a busy clinical practice, it is helpful to have reliable summaries of research for academic–clinical integration. These summaries appear in our profession in the form of systematic reviews and meta-analyses.

The prefix "meta-" refers to the ability to view, observe, and assess other processes; the concept of metacognition can be defined as thinking about thinking. Subsystems would include metamemory, metalinguistics, and metacomprehension. Metacognition is also used for self-monitoring and self-control during an activity. Meta-analysis of a systematic review means that the authors assessed and interpreted the results of the literature review. A meta-analysis is a statistical method to estimate effect sizes of an individual factor. For example, Rudolph (2017) used meta-analyses to determine the statistical significance of risk factors associated with specific language impairment.

Recent systematic reviews that are designed to provide clinical and research guidelines follow the protocol of the Preferred Reporting Items for Systematic Reviews and Meta-Analyses (PRISMA; Moher, Liberati, Tetzlaff, Altman, & Group, 2009). The PRISMA Statement includes a 27-item checklist and a four-phase flow diagram. The checklist evaluates the title, abstract, introduction, methods, results, discussion, and funding of reports that are systematic reviews, meta-analyses, or both. The flow diagram shows how information should appear in a systematic review, from the number of records identified when duplicates are removed → records screened → articles assessed for eligibility → studies included. It is hoped that a standard protocol for evaluation of systematic reviews and meta-analyses will reduce the confusion that has led to disagreements in the past. For example, Whurr, Lorch, and Nye (1992; see also Nye, Lorch, & Whurr, 1997) reviewed and analyzed early studies of efficacy of aphasia therapy from 1946 to 1988 and found a lack of internal and external validity in the efficacy studies but a robust and significant positive effect of treatment on meta-analysis. Robey (1994) criticized both the effect sizes and the strategy for analysis in the Whurr et al. (1992) findings, but both discussions ultimately arrived at the same conclusions. Robey (1998) had the last word and it seemed to this reader that, in the end, the differences that caused the ruckus were trivial.

In the area of medical speech-language pathology, the systematic reviews were undertaken largely by subcommittees of the Academy of Neurologic Communication Disorders and Sciences (ANCDS; http://www.ancds.org), and many of the reports were published in the *Journal of Medical Speech-Language Pathology*, a fine publication that is, unfortunately, now discontinued. The reviews were completed through evidence-based guidelines that included searching through electronic databases, conducting hand searches, and providing exhaustive literature reviews.

The purposes of ANCDS reviews were to assess levels of evidence based on objective criteria agreed on by the committee. The committee would then write guidelines based on the reviews and assessments of levels of scientific evidence, make the information available to practicing clinicians, and determine areas where further research is needed. Evaluating research related to interventions considered the purpose of the study; characteristics of the participants; control of threats to internal, external, and content validity; and characteristics of dosage of treatments, including frequency, intensity, and duration. The reports concluded with measures of outcomes, results, and methodology.

Ellis (2009) reviewed articles related to adult neurogenic communication disorders in the *American Journal of Speech-Language Pathology* (AJSLP) and the *Journal of Speech, Language, and Hearing Research* (JSLHR) from 1997 through 2007 and reported the race/ethnicity of the participants. He concluded that because few studies report race/ethnicity or consider how race/ethnicity has the potential to confound the results and conclusions drawn, the generalization of the reported findings may be limited. He further stated that reporting race/ethnicity is likely critical to the external validity (generalizability) of studies in adult neurogenic communication disorders, and when available can enhance the relevance of the findings reported. Chapter 7 includes more information on the inclusionary and exclusionary criteria that should be reported in experimental research.

The ANCDS has conducted systematic reviews of published literature on the five topics of aphasia, acquired apraxia of speech, dysarthria, dementia, and cognitive-communication disorders after traumatic brain injury. The findings of these systematic reviews will be detailed later in this chapter. The reports made clinical practice recommendations based on the levels of research evidence found in the systematic review (Ehlhardt et al., 2008, p. 8; Halpern & Goldfarb, 2013, p. 2). Box 2–1 summarizes these levels. Evidence-based practice (EPB) depends on understanding levels of research evidence and using the best evidence to inform treatment methods. However, EBP is currently taught primarily in graduate-level courses in Research Methods and students may not develop adequate skills in the EBP process or may lose them when they start professional practices. Anema (2014) detailed both undergraduate and graduate EBP protocols to facilitate the development of EBP for treatment of disorders of fluency.

A review of levels of evidence in more than 2,500 articles in four major otolaryngology journals (Wasserman, Wynn, Bash, & Rosenfeld, 2006) indicated that more than half were at a weak level (case studies or therapy studies; retrospective study or nonindependent reference standard for diagnostic studies). Studies of therapy had the weakest evidence, and assessments of diagnostic tests had the strongest evidence. Newer studies had stronger evidence than older ones. The definitions of the levels varied slightly from the ones described in Box 2–1, and a fifth category, expert opinion without critical appraisal, was added.

The levels of evidence required by physicians and health agencies may be higher than the level of evidence required for education and intervention. For example, the following groups may be stakeholders in establishing a policy of universal newborn hearing screening (UNHS): the general public; families with children who are deaf or hard of hearing; the Deaf and hard of hearing communities; hospital administrators; various physician specialists; managed care, Medicaid, and insurance agencies; and politicians (Yoshinaga-Itano, 2004, p. 452). The groups involved in medical safety and cost may require higher levels of evidence to persuade them to intervene or implement a social policy, whereas parents of children with hearing loss may be more easily persuaded to support a UNHS policy.

The gold standard of research (Level I and, to some extent, Level II studies) is not without controversy, especially because no-treatment control groups may be included. If the control group is composed of individuals who are matched to the treatment group on variables other than a communication disorder, then that is ideal, but it is unethical to withhold treatment from someone who has a communication disorder and wants therapy.

Federal law prohibits randomly assigning patients to treatment and no-treatment control groups, in terms of both when to start treatment and in the type of treatment, making this kind of random assignment to groups illegal as well as unethical. Researchers and practitioners are prohibited by law from withholding relevant information, such as presence of hearing loss in children, in order to have a child randomly assigned to a no-treatment control group (Yoshinaga-Itano, 2004, p. 457).

Patients and family members advocating for children have the right to accept or refuse clinical intervention and to request the type of intervention they want. Competent adults and advocates for individuals in protected classes (see Chapter 3 for information about protected classes) may refuse treatment so they can legally and ethically be members of a no-treatment control group. However, there are research design problems even under these conditions. Participants in the experimental group are likely to be individuals who are more highly motivated and more apt to be compliant than participants in the self-selecting no-treatment control group, biasing results in favor of the group that sought treatment.

International Classification of Functioning, Disability, and Health

Research evidence can also follow an internationally recognized protocol. The International Classification of Functioning, Disability, and Health, abbreviated in the literature as ICF, complements the World Health Organization's International Classification of Diseases (ICD; WHO, 1992). Developed by the WHO (2002), the purpose of the ICF is to establish a universally accepted set of terms for classifying health. The three categories in the ICF classification system are body functions (and its impairments), activity (and its limitations), and participation (and its restrictions). These terms are defined in Box 2–3.

In a tutorial on implementing ICF in assessment and intervention for school-age children with language disorders, Westby and Washington (2017) demonstrate how the language impairment affects daily functioning and how language intervention has effects that integrate with other aspects of the child's life. The authors show how integrating ICF with the Individuals with Disabilities

Box 2–3. Definitions of Terms in the ICF Classification System

- *Function:* Applies to an individual's typical environment, as well as to one defined as standard, and accounts for environmental and personal factors. There are three levels of functioning: body or body part, person, and person in an environment or social context.
- *Body structures:* Refers to organs, limbs, and their components; in other words, the anatomical composition of the body.
- *Impairments:* Refers to significant deviation or loss caused by problems in body function or structure.
- *Activity:* Refers to execution of an action or a task by an individual, who may have *activity limitations.*
- *Participation:* Refers to involvement in a life situation, where the individual may have *participation restrictions.*
- *Environmental factors:* Refers to the individual's physical and social environment, as well as attitudes toward these environments.

Education Act (IDEA, 2004) can support individualized education plans (IEPs) in terms of current skill levels; annual goals; alternative assessments; measuring progress; description of services; and program modifications, accommodation, or supports for school personnel (Westby & Washington, 2017, p. 141).

Using the ICF model, research on the *body functions* that result in language disorders in children focuses primarily on the brain and secondarily on ear structures. Research on the *activity* level and its limitations focuses on standardized diagnostic testing. This is required by most school districts to qualify a student for speech and language services. Westby and Washington (2017, p. 142) highlight a protocol for the *participation* portion of the ICF called The Focus on the Outcomes of Children Under Six (FOCUS; Thomas-Stonell, Oddson, Robertson, & Rosenbaum, 2010) that is used for children 12 months to 6 years. It is a questionnaire that parents and clinicians use to rate children on a 7-point Likert scale.

Clinical Trials

Clinical trials go through four stages, or phases. A Phase I trial is in its early stages. It is nonrandomized (i.e., there is only one group that receives treatment) and provides the least influence on evidence compared to the subsequent stages. Phase II clinical trials establish more compelling evidence. While they are normally nonrandomized, some Phase II trials may be randomized. This means that there is more than one group in the study—a control group that does not receive the treatment and an experimental group that does. Considered the "gold standard" of clinical research, Phase III trials are randomized to enable collection of the most convincing evidence regarding a treatment. Lastly, a Phase IV trial determines how well the particular treatment being studied works when used by clinicians in their everyday practice (Onslow, 2017, pp. 117–121).

Levels of evidence in medical speech-language pathology research are described in the following section on systematic reviews and meta-analyses.

Aphasia

An example is a systematic review and meta-analysis that addressed treatment of aphasia. Beeson and Robey (2006) reviewed more than 600 articles published over the past 50 years, where 288 articles used group studies to examine effects of treatment and 332 were single-subject case reports or experiments. Studies of efficacy of aphasia therapy included group studies and single-participant experimental studies. The group studies assessed effects of aphasia therapy in its various forms as opposed to no therapy or deferred therapy, effects of therapy administered by SLPs as opposed to trained volunteers, and the ability to generalize findings to the greater population. Single-subject experimental studies evaluated effectiveness of a specific therapy for one patient over time, checked at designated intervals. Findings were applicable only to the individual participant and could not be generalized to other individuals with aphasia.

The ANCDS authors reported that the committee had difficulties in assessing efficacy of various treatments and in synthesizing findings in a meaningful way.

Meta-analyses revealed that outcomes from group studies suggest therapy for aphasia results in improved language relative to an untreated group, but that these analyses were not appropriate for single-participant ($N = 1$) research.

Some suggestions (Beeson & Robey, 2006) for evaluating single-participant research include focusing on the following types of studies:

- Studies with large effect size, where the treatment effect diverges from the null state, that is, where the outcome is more or less than zero
- Studies that present testable hypotheses, either in pretreatment versus posttreatment or treatment versus no treatment conditions
- Studies that can be grouped because they address a common dependent variable, such as lexical retrieval, speech fluency, or auditory comprehension

Dementia

A review of about thirty years of electronic databases (Zientz et al., 2007) yielded six studies that specifically assessed the effect of educational interventions in communication strategies on families and caregivers of individuals with Alzheimer disease and dementia. There were five trends that emerged regarding educating caregivers in communication strategies: more successful conversational exchanges, both reduced and increased caregiver burden, improved quality of life, maintenance of language abilities of individuals with Alzheimer disease, and increased understanding by caregivers of communication breakdown and Alzheimer disease in general.

The literature reviewed (Zientz et al., 2007) was not helpful regarding optimal therapy dose characteristics (frequency, intensity, and duration of treatment), which varied widely. The content of the training programs was predictable: impact of Alzheimer disease on communication, both verbal and nonverbal communication strategies, and opportunities for practice with individualized feedback. Expected outcomes of caregiver education reflected the training: increased knowledge of communication problems in Alzheimer disease and better use of and satisfaction with communication strategies. The literature did not provide evidence to support conclusions about effects of caregiver training on attitudes, symptoms, or communication skills of individuals with Alzheimer disease.

The ANCDS writing committee for dementia (Bayles et al., 2006) reviewed more than thirty years of literature in nine databases, as well as manual searches of textbooks and other articles, and identified five papers on one type of therapy: SimPres. (simulated presence therapy), where a family member or caregiver makes an audiotape about positive events to simulate their presence in the life of an individual with dementia. The data did not provide evidence of how long positive effects lasted, or whether SimPres was better than usual care.

Traumatic Brain Injury

In establishing guidelines for clinical assessments of traumatic brain injury (TBI), more recently classified as acquired brain injury (ABI), the ANCDS committee

(Turkstra, Ylvisaker, et al., 2005, pp. 9–10) focused on two questions:

- What tests can or should be used by SLPs for evaluating and assessing communication abilities in individuals with TBI?
- What unique contribution does the SLP make in the process of interdisciplinary evaluation?

The committee gathered information by surveying SLPs engaged in clinical practice with individuals with TBI, surveying test publishers and distributors, reviewing test manuals, reviewing published literature appearing in four databases, and reviewing published expert opinion.

Most tests showed strengths in content and face validity, but weaknesses in other elements of reliability (consistency) and validity (truthfulness and generalizability). For example, a majority of tests did not meet strict criteria for interrater reliability, internal consistency, and test–retest reliability. They were also much more likely to show concurrent validity (where the test is comparable to another, similar test) than predictive validity (where future performance is estimated). Overall, despite some strength in content validity, many of the tests designed for and administered to individuals with TBI were weak psychometrically, lacking established relationships between test scores and important measures of outcomes (Turkstra, Ylvisaker, et al., 2005, p. 23). Validity and reliability are explored further in Chapters 7, for journal articles, and 8, for diagnostic tests.

Assessing cognitive-communication disorders in individuals after TBI is challenging for SLPs. The clinical population tends to be heterogeneous, showing complex constellations of strengths and limitations (Turkstra, Coelho, & Ylvisaker, 2005, p. 216). Evaluation addressed the following questions:

- Does the individual with TBI have a cognitive-communication problem?
- If there is such a problem, what are its characteristics?
- What are the implications of the test results?
- How do the test results inform treatment?

The ANCDS writing committee (Turkstra, Coelho, et al., 2005) reviewed 84 tests recommended by practicing SLPs and 40 tests recommended by publishers and distributors. After eliminating tests that did not mention TBI in the test manual, 31 tests for children, adolescents, and adults remained.

Most experts agreed that standardized tests constitute only one component of an evaluation, leading the committee (Turkstra, Coelho, et al., 2005, p. 220) to make the following recommendations:

- use caution when using existing standardized tests to evaluate individuals with TBI;
- in addition to standardized testing, evaluate the individual's preinjury characteristics (based on a reliable informant), stage of development and recovery, and demands and contexts for communication in the individual's activities of daily living; and
- collaborate with other professionals when considering how to interpret cognitive impairment level based on tests.

A review (Kennedy et al., 2008) focused on intervention for improving everyday problem solving, planning, organizing, and multitasking. Using several databases, more than 2,500 published articles were identified in these areas. Most were excluded because they were not intervention studies with objective outcomes, leaving 15 quantitative intervention studies. The strength of evidence was evaluated as Class I for five studies, Class II for three studies, and Class III for seven studies. Treatment dosage varied from two 15-min sessions to 48 hr, with therapy provided individually in most cases (87%). Treatment outcomes were classified according to the International Classification Framework for Enablement, included in ICF (WHO, 2001) at the impairment level and at the activity/participation level.

Goals of intervention varied according to the aspect of executive function targeted. All studies focused on some aspect of problem solving, planning, organizing, and multitasking, but some specifically addressed social or behavioral problem solving, time management, goal management, decision making, self-regulation, verbal reasoning, complex activities with cues, organization strategies during functional activities, or dual-task training. Intervention approaches tended to include metacognitive strategy instruction, including self-monitoring, self-recording of performance, basing strategy decisions on goals, and adjusting or modifying plans based on self-assessment or external feedback (Kennedy et al., 2008, p. 35).

Nearly all studies reported positive treatment outcomes immediately following the experimental interventions. Positive activity/participation treatment effects were also reported in most studies. A majority of studies (60%) also reported positive maintenance effects, that is, generalization to untrained tasks and contexts. In other words, there was strong evidence of efficacy of treatment.

Dysarthria

The ANCDS writing committee on dysarthria searched 30 years of databases covering 5,800 journals using key words paired with the term *dysarthria*, and identified 51 intervention studies focusing on loudness ($N = 21$), speaking rate ($N = 19$), prosody ($N = 10$), and general instructions ($N = 6$), with some articles placed in more than one category. In general, statistically significant improvement in loudness was found for participants with Parkinson disease who completed the 16-session protocol for the Lee Silverman Voice Treatment (LSVT; Yorkston, Hakel, Beukelman, & Fager, 2007, p. 19). Although statistical analysis related to acoustic variables, there were also improvements noted on physiologic and perceptual measures. Rate control treatments included delayed auditory feedback (DAF), pacing board, metronome, computer training, behavioral instructions, and biofeedback. Outcome measures were most often based on perceptual ratings of such variables as intelligibility. The research generally supports a relationship between reduced speaking rate and increased intelligibility.

Prosodic or suprasegmental features studied in the literature included stress patterning, intonation, and rate/rhythm. Prosodic disturbances are particularly noted in ataxic dysarthria, and refer to a complex interaction of rate loudness and pitch adjustments (Yorkston et al.,

2007, p. 26). Acoustic parameters of fundamental frequency contours, intensity, and duration of speech production were the most frequent outcome measures analyzed in prosodic studies. Interpretation of outcomes was limited by the heterogeneity of the individuals in treatment, the small number of studies, and the fact that most investigations were case reports.

The final category of general instructions included many techniques telling patients to produce clear speech and providing feedback about the clarity of utterances. Perceptual ratings of clarity, intelligibility, and precision of articulation were the outcomes in the great majority of studies. Results do not provide strong evidence that there is an important benefit of instructing individuals with dysarthria to speak clearly.

Apraxia of Speech

A committee of the ANCDS was charged with developing evidence-based treatment guidelines for acquired apraxia of speech (AOS). They reported (Wambaugh, 2006) the following concerns about diagnosis and description of individuals in the AOS treatment literature:

- description of participants in investigations was cited as a particularly problematic area;
- published reports did not include enough information about AOS diagnosis, the speech behaviors of participants, severity levels of impairment, and other speech-language disorders that co-occurred with AOS;
- the profession does not yet agree on diagnostic standards for AOS; and
- more than half of the published reports of AOS were case studies, which lack scientific controls for internal and external validity.

Accordingly, the committee recommended that researchers detail the behaviors that characterize and support their diagnosis of AOS, and include the level of severity of the disorder.

When aphasia co-occurs with AOS, investigators need to provide information about the language disorder and its impact on verbal production.

The ANCDS writing committee on apraxia of speech (Wambaugh, Duffy, McNeil, Robin, & Rogers, 2006, p. 36) identified five general categories of treatments:

- articulatory kinematic;
- rate/rhythm;
- intersystemic facilitation/reorganization;
- AAC; and
- other.

Verbal production was a requisite goal for the 30 studies of articulatory kinematics to improve speech production. Most treatments used modeling/repetition, also called "integral stimulation," to elicit desired speech behaviors. In integral stimulation, the patient is instructed to "watch me, listen to me, and say it with me" (Wambaugh et al., 2006, p. 36). In many studies, articulatory placement cues are also used to correct sounds produced in error. Other forms of stimulation include prompts for restructuring oral and muscular phonetic targets (PROMPT), which obliges the clinician to obtain specialized training, and written cues.

There were seven studies of rate or rhythm control for treatment of AOS. In all investigations, there was an external source of control, including metronomic pacing, computerized control using visual displays, and a pacing board. The present author has found that it is easy to create a pacing board by wrapping rubber bands around the inch markers of a six-inch ruler, and much less expensive than buying commercially available types.

There were eight investigations of effects of intersystemic facilitation/reorganization treatments. The most frequently studied type of treatment was gestural reorganization, often employing American Indian Hand Talk (Amer-Ind), with most treatments requiring vocalizations paired with the gestures. The code developed by Native Americans (Skelly, 1979) appears elsewhere in this section. There is some overlap between rate/rhythm and intersystemic facilitation/reorganization treatments, such as in singing and in vibrotactile stimulation.

The eight treatment studies that employed augmentative and alternative communication (AAC) focused on improving communication without using speech. An additional five studies that could not fit into the other categories of treatment included a focus on communication partners, work on segmental and suprasegmental aspects of speech productions paired with head movements, and treatment that appeared to combine several approaches.

The ANCDS writing group (Wambaugh et al., 2006, p. 42) concluded that articulatory kinematic approaches were probably effective, rate/rhythm control approaches and intersystemic approaches were possibly effective, and AAC approaches could not be rated regarding likelihood of benefit because of insufficient data.

Augmentative and Alternative Communication

Systematic reviews and meta-analyses remain fruitful ways of exploring large numbers of publications in a given subject to look for important findings. In terms of AAC, a more recent meta-analysis (Kent-Walsh, Murza, Malani, & Binger, 2015) using electronic database searches yielded 17 single-case design studies that included 53 individuals who met the inclusion criteria. The purposes of this meta-analysis were to determine the overall effects of communication partner interventions on the communication of individuals using AAC, and to determine if these effects might differ by participant, intervention, and/or outcome characteristics. Mean effect size aggregated across the studies was very large, as were semantic and morpho-syntactic measures; the pragmatic outcome measure yielded a moderate effect size rating. The review concludes that the evidence analyzed consistently indicates that instructing communication partners positively affects communication performance of individuals using AAC. The authors concluded that it is helpful to include communication partner instruction in AAC intervention plans with the goal of improving communication skills of individuals with complex communication needs.

Specific Language Impairment

Systematic reviews and meta-analyses of literature on language disorders in children have also been conducted. Rudolph

(2017) examined the literature on risk factors for specific language impairment (SLI) in young children, a condition seen in just over 1 in 14 in children 5 years old. That is, there will likely be one or two children with SLI in a given kindergarten class. The epidemiological data on risk factors indicated that the inability to combine words at 24 months together with a family history of reading or communication disorders accounted for 90% of children with SLI. Rudolph (2017) noted that an SLI screening tool should include the strongest and most clinically relevant risk factors that predict the disorder.

A literature search of 2,529 references was ultimately narrowed down to eight studies of more than 200,000 children between ages 4 and 8, where more than 6,000 had SLI. A total of 122 risk factors with varying effect sizes were narrowed down to nine statistically significant risk categories, with five of the nine categories having at least one combined effect size (at least two effect sizes are required to perform meta-analyses). Rudolph (2017) concluded that the children who had mothers with less than a high school education, were male, had a very low 5-min Apgar score, or were later born (as opposed to full-term or premature) were at as high a risk for developing SLI as those who were late talkers.

Autism Spectrum Disorders

A diagnostic evaluation for autism spectrum disorders (ASD) includes a comprehensive assessment of communication. However, individuals with autism may communicate in a self-directed or context-specific way and may not demonstrate their communication abilities adequately in a formal assessment. Because assessment drives treatment (what you do about the communication problem in autism depends on what you think it is), then proper diagnosis is needed for best practices in intervention. A recent systematic review of assessment of the speech of children with ASD (Broome, McCabe, Docking, & Doble, 2017) yielded 2,687 articles from eight databases. Nearly half the articles were duplicates, and the 1,484 remaining articles were winnowed to 116 when all filtering criteria were met. A final 21 articles met all inclusion and search criteria as well as confidence in ASD diagnosis.

The assessment methods included connected speech samples, speech imitation, and single-word naming tasks. However, some studies included prelinguistic children and others assessed children who were verbal. The heterogeneity of the populations made it difficult for Broome et al. (2017) to identify trends across the 21 studies.

Stuttering

A systematic review of behavioral interventions for stuttering (Nye et al., 2013) shows how rare it is to find the highest level of evidence (randomized controlled trials, or RCTs) in studies of therapy. Eight electronic database searches yielded a total of 3,271 titles. After eliminating 2,959 studies because they did not meet inclusion criteria, the remaining 312 citations were evaluated by two independent reviewers to see if the studies met all inclusion criteria. This further review established that only nine studies met all four inclusionary criteria of domain, age, design, and outcomes, and eight of the studies were RCTs. Four of these RCTs assessed one behavior modification treatment to enhance fluency in young children who stuttered: the Lidcombe Program that was itself the focus of a systematic review and meta-analysis (Ingham, 2016). For a comprehensive look at systematic reviews of stuttering intervention, see Yairi and Seery (2015).

Voice Disorders

Sometimes critical reviews of a body of literature are followed by a critique of the reviews in the form of a meta-analysis. Twenty years of studies of vocal fold function after thyroidectomy procedures that resulted in either unilateral vocal fold paralysis (UVFP) or bilateral vocal fold paralysis (BVFP) (see, for example, Rosenthal, Benninger, & Deeb, 2007) included 39 published studies (13 for UVFP and 26 for BVFP) that included 1,798 patients. Injection laryngoplasty followed by voice therapy was found to be a significantly better treatment option than neurolysis for UVFP in terms of vocal function measurements. For BVFP, cordectomy only was a significantly better treatment option than vocal fold laterofixation and arytenoidectomy with cordectomy. However, Watts (2016) raised methodological concerns about the analysis that readers should consider before accepting the evidence provided by Rosenthal et al. (2007). The principal concern raised by Watts was the lack of specificity of the outcome measurements that formed the basis of statistical analysis.

BEST PRACTICES AND EVIDENCE-BASED PRACTICE

The following is the American Speech-Language-Hearing Association's (ASHA) position statement on evidence-based practice in communication disorders (ASHA, 2005; reprinted with permission):

> It is the position of the American Speech-Language-Hearing Association that audiologists and speech-language pathologists incorporate the principles of evidence-based practice in clinical decision making to provide high quality clinical care. The term *evidence-based practice* refers to an approach in which current, high-quality research evidence is integrated with practitioner expertise and client preferences and values into the process of making clinical decisions. In making clinical practice evidence based, audiologists and speech-language pathologists:
>
> A. recognize the needs, abilities, values, preferences, and interests of individuals and families to whom they provide clinical services, and integrate those factors along with best current research evidence and their clinical expertise in making clinical decisions;
>
> B. acquire and maintain the knowledge and skills that are necessary to provide high quality professional services, including knowledge and skills related to evidence based practice;
>
> C. evaluate prevention, screening, and diagnostic procedures, protocols, and measures to identify maximally informative and cost-effective diagnostic and screening tools, using recognized appraisal criteria described in the evidence-based practice literature;
>
> D. evaluate the efficacy, effectiveness, and efficiency of clinical protocols

for prevention, treatment, and enhancement using criteria recognized in the evidence-based practice literature;

E. evaluate the quality of evidence appearing in any source or format, including journal articles, textbooks, continuing education offerings, newsletters, advertising, and Web-based products, prior to incorporating such evidence into clinical decision making; and

F. monitor and incorporate new and high quality research evidence having implications for clinical practice.

Evidence of the efficacy of therapy tends to be stronger when the treatment protocol follows the scientific method (see Chapter 4), where therapy is seen as a means of testing hypotheses. We understand the term *hypothesis* to be a proposed explanation that serves as a starting point for further investigation. Hypotheses are usually based on limited evidence; when a large body of evidence has been collected, the proposed explanation may be described as a *theory*. Hypotheses or theories are never proven correct 100% of the time, because only a fraction (not 100%) of the relevant population is tested. However, hypotheses may be falsified. For example, if you propose the hypothesis that birds can fly, then you must falsify this hypothesis after you visit the sanctuary for flightless birds in New Zealand. In terms of clinical practice, if the hypothesis underlying your clinical intervention is falsified, then the therapy can be abandoned and another therapeutic hypothesis can be tested. In an educational model, a curriculum is meant to be followed without critical evaluation. If it doesn't work, there are few alternatives. Evidence-based practice supports the hypothesis-testing model.

Individual therapy can model an experiment where $N = 1$. However, there are problems with single-subject treatment research that involve statistical interpretation (described in detail in Chapter 6). Any attempt to generalize findings will necessarily suffer from a lack of statistical power. With low statistical power, you may not detect an effect of your therapy, even though there is one that would be detected if you had an adequate sample of participants on whom to test the effect.

ASHA's (2005) use of the term *evidence-based practice* refers to an approach in which current, high-quality research evidence is integrated with practitioner expertise and client preferences and values into the process of making clinical decisions. However, the ASHA guidelines don't explain *how* to weigh the evidence. We use critical thinking to make evidence-based decisions. Practitioners and researchers rely on critical thinking, defined as the ability and willingness to assess claims and make objective judgments on the basis of well-supported reasons and evidence, rather than on emotion or anecdote. The purpose of weighing the evidence using critical thinking is to identify flaws in an argument, evaluate explanations for events, determine implications of research findings, apply new knowledge to clinical or research questions and problems, and resist claims that have no support (Wade, Tavris, & Garry, 2015).

Critical thinking underlying evidence-based case management is apparent in three case studies of the dilemmas faced by SLPs making decisions about dysphagia management (Coyle, Easterling, Lefton-Greif, & Mackay, 2007). Many fragile patients in acute care settings have other conditions, such as pneumonia and even terminal illnesses, in addition to difficulty swallowing. One role of the SLP is to prevent further adverse health outcomes by using critical thinking and clinical expertise in making the appropriate decision regarding oral feeding while considering quality of life consequences for the patient.

A MODEL OF THERAPY

Goldfarb and Santo Pietro (2012) proposed a model for evaluation and treatment of communication disorders based on set theory. A set is a collection of things where we regard the collection as a single object. We are all members of the set of human beings and may also be members of subsets, such as adults and scholars, but we are not all members of the subset of females. In linguistics, the meaning of a predicate is a set. For example, the predicate *is large* refers to all things that are large. In addition, if we consider that large is a size, then we can think of a set containing all things in all sizes.

Overlaps between two collections yield more familiar applications of set theory. We use braces to denote sets, so {0, 1} is the set containing the elements 0 and 1. Santo Pietro and Goldfarb (1995) used this language of sets to demonstrate treatment strategies for aphasia. An example of one such treatment strategy follows.

A patient receiving treatment for aphasia and a clinician are each asked, independently, to list their five most important goals for language rehabilitation. The patient indicates the desire to improve the following abilities:

Set A

1. recite hymns and prayers in church;
2. state bids while playing games of bridge;
3. retrieve names and relationships of family members;
4. verbalize activities of daily living; and
5. speak and understand conversational speech on the telephone.

The clinician's goals for the patient are to improve the following abilities:

Set B

3. retrieve names and relationships of family members;
4. verbalize activities of daily living;
5. speak and understand conversational speech on the telephone;
6. read and understand the newspaper; and
7. write legibly with the left hand.

Selecting appropriate target goals can be aided by examining the two sets of goals arithmetically. If Set A = {1,2,3,4,5} and Set B = {3,4,5,6,7}, then the intersection of these two sets of goals is {3,4,5}, or Set C. Expressed in symbols, $A \cap B = C$, or $\{1,2,3,4,5\} \cap \{3,4,5,6,7\} = \{3,4,5\}$, where $\cap$ (read "cap") is the symbol for intersection. The three goals in Set C {3,4,5} might be expected to elicit maximal motivation and cooperation between patient and clinician.

John Venn (1834–1923) is best known for his development of diagrams, later named after him, depicting relationships between sets. The logo for the Olympic Games is a Venn diagram. Venn diagrams also illustrate strategies of clinical intervention in individuals with communication disorders following Alzheimer disease (Ostuni & Santo Pietro, 1991), aphasia (Santo Pietro & Goldfarb, 1995), and stuttering (Goldfarb, 2006).

Figure 2–1 shows a Venn diagram of a person (P) with a language impairment (I) communicating (C) with a communication partner (CP) within an environment (E). None of the components should be treated independently of the others. The clinician who works only to build skills lost as a result of the neurological impairment (treating to deficit) is addressing only (I). However, (I) is contained completely within the set of the person (P), who is contained completely within an environment (E). It also intersects the communication (C) between the person and the communication partner (CP) as well as the communication partner alone. Rebuilding skills lost or absent through impairment will have a direct effect on the total person (P), the person's communication partner (CP), the level of communication between them (C), and their shared environment (E). Conversely, (P), (CP), (C), and (E) will have a direct effect on level of impairment as the skill-(re)building proceeds.

To be effective, therapy must address all intersections to maximize the person's unimpaired communication skills (treating to strength), repair communication acts between persons and communication

Figure 2–1. *A model for therapy using a Venn diagram.* Source: *Goldfarb, R., and Santo Pietro, M. J. (2012). The use of sets in SLP diagnosis and treatment. In R. Goldfarb (Ed.),* Translational speech-language pathology and audiology *(pp. 313–318). San Diego, CA: Plural Publishing, Inc.*

partners, educate and support the partners, repair the communication-impaired environment to provide opportunities for communication, and treat the whole person to reduce psychosocial handicap.

Set theory may also apply to diagnosis and evaluation. Recently (Goldfarb & Serpanos, 2020), we identified five rules for diagnosis: (1) Say what the client does, not what the client is; (2) Be an educated consumer of tests and measures; (3) Beware of "clinicese," where clients may exhibit behaviors in the clinic that they do not generalize outside of the speech and hearing center; (4) Do differential diagnosis when appropriate; and (5) Obey the limits of our scope of practice.

The third and fourth rules, in particular, express aspects of set theory. Regarding rule 3, a working hypothesis for carryover (or generalization of linguistic skills acquired in therapy to other communication environments) might be for the two sets of clinical communication and communication in another environment to approximate the same set or cardinal number. Deciding where among diagnostically related groups the observed language behavior best fits (rule 4) offers the opportunity to examine intersections along a continuum (see Chapter 8 for an example of the difficulty of differential diagnosis).

The Venn diagram in Figure 2–1 also illustrates two major points of applying set theory to diagnosis and evaluation of fluency disorders (Goldfarb, 2006, p. 25). (1) Diagnosis must be comprehensive. The whole person as well as the communication partners and environment must be considered. And (2) The individual's needs and wishes must be an integral component in determining approaches to treatment.

SOME CLINICAL RESEARCH CONCERNS

How often should we schedule therapy? Is intensive treatment most effective? How many trials should each therapy session contain? Should treatment tasks be grouped together as massed practice or spread out across the therapy session as distributed practice? How large, bold, or colorful should therapy stimuli be? What warrants immediate placement, follow-up, or watchful waiting? What are the criteria that motivate discharge from clinical intervention? What should we do when our clients do not comply with therapy procedures?

Dosage of Therapy

Determining efficacy of clinical intervention requires examination of both effectiveness (Does the therapy work?) and efficiency (Does it take less time and/or cost less than comparable therapies?) of treatment, with both related to dosage of therapy. In an attempt to quantify the complicated impact of intensity of therapy, Yoder, Fey, and Warren (2012) created a formula called *cumulative intensity* that depends on understanding the operational definitions of several terms:

- *Dose* refers to the number of clinically appropriate therapy trial episodes (the authors use the term "teaching episodes" that I find confusing) in one intervention session. It is quantified as the number of trials per minute, or the rate of correct trials.
- *Dose form* refers to the task or activity that frames the therapy episodes.

These forms can be highly structured (drill and practice) or contextually embedded (activity based). Usually activity-based treatments result in fewer trials or a smaller dose than drill and practice approaches.

- *Dose frequency* refers to the number of therapy sessions per day or per week. For example, Yoder et al. (2012) implemented a milieu communication teaching (MLC) program to toddlers with intellectual disabilities. MLC was administered either for 1 hr once a week or 1 hr five times a week for 9 weeks. The authors did not find a main effect of dose frequency on communication and language development.
- *Cumulative intensity* refers to the result of multiplying dose × dose frequency × duration of therapy (Yoder et al., 2012, p. 410).

Other concerns about dosage might be called *dose duration* that refers to the length of one therapy session; *dose environment* that refers to an individual or group therapy session; and *dose schedule* that refers to the time of day of the therapy session, an important consideration when the client is taking medication. All need further research validation.

Much of the literature on dosage of SLP treatment comes from studies of aphasia therapy. In an evidence-based systematic review that focused on one type of aphasia treatment (constraint-induced language therapy [CILT]), the authors (Cherney, Patterson, Raymer, Frymark, & Schooling, 2008) examined effects of intensity of treatment. CILT is based on constraint-induced movement therapy (CIMT), where use of the unimpaired or less-impaired arm and hand is restrained. While efficacy of CIMT is well documented in physical and occupational therapy, the jury is still out on whether CILT works as an aphasia therapy and what the intensity of CILT treatment should be. A review of dose parameters in some aphasia studies of different designs (randomized controlled trial, descriptive study, crossover study, case series, between groups, and retrospective crossover designs; Cherney, 2012) focused on a definition of aphasia treatment intensity. When studies provided information about dose, then intensity of intervention could be calculated (total number of sessions × dose). However, many studies did not give dose information, especially when therapy targeted multiple modalities and used several different strategies (Cherney, 2012, p. 428). Cherney (2012, p. 430) concluded that there is no standard definition of intensity and that a "more is better" conclusion about therapy is not consistently supported by evidence.

Other studies of dosage and intensity of aphasia treatment considered a meta-analysis supporting the conclusion that the number of sessions is important for aphasia recovery (Basso, 2005) as well as intensive speech-language intervention for chronic aphasia (Breitenstein et al., 2017), anomia (Laganaro, Di Pietro, & Schnider, 2006), apraxia of speech (Wambaugh, Nessler, Cameron, & Mauszycki, 2013), and finally, clinician perspectives about intensity of aphasia therapy (Gunning et al., 2017).

Our professions do not yet have the communication equivalent of "Take two aspirin and call me in the morning," but pharmacological dosage concepts may have limited utility for SLPs. Kamhi (2012) examined the possibility of finding what he considered the active ingredients of an ideal or optimal dose of treatment. In acknowledging that SLPs can provide effective intervention without knowing the ideal treatment intensity, Kamhi (2012) added that insisting on fixed, ideal dosages may be inconsistent with evidence-based practice in SLP, where treatment may need to be flexible and individualized. This conclusion was supported by Baker (2012) who claimed that the active ingredients of a teaching episode must be considered when constructing a definition of intensity of treatment. Togher (2012) cited two conditions where technology needs to be assessed when it enables SLPs to increase dosage of therapy: the first is that treatment must address the client's needs in everyday life; and the second is that SLPs need to measure the client's perceptions of treatment outcomes in addition to standardized assessments. Qualitative analysis should be added to quantitative analysis of the efficacy of therapy.

Should Exercises and Practice be Massed or Distributed?

The controversy in the present question refers to a learning principle called the spacing effect. Do we learn better when information is distributed across a period of time or when presented in bulk at one time? For example, if the clinician has a goal for a client with aphasia to retrieve the target word 20/25 times (80% correct), should the 25 trials be presented all at once or should five trials be spaced apart at five different times during the therapy session? The massed versus distributed practice question can also apply to the total number of therapy sessions. For example, a student clinician has a goal of increasing eye gaze behavior of a middle school child with autism spectrum disorder who avoids eye contact. Is it better to work on eye gaze tasks intensively in the first few sessions or addressed less intensively over the entire semester (assuming that the total number of eye-gaze tasks is held constant)?

A review of the literature (Green & Bavelier, 2008) suggested that distributed practice improves both memory and verbal learning for a variety of tasks. The effect of distributed practice includes the lag effect, or the effect of the interstudy interval on learning (see, for example, the meta-analysis by Cepeda, Pashler, Vul, Wixted, & Rohrer, 2006). Longer interstudy intervals seem to improve learning of verbal information and working memory.

However, a recent study (Tye-Murray, Spehar, Barcroft, & Sommers, 2017) examined distributed practice and the spacing effect on auditory perceptual learning that involved recognizing a degraded auditory signal, a task that is qualitatively different from verbal learning and working memory. Tye-Murray et al. found that there was no difference in retention of benefits between massed and distributed practice for their auditory training tasks. Children with specific language impairment (SLI) demonstrated improved sequential learning and retention when the training sessions on a serial reaction time task were distributed over 1 week, rather than massed in immediate succession in 1 day (Desmottes, Meulemans, Patinec, & Maillart, 2017). However, there was no difference between massed and distributed practice for typically developing children undertaking the same task.

In evaluating effects of motor learning in stroke rehabilitation, Krakauer (2006,

p. 84) identified differences between kinematics, defined as the geometry and speed of a movement, and dynamics, defined as the forces needed to generate the movement. He discussed the motor-learning mechanisms of kinematics and dynamics in various rehabilitation approaches, including CIMT. While CIMT usually refers to the physical and occupational therapy approaches to stroke rehabilitation, a focus on kinematics and dynamics can also be part of the treatment of dysarthria and acquired apraxia of speech. Regarding training schedules, the strategy of distributed practice that introduces frequent rest periods between repetitions improved performance and learning more than massed practice, the strategy that uses a single task of a block of repetitions.

In a tutorial acknowledging that studies of motor control and learning are lacking in CSD, Maas et al. (2008, p. 279) refer to Schema Theory. Rapid discrete movements, such as those needed for speech, use motor programs retrieved from memory and adapted for the required task. Even though these movements are never produced exactly the same, their essential characteristics are maintained. Schema Theory assumes that motor programs generalize the aspects of movements that are invariant. The academic–clinical integration question is determining the training schedule that best facilitates this generalization. Maas et al. (2008) recommend a period of prepractice to make sure clients understand the instructions and are motivated to perform a large number of trials. They support using distributed practice over massed practice, and also offer evidence to support variable versus constant practice. Variable practice targets more than one variant of a given movement. Maas et al. (2008, p. 284) use the example of practicing a golf swing from varying distances from the hole. Constant practice works on only one variant of a movement. Variable practice results in a more reliable schema that is more capable of generalization to untrained movements.

In a meta-analysis of 63 studies (Donovan & Radosevich, 1999), effect sizes supported spaced practice over massed practice conditions. However, effect sizes varied widely, and the largest effect sizes appeared in studies with poorer methodological rigor. Studies in CSD are inconsistent in supporting the clinical use of spaced practice. To improve word finding in adults with naming impairments secondary to aphasia, spaced practice worked better than both massed practice and errorless learning strategies (Middleton, Schwartz, Rawson, Traut, & Verkuilen, 2016). Regarding retention of learning effects, distributed practice was better than a massed practice schedule in addressing language recovery in adults whose brains were reorganizing following aphasia (Raymer et al., 2008, p. S263), but massed practice was advocated for CILT treatment of adults with chronic aphasia (Pulvermüller & Berthier, 2008).

The Adequate Stimulus

Many years ago, we built temporary walls out of dark green felt that we put over the existing walls when we wanted to limit distractions in the therapy room. The purpose was to help the client pay attention only to the stimuli we presented. Around the same time, we were influenced by Slobin's (1973, p. 412) operating principle, "Pay attention to the ends of words" to emphasize how important it is for language learners to focus on a word's final sounds. Earlier, Schuell, Jenkins, and Jimenez-Pabon (1964) wrote about the importance of the adequate stimulus in language intervention for adult aphasia.

What do we mean when we refer to the adequate stimulus? Does it have to do with the size, boldness, and color saturation of words or pictures? Is it the speed or modality of stimulus presentation? Might it relate to word parameters, such as part of speech, word length, abstraction level, or frequency of occurrence? Here, as elsewhere in this chapter, many of the suggested answers lie in the research literature about language intervention in adult aphasia.

In a classical study that looked at effects of certain stimuli on language comprehension as well as word retrieval and naming in aphasia, Gardiner and Brookshire (1972) found that combining auditory and visual presentation of stimuli was better than presenting either modality alone, and that the auditory modality alone was better than the visual modality alone. However, there may be different types of representations for speech, with stronger weight in the auditory modality, than for nonspeech stimuli, with more processing in the visual modality (Schmid, Thielmann, & Zieglerm, 2009). There are clinical implications in that individuals with apraxia of speech made more errors in imitation of bimodal nonspeech gestures, while neurotypical controls made more errors in imitation of auditory nonspeech stimuli compared to visual and bimodal stimuli. For both groups, most errors in the speech domain were made in response to visual stimuli. The patients with aphasia, oral apraxia, and apraxia of speech seemed to rely heavily on the acoustic signal (Schmid et al., 2009, p. 219). Finally, multisensory stimulation had positive effects on the care of elderly individuals with dementia (Milev et al., 2008). The beneficial effects on behavior as opposed to care as usual persisted for 12 additional weeks after treatment ended.

A multidimensional approach to therapy also applies to augmentative and alternative treatment of adults with motor speech disorders. An examination of multimodal supplementation (Hanson, Beukelman, & Yorkston, 2013) looked at alphabet, topic, syntactic, and gestural supplementation because these strategies, whether used singly or in combination, have been reported to help a communication partner decode unintelligible speech signals (Hanson et al., 2013, p. 310). The authors concluded that the evidence basis for speech supplementation is robust, and that the future of clinical practice is multidimensional (Hanson et al., 2013, p. 320).

Regarding manipulation of speed of stimulus presentation, Goldfarb and Halpern (1981) found that slower rates of stimulus presentation through auditory or visual modalities resulted in more appropriate word association responses by adults with aphasia. They also reported that adjectives and nouns, rather than verbs; frequent rather than infrequent words; longer rather than shorter words; and concrete rather than abstract stimuli resulted in more appropriate word association responses. However, Brookshire and Nicholas (1984) did not find consistent effects of speed of stimulus presentation on sentence comprehension by adults with aphasia.

More recently, McKelvey, Hux, Dietz, and Beukelman, (2010) asked if adults with aphasia would match a printed word to a photograph that was personally relevant and contextually appropriate more than to a photo that was not personally relevant but contextually appropriate or to images that were not contextualized. Their findings support the use of personally relevant, contextualized photographs as opposed to noncontextualized, iconic symbol systems in language therapy with adults when aphasia is severe enough to impede sole reliance on natural speech (Mckelvey et al., 2010, p. 31). Heuer, Ivanova, and Hallowell (2017) were interested in learning if adults with aphasia choose the wrong option in a multiple-choice task because of a comprehension deficit or because of the characteristics of the stimuli. They looked at eye fixations of 41 people with aphasia who were asked to choose an image that corresponded best with a verbal stimulus. The participants had longer visual fixations on images that were considered singletons (defined as differing from the majority images by one image characteristic) rather than majority images, regardless of which one was the target response. The authors concluded that regardless of presence or severity of language deficits, physical image characteristics influence visual attention.

The literature seems to support the following conclusions in terms of the adequate stimulus:

- *Stimulus modality:* Multimodal stimulus presentation may be better than unimodal, and the auditory modality alone is preferable to the visual modality alone for treatment of aphasia in adults. Multidimensional speech supplementation is likely to be more effective in improving comprehensibility of adults with motor speech disorders than a single augmentative and alternative supplemental strategy.
- *Stimulus presentation:* Slowing the speed of stimulus presentation may or may not be better than normal speed, but slower speech will certainly not hurt.
- *Stimulus saliency:* If photographs are used, make sure that they are personally relevant and contextually appropriate. Visual characteristics of stimuli may be manipulated in assessment and treatment materials to maximize visual attention on a client-centered basis.

Implications of Noncompliance

Noncompliance is a serious problem for both the clinical researcher and the patient or client. In Chapter 3, the issue of privacy and security of medical information is noted to have ethical and legal ramifications. Clinicians have to become familiar with best practices of complying with local, state, and federal regulations governing security of patient information, or they will be at risk for civil and criminal penalties (Jobes, White, & Antonelli, 2002).

Patient noncompliance comes in different forms. For example, the patient with impaired executive functioning following acquired brain injury may not have the capacity to follow rules. Tate (1999) assessed 30 adults with traumatic damage to frontal lobe areas and their connections, as well as 30 close relatives and 30 nonbrain damaged control participants to examine aspects of executive dysfunction and changes in character. Posttraumatic loss of emotional control led to rule-breaking errors, as observed by relatives.

Frequent noncompliance with prescribed medications and diets are seen in patients with gastro-esophageal reflux disease (GERD; Floch, 2000). Spaeth (1995, p. 189) claimed that the fact that one-third to one-half of patients do not take their prescribed medications represents a serious misunderstanding of health and how to achieve it.

In audiology, noncompliance has been reported in follow-up after neonatal hearing impairment identification (Folsom et al., 2000). In speech-language pathology, in reports of noncompliance when parents were enlisted as therapy assistants in the Lidcombe program for stuttering that was delivered as a telehealth adaptation (Wilson, Onslow, & Lincoln, 2004); in reports of noncompliance and sporadic attendance in voice therapy (Portone, Johns, & Hapner, 2008; Santos et al., 2013; Starmer, Liu, Akst, & Gourin, 2014); and in many reports of noncompliance in dysphagia management.

In interviews (Colodny, 2005), dysphagia patients who were feeding independently reported why they were not compliant with the SLP's recommendations. The most frequently cited reasons were open denial of impairment, followed by dissatisfaction with thickened liquids or other products, and willingness to accept the calculated risk of noncompliance. In another study, SLPs reported reasons for patient noncompliance in dysphagia treatment (King & Ligman, 2011). All patients who were noncompliant were dissatisfied with diet modifications. Some did not acknowledge that they had a swallowing impairment; said they were willing to take a chance or a calculated risk about swallowing unsafely; agreed that they had a swallowing problem but minimized it; and other reasons that were cited by fewer patients. Finally, a retrospective study of patients who had videofluoroscopic studies done in New Zealand (Low, Wyles, Wilkinson, & Sainsbury, 2001, p. 123) revealed the degree to which noncompliance was associated with chest infections, aspiration pneumonia, and readmission to the hospital. More than one-fifth of the patients were never compliant and had a higher rate of hospital readmission because of chest infections or aspiration pneumonia.

There are many questions about noncompliance, and several answers. We know who is noncompliant; how, and to some extent, when they are noncompliant; and what types of disorders and treatments are more likely to lead to noncompliance. The literature gives us some idea of why people are noncompliant and what the SLP and A can do to improve compliance. In a qualitative retrospective study of 10 people who did not comply with speech therapy in a primary care facility in Brazil, Paro, Vianna, Marconi, and Lima (2013, p. 1320) found several trends for noncompliance:

- incompatibility of time;
- the dynamics of speech therapy visits;
- noted improvement/resolution of the case;
- the need for pretreatment in another area; and
- patient's lack of interest.

In another study from Brazil (Duarte de Almeida, Santos, Bassi, Teixeira, & Gama, 2013) of female teachers with dysphonia, the abandonment rate of about one-third of the group was lower than the internationally reported rate of about two-thirds of voice patients who stop voice therapy. In the present study, patients with a lower perception of quality of life abandoned therapy more than those with a more positive perception. The study was limited in that the participants whose dysphonia persisted were in a position to experience significant job loss.

There are some recommendations for specific communication disorders. In a 10-year study of pure tone and tympanometric screening of nearly 35,000 preschool children, Serpanos and Jarmel (2007, p.10) found some trends among caregivers who did and did not follow up on professional recommendations. Those who were compliant praised the screening program and were grateful for the follow-up inquiry. Those who were not compliant included physicians who thought that the child was too young to be treated, that the child was being treated for a middle ear disorder at the time of screening, or that there was no problem with hearing, as well as parents who indicated that the child was being treated for a middle ear disorder at the time of screening or who did not suspect a hearing problem. The authors concluded that the physician's role is of utmost importance and may influence parental noncompliance. Regarding speech-language pathology, Starmer et al. (2014) reported that when the SLP who was part of an interdisciplinary voice clinic was included in the initial patient visit, as opposed to the otolaryngologist visiting the patient alone, subsequent participation in voice therapy and compliance with therapeutic recommendations improved.

ADVANCED STUDY

The author proposes that academic–clinical integration skills are necessary for an individual to be granted power of professor. With new generations of scholars and researchers needed every 10 years, professors and master clinicians have an obligation to prepare individuals with adequate knowledge and skills to undertake the tasks of scholarship and research, and academic–clinical integration is a key component. For evidence of the requisite academic–clinical integration skills, complete the following, and have your instructor, academic adviser, mentor, or CSD department chair review that you have completed the requirements and sign and date where indicated.

Student's Name:____

1. List and explain four levels of research evidence.
2. List and explain six terms in the ICF classification system.
3. Write a paragraph or two explaining what is meant by systematic reviews and meta-analyses.
4. Write a paragraph or two explaining the ASHA position on evidence-based practice.
5. Using the set theory model of therapy, explain why it is important to treat to strength and not just treat to deficit.
6. What are some variables to consider regarding dose of therapy?
7. Why is distributed practice better than massed practice?
8. What does the literature on language and motor speech disorders in adults tell us about the adequate stimulus?
9. What are three consequences of noncompliance in speech-language pathology and/or audiology?
10. Write a paragraph or two explaining how academic–clinical integration of research will affect your professional practice.

Date of Completion: ____________________________________

Faculty/Supervisor Signature: ______________________________

REFERENCES

Ackley, B. J., Swan, B. A., Ladwig, G., & Tucker, S. (2008). *Evidence-based nursing care guidelines: Medical-surgical interventions* (p. 7). St. Louis, MO: Mosby Elsevier.

Anema, I. (2014). Integrative learning and evidence-based practice: Mastering the process. *Contemporary Issues in Communication Science and Disorders, 41*, 1–11.

American Speech-Language-Hearing Association. (2005). *Evidence-based practice in communication disorders* [Position statement]. Retrieved from http://www.asha.org/docs/html/PS2005-00221.html

Baker, E. (2012). Optimal intervention intensity. *International Journal of Speech-Language Pathology, 14*, 401–409.

Basso, A. (2005). How intensive/prolonged should an intensive-prolonged treatment be? *Aphasiology, 19*(10–11), 975–984.

Bayles, K., Kim, E., Chapman, S., Zientz, J., Rackley, A., Mahendra, N., . . . Cleary, S. (2006). Evidence based practice recommendations for working with individuals with dementia: Simulated presence therapy. *Journal of Medical Speech-Language Pathology, 14*, 13–21.

Beeson, P. M., & Robey, R. R. (2006). Evaluating single-subject treatment research: Lessons learned from the aphasia literature. *Neuropsychology Review, 16*, 161–169.

Breitenstein, C., Grewe, T., Flöel, A., Ziegler, W., Springer, L., Martus, P., . . . Baumgertner, A. (2017). Intensive speech and language therapy in patients with chronic aphasia after stroke: A randomised, open-label, blinded-endpoint, controlled trial in a health-care setting. *Lancet, 389*, 1528–1538.

Brookshire, R. H., & Nicholas, M. E. (1984). Consistency of effects of slow rate and pauses on aphasic listeners' comprehension of spoken sentences. *Journal of Speech and Hearing Research, 27*, 323–328.

Broome, K., McCabe, P., Docking, K., & Doble, M. (2017). A systematic review of speech assessments for children with autism spectrum disorder: Recommendations for best practice. *American Journal of Speech-Language Pathology, 26*, 1011–1029.

Cepeda, N. J., Pashler, H., Vul, E., Wixted, J. T., & Rohrer, D. (2006). Distributed practice in verbal recall tasks: A review and quantitative synthesis. *Psychological Bulletin, 132*, 354–380.

Cherney, L. R. (2012). Aphasia treatment: Intensity, dose parameters, and script training. *International Journal of Speech-Language Pathology, 14*, 424–431.

Cherney, L. R., Patterson, J. P., Raymer, A., Frymark, T., & Schooling, T. (2008). Evidence-based systematic review: Effects of intensity of treatment. *Journal of Speech, Language, and Hearing Research, 51*, 1282–1299.

Colodny, N. (2005). Dysphagic independent feeders' justifications for noncompliance with recommendations by a speech-language pathologist. *American Journal of Speech-Language Pathology, 14*, 61–70. Retrieved from https://search-proquest-com.libproxy.adelphi.edu:2443/comdisdome/docview/67945737/2F8C6E8B6D5E4BA9PQ/2?accountid=8204

Coyle, J. L., Easterling, C., Lefton-Greif, M., & Mackay, L. (2007). Evidence-based to reality-based dysphagia practice: Three case studies. *The ASHA Leader, 12*, 10–32.

Desmottes, L., Meulemans, T., Patinec, M-A., & Maillart, C. (2017). Distributed training enhances implicit sequence acquisition in children with specific language impairment. *Journal of Speech, Language, and Hearing Research, 60*, 2636–2647.

Donovan, J. J., & Radosevich, D. J. (1999). A meta-analytic review of the distribution of practice effect: Now you see it, now you don't. *Journal of Applied Psychology, 84*, 795–805.

Duarte de Almeida, L., Santos, L. R., Bassi, I. B., Teixeira, L. C., & Gama, A. C. C. (2013). Relationship between adherence to speech therapy in patients with dysphonia and quality of life. *Journal of Voice, 27*, 617–621.

Ehlhardt, L. A., Sohlberg, M. M., Kennedy, M., Coelho, C., Ylvisaker, M., Turkstra, L., & Yorkston, K. (2008). Evidence-based practice guidelines for instructing individuals with neurogenic memory impairments: What have we learned in the past 20 years? *Neuropsychological Rehabilitation, 1*, 1–43.

Ellis, C. (2009). Does race/ethnicity really matter in adult neurogenics? *American Journal of Speech-Language Pathology, 18*, 310–314.

Floch, N. R. (2000). Surgical therapy for atypical symptoms of GERD: Patient selection and preoperative evaluation. *Journal of Clinical Gastroenterology, 30*, S45–S47.

Folsom, R. C., Widen, J. E., Vohr, B. R., Cone-Wesson, B., Gorga, M. P., Sininger, Y. S., & Norton, S. J. (2000). Identification of neonatal hearing impairment: Recruitment and follow-up. *Ear and Hearing, 21*, 462–470.

Gardiner, B. J., & Brookshire, R. H. (1972). Effects of unisensory and multisensory presentation of stimuli upon naming by aphasic subjects. *Language and Speech, 15*, 342–357.

Goldfarb, R. (2006). Diagnosis. In R. Goldfarb (Ed.), *Ethics: A case study from fluency* (pp. 12–29). San Diego, CA: Plural Publishing.

Goldfarb, R., & Halpern, H. (1981). Word association of time-altered auditory and visual stimuli in aphasia. *Journal of Speech and Hearing Research, 24*, 234–247.

Goldfarb, R., & Santo Pietro, M. J. (2012). The use of sets in SLP diagnosis and treatment. In R. Goldfarb (Ed.), *Translational speech-language pathology and audiology* (pp. 313–318). San Diego, CA: Plural Publishing.

Goldfarb, R., & Serpanos, Y. (2020). *Professional writing in speech-language pathology and audiology* (3rd ed.). San Diego, CA: Plural Publishing.

Green, C. S., & Bavelier, D. (2008). Exercising your brain: A review of human brain plasticity and training-induced learning. *Psychology and Aging, 23*, 692–701.

Gunning, D., Wenke, R., Ward, E. C., Chalk, S., Lawrie, M., Romano, M., . . . Cardell, E. (2017).

Clinicians' perceptions of delivering new models of high intensity aphasia treatment. *Aphasiology, 31*, 406–426.

Halpern, H., & Goldfarb, R. (2013). *Language and motor speech disorders in adults* (3rd ed.). Burlington, MA: Jones & Bartlett Learning.

Hanson, E. K., Beukelman, D. R., & Yorkston, K. M. (2013). Communication support through multimodal supplementation: A scoping review. *Augmentative & Alternative Communication, 29*, 310–331.

Harris, C., & Turner, T. (2011). *Evidence-based answers to clinical questions for busy clinicians*. Melbourne, Australia: The Centre for Clinical Effectiveness, Monash Health.

Heuer, S., Ivanova, M. V., & Hallowell, B. (2017). More than the verbal stimulus matters: Visual attention in language assessment for people with aphasia using multiple-choice image displays. *Journal of Speech, Language, and Hearing Research, 60*, 1–14.

Individuals with Disabilities Education Act of 2004, 20 U.S.C. § 300.1 (2004).

Ingham, J. C. (2016). Some things haven't changed: Lidcombe program for the treatment of early childhood stuttering is effective, and more research is still needed. *Evidence-Based Communication Assessment and Intervention, 9*, 91–95.

Jobes, K. E., White, E. R., & Antonelli, P. J. (2002). Privacy and security of medical information. *Otolaryngologic Clinics of North America, 35*, 1203–1209.

Kamhi, A. (2012). Pharmacological dosage concepts: How useful are they for educators and speech-language pathologists? *International Journal of Speech-Language Pathology, 14*, 414–418.

Kennedy, M., Coelho, C., Turkstra, L., Ylvisaker, M., Sohlberg, M., Yorkston, K., . . . Kan, P-F (2008). Intervention for executive functions after traumatic brain injury: A systematic review, meta-analysis and clinical recommendations. *Neuropsychological Rehabilitation, 1*, 1–43.

Kent-Walsh, J., Murza, K. A., Malani, M. D., & Binger, C. (2015). Effects of communication partner instruction on the communication of individuals using AAC: A meta-analysis. *Augmentative Alternative Communication, 31*, 271–284.

King, J. M., & Ligman, K. (2011). Patient noncompliance with swallowing recommendations: Reports from speech-language pathologists. *Contemporary Issues in Communication Science and Disorders, 38*, 53–60.

Krakauer, J. W. (2006). Motor learning: Its relevance to stroke recovery and neurorehabilitation. *Current Opinion in Neurology, 19*, 84–90.

Laganaro, M., Di Pietro, M., & Schnider, A. (2006). Computerised treatment of anomia in acute aphasia: Treatment intensity and training size. *Neuropsychological Rehabilitation, 16*(6), 630–640.

Low, J., Wyles, C., Wilkinson, T., & Sainsbury, R. (2001). The effect of compliance on clinical outcomes for patients with dysphagia on videofluoroscopy. *Dysphagia, 16*, 123–127.

Maas, E., Robin, D. A., Austermann Hula, S. N., Freedman, S. E., Wulf, G., Ballard, K. J., & Schmidt, R. A. (2008). Principles of motor learning in treatment of motor speech disorders. *American Journal of Speech Language Pathology, 17*(3), 277–298.

McKelvey, M. L., Hux, K., Dietz, A., & Beukelman, D. R. (2010). Impact of personal relevance and contextualization on word-picture matching by people with aphasia. *American Journal of Speech-Language Pathology, 19*, 22–33.

Middleton, E. L., Schwartz, M. F., Rawson, K. A., Traut, H., & Verkuilen, J. (2016). Towards a theory of learning for naming rehabilitation: Retrieval practice and spacing effects. *Journal of Speech, Language, and Hearing Research, 59*, 1111–1122.

Milev, R. V., Kellar, T., McLean, M., Mileva, V., Luthra, V., Thompson, S., & Peever, L., (2008). Multisensory stimulation for elderly with dementia: A 24-week single-blind randomized controlled pilot study. *American Journal of Alzheimer's Disease and Other Dementias, 23*, 372–376.

Moher, D., Liberati, A., Tetzlaff, J., Altman, D. G., & Group, P. (2009). Preferred reporting items for systematic reviews and meta-analyses: The PRISMA statement. *Journal of Clinical Epidemiology, 62*, 1006–1012.

Nye, C., Lorch, M. P., & Whurr, R. (1997). The utility of meta-analysis in the determination of efficacy of treatment in aphasia: A reply to Robey (1994). *Brain and Language, 57*, 280–282.

Onslow, M. (2017). *Stuttering and its treatment: Eleven lectures.* Sydney, Australia: Australian Stuttering Research Centre.

Ostuni, E., & Santo Pietro, M. J. (1991). *Getting through: Communicating when someone you care for has Alzheimer's disease.* Vero Beach, FL: The Speech Bin.

Paro, C. A., Vianna, N. G., Marconi, P., & Lima, M. C. (2013). Investigating the compliance with speech therapy service in the context of primary care. *Revista CEFAC, 15,* 1316–1324.

Portone, C., Johns, M. M., & Hapner, E. R. (2008). A review of patient adherence to the recommendation for voice therapy. *Journal of Voice, 22,* 192–196.

Pulvermüller, F., & Berthier, M. L. (2008). Aphasia therapy on a neuroscience basis. *Aphasiology, 22*(6), 563–599.

Raymer, A. M., Beeson, P., Holland, A., Kendall, D., Maher, L. M., Martin, N., . . .Gonzalez-Rothi, L. J. (2008). Translational research in aphasia: From neuroscience to neurorehabilitation. *Journal of Speech, Language, and Hearing Research, 51,* S259–S297.

Robey, R. R. (1994). The efficacy of treatment for aphasic persons: A meta-analysis. *Brain and Language, 47,* 582–608.

Robey, R. R. (1998). On Nye, Lorch, and Whurr (1997). *Brain and Language, 61,* 145–146.

Rosenthal, L. H., Benninger, M. S., & Deeb, R. H. (2007). Vocal fold immobility: A longitudinal analysis of etiology over 20 years. *Laryngoscope, 117,* 1864–1870.

Rudolph, J. M. (2017). Case history risk factors for specific language impairment: A systematic review and meta-analysis. *American Journal of Speech-Language Pathology, 26,* 991–1010.

Santo Pietro, M. J., & Goldfarb, R. (1995). *Techniques for aphasia rehabilitation: Generating effective treatment (TARGET).* Vero Beach, FL: The Speech Bin.

Santos, L. R., Almeida, L., Teixeira, L. C., Bassi, I., Assunção, A. A., & Gama, A. A. C. (2013). Adherence of the dysphonic teachers in speech therapy. *CoDAS, 25,* 134–139. https://doi.org/10.1590/S2317-17822013000200008

Schmid, G., Thielmann, A., & Zieglerm, W. (2009). The influence of visual and auditory information on the perception of speech and nonspeech oral movements in patients with left hemisphere lesions. *Clinical Linguistics & Phonetics, 23,* 208–221.

Schuell, H., Jenkins, J., & Jimenez-Pabon, E. (1964). *Aphasia in adults: Diagnosis, prognosis, and treatment.* New York, NY: Hoeber Medical Division, Harper.

Serpanos, Y., & Jarmel, F. (2007). Quantitative and qualitative follow-up outcomes from a preschool audiologic screening program: Perspectives over a decade. *American Journal of Audiology, 16,* 4–12.

Skelly, M. (1979). *Amer-Ind gestural code based on universal Americal Indian hand talk.* New York, NY: Elsevier North-Holland.

Slobin, D. I. (1973). Cognitive prerequisites for the development of grammar. In C. A. Ferguson & D. I. Slobin (Eds.), *Studies of child language development.* New York, NY: Holt, Rinehart, & Winston.

Spaeth, G. L. (1995). "Noncompliance"—not a patient problem, but rather a sign of a sick doctor-patient relationship. *Ophthalmic Surgery, 26,* 189–193.

Starmer, H. M., Liu, Z., Akst L. M., & Gourin, C. (2014). Attendance in voice therapy: Can an interdisciplinary care model have an impact? *Annals of Otology, Rhinology, and Laryngology, 123,* 117–123.

Tate, R. L. (1999). Executive dysfunction and characterological changes after traumatic brain injury: Two sides of the same coin? *Cortex, 35,* 39–55.

Thomas-Stonell, N., Oddson, B., Robertson, B., & Rosenbaum, P. (2010). Development of the FOCUS (FOCUS on the Outcomes of Communication Under Six), a communication outcome measure for preschool children. *Developmental Medicine and Child Neurology, 52,* 47–53.

Togher, L. (2012). Challenges inherent in optimizing speech-language pathology outcomes: It's not just about counting the hours. *International Journal of Speech-Language Pathology, 14,* 438–442.

Turkstra, L., Coelho, C., & Ylvisaker, M. (2005). The use of standardized tests for individuals with cognitive-communicative disorders. *Seminars in Speech and Language, 26,* 215–222.

Turkstra, L., Ylvisaker, M., Coelho, C., Kennedy, M., Sohlberg, M., Avery, J., & Yorkston, K. (2005). Practice guidelines for standardized assessment for persons with traumatic brain injury. *Journal of Medical Speech-Language Pathology, 13,* 9–38.

Tye-Murray, N., Spehar, B., Barcroft, J., & Sommers, M. (2017). Auditory training for adults who have hearing loss: A comparison of spaced versus massed practice schedules. *Journal of Speech, Language, and Hearing Research, 60*, 2337–2345.

Wade, C., Tavris, C., & Garry, M. (2015). *Invitation to psychology* (6th ed.). New York, NY: Pearson Higher Ed.

Wambaugh, J. (2006). Treatment guidelines for apraxia of speech: Lessons for future research. *Journal of Medical Speech-Language Pathology, 14*, 317–321.

Wambaugh, J., Duffy, J., McNeil, M., Robin, D., & Rogers, M. (2006). Treatment guidelines for acquired apraxia of speech: Treatment descriptions and recommendations. *Journal of Medical Speech-Language Pathology, 14*, 35–67.

Wambaugh, J. L., Nessler, C., Cameron, R., & Mauszycki, S. C. (2013). Treatment for acquired apraxia of speech: Examination of treatment intensity and practice schedule. *American Journal of Speech-Language Pathology, 22*(1), 84–102.

Wasserman, J. M., Wynn, R. W., Bash, T. S., & Rosenfeld, R. M. (2006). Levels of evidence in otolaryngology journals. *Otolaryngology–Head and Neck Surgery, 134*, 717–723.

Watts, C. R. (2016). Treatment modality and timing influence voice outcomes for vocal fold paralysis after thyroidectomy: A recommendation for guarded generalizations from a meta-analysis. *Evidence-Based Communication Assessment and Intervention, 10*, 20–24.

Westby, C., & Washington, K. N. (2017). Using the International Classification of Functioning, Disability and Health in assessment and intervention of school-aged children with language impairments. *Language, Speech, and Hearing Services in Schools, 48*, 137–152.

Whurr, R., Lorch, M., & Nye, C. (1992). A meta-analysis carried out between 1946 and 1988 concerned with efficacy of speech and language therapy treatment for aphasic patients. *European Journal of Disorders of Communication, 27*, 1–17.

Wilson, L., Onlow, M., & Lincoln, M. (2004). Telehealth adaptation of the Lidcombe program of early stuttering intervention: Five case studies. *American Journal of Speech-Language Pathology, 13*, 81–93.

World Health Organization. (1992). *ICD-10 classifications of mental and behavioural disorder: Clinical descriptions and diagnostic guidelines*. Geneva, Switzerland: Author.

World Health Organization. (2002). *Towards a common language for functioning, disability and health: ICF*. Geneva, Switzerland: Author.

Yairi, E., & Seery, C. H. (2015). *Stuttering: Foundations and clinical applications*. Upper Saddle River, NJ: Pearson Education.

Yoder, P., Fey, M. E., & Warren, S. F. (2012). Studying the impact of intensity is important but complicated. *International Journal of Speech-Language Pathology, 14*, 410–413.

Yorkston, K. M., Hakel, M., Beukelman, D. R., & Fager, S. (2007). Evidence for effectiveness of treatment of loudness, rate, or prosody in dysarthria: A systematic review *Journal of Medical Speech-Language Pathology, 15*, 11–36.

Yoshinaga-Itano, C. (2004). Levels of evidence: Universal newborn hearing screening (UNHS) and early hearing detection and intervention systems (EHDI). *Journal of Communication Disorders, 37*, 451–465.

Zientz, J., Rackley, A., Chapman, S. B., Hopper, T., Mahendra, N., Kim, E. S., & Cleary, S. (2007). Evidence-based practice recommendations for dementia: Educating caregivers on Alzheimer's disease and training communication strategies. *Journal of Medical Speech-Language Pathology, 15*, 53–64.

3

Ethics of Research

INTRODUCTION: PRINCIPLES OF RESEARCH

When is it ethically permissible to conduct research? An ethical decision is a moral one, not only a legal one. The standard for ethical behavior is higher than that for legal behavior. For example, it may be legal to implement an outdated therapy, but it is not ethical to do so. There are ethical standards, described in this chapter, that guide us, and there are ethical principles that need to be considered.

Learning Objectives

After reading this chapter, the student will be able to

- describe the rules of ethics;
- infuse the highest ethical standards in research and clinical practice;
- comply with standards for best practices; and
- prepare for the Praxis II examination in speech-language pathology and audiology.

THE RULES OF ETHICS

The seven ethical rules or principles described in Box 3–1 have been defended as being essential to the protection of human research participants. The practice of being skeptical and challenging the logic of the rules in no way invalidates them. As in every aspect of the endeavor of consuming and producing research, it is important to raise legitimate, thoughtful questions. One question refers to the terms we use in research. That we now refer to humans in research studies as participants instead of subjects is not a trivial matter. As is discussed in the following text, individuals who are regarded as *subjects* in research need the protection of the ethical principles and applications in the Belmont Report. Community-engaged researchers enlist participants from that community

Box 3–1. Rules of Ethics

Rule	*Name*	*Key Concepts*
1	Equipoise	Not sure which of a set of interventions are best May treat or test any intervention in the set
2	Valid Design	Study is designed in scientifically valid ways Study conforms to accepted scientific principles
3	Risk Minimization	Minimize risk and maximize benefit Do no harm
4	Posttrial Access	Participant has the right to be informed about the outcome of the study Participant shares in any subsequent benefit
5	Risk Payment	Money is not a benefit Risks to participants can be offset by the benefit of social value
6	Undue Inducement	Prevents participants from acting against their better judgment
7	Right of Withdrawal	Participant may choose to leave the study any time Participant has no penalty or loss of benefits for leaving

and the organizations that represent them as research partners (Bromley, Mikesel, Jones, & Khodyakov, 2015). Being a "subject" can signal exploitation instead of ethical protection, as it is seen to connote passive acquiescence. Those of us who, by virtue of our specialized interests, are involved with such communities as the National Aphasia Association, the Stuttering Association for Youth, or the Deaf community have already made the transition from viewing research participants as "aphasics," "stutterers," or "cochlear implant users" to seeing whole human beings who also happen to have communication disorders.

Rule I: Equipose

The first ethical principle or rule is equipoise (London, 2017). We define research equipoise as an ethical basis for assigning participants to different treatments in a clinical trial. If expert opinion about a treatment is uncertain or based on conflicting findings regarding a set of interventions, then it is ethical to implement treatment from any intervention in the set. For example, some physicians claim that video laryngoscopy for orotracheal intubation in the intensive care unit (ICU) is better than direct laryngoscopy, while others maintain that there is not enough evidence for or against this approach. The principle of equipoise states that the uncertainty or conflicting evidence permits the ethical use of randomized clinical trials to generate new knowledge.

However, there are two conflicting ethical imperatives in health care research that are not resolved by the principle of equipoise. The first is that health care research involving human participants must generate scientifically sound and clinically relevant information. The second is that the rights and interests of research participants must be respected.

The principle of equipoise does not resolve potential individual ethical concerns. A clinician may be asked to participate in randomized trials to see if one intervention is more effective and efficient than another. Based on clinical experience, a practitioner may be convinced that one of the interventions assures the best interests of the patient. Using the example of intubation in the ICU, a procedure with potentially serious side effects, those practitioners who are convinced that video laryngoscopy is better might consider it unethical to use the inferior approach of direct laryngoscopy, if asked to perform the latter procedure in a randomized study. Speech-language pathologists (SLPs) whose clinical experience makes them favor oral-motor exercises for dysarthria, even though research evidence is lacking, may be similarly ethically conflicted if they are asked to forgo this treatment in a randomized clinical trial.

There are six other ethical rules. Sachs (2011) identified three criteria by which ethical rules or principles need to be judged before they are considered canonical or well established. These include the following: (1) the rule or principle is widely known by those who will apply it and by those to whom it will apply; (2) most people agree that it is valid; and (3) those who disagree do not ignore it, but feel compelled to justify any infringement on it. However, establishing canonicity does not prohibit unethical behaviors. They seem driven only by consensus to follow the rule or justify its infringement. Sachs considered the following six ethical rules to be canonical. The six rules have been expressed in documents that are canonical themselves, including, among others, the Nuremburg Report (http://ohsr.od.nih.gov/guidelines/nuremberg.html), the Declaration of Helsinki (http://www.wma.net/e/policy/b3.htm), and the Belmont Report (http://ohsr.od.nih.gov/guidelines/belmont.html). We are about to wade in muddy ethical waters here, so keep an open mind and draw your own conclusions.

Rule 2: Valid Design

Valid design stipulates that investigators ensure that studies are designed in scientifically valid ways and conform to accepted scientific principles. In other words, there is an expectation by a potential research participant that generalizable knowledge will result from the research. But consider this scenario: An audiologist in clinical practice designs a research protocol, submits it to an Institutional Review Board (IRB), and acts according to the IRB's recommendations. (An IRB is a committee that has been formally charged to approve, monitor, and review biomedical and behavioral research.) The audiologist's proposal demonstrates that the risks are minimal or justified by the benefits of the research. Included is a consent form that specifies what kind of generalizable knowledge will be gained from the study. The potential research participant is given the impression that the audiologist is a scientist only when doing the kinds of things that scientists do. When the audiologist administers a complete audiological evaluation in a clinical setting, there is no expectation that generalizable knowledge will ensue. The behaviors that give rise to a reasonable expectation that real science is being done are the very behaviors (submission to the IRB, etc.) that meet those same expectations. So there are no potentially unethical behaviors to prohibit, and the rule of valid design is superfluous (Sachs, 2011, p. 11). The argument against this conclusion is that it the valid design rule ensures that any findings are useful and not limited by potentially addressable confounds.

Rule 3: Risk Minimization

Risk minimization is self-explanatory. Research should always strive to minimize risk and maximize benefit. However, a requirement to do no harm is not the same as a requirement to do good. If the goal is to avoid malfeasance, then a study that is not consequential is ethical because no harm is done. This argument ignores what Sachs (2011, p. 12) refers to as the transformative power of consent. However, risk is not being transformed; in the following example, aspiration is still a risk. Consider this scenario: An individual with dysphagia is asked to participate in research that examines the effect of various textures of food on swallowing ability. There is clearly a risk of aspiration, but the participant consents. In much of dysphagia research, the injunction to do no harm would result in the study never being done.

There are only two ways that a competent adult's consent is not transformative.

In the first, the participant's consent harms a third party. In Milgram's (1963) experiment, a participant, identified as the teacher in a teacher–learner dyad, was told by an authority figure to administer electric shocks to learners every time they made mistakes. The study modeled a situation where the participant thought that a third party would be harmed, although the third party was part of the experiment and was unharmed. The study examined the conflict between obeying an authority figure and personal conscience. Had the "learner" not been part of the experiment and was actually exposed to harm, then the participant's consent would not have been transformative in overriding the exposure to risk.

In current experiments, an investigator–participant interaction will rarely harm a third party. In the second exception to the transformative power of consent, the participant consents to letting the experimenter do something that is inherently objectionable (the example that Sachs, 2011, uses is slavery). This exception is specious, as it does not seem to apply to current investigator–participant relationships. The Tudor Study from 1939, discussed in the following text, is another example of the second exception that forbids inherently objectionable research.

Rule 4: Posttrial Access

In posttrial access, a participant has the right to be informed about the outcome of the study and share in any resulting benefit; otherwise, the investigator–participant relationship is exploitative. However, we as SLPs and audiologists (As) routinely find ourselves in a relationship where the person we work with is vulnerable. (Just because we are paid for our interventions does not mean that we have exploited the client's vulnerabilities.) In this situation, an advocate's consent for the vulnerable person to participate, as well as posttrial access, is required. Proportionality and fairness in an interaction, whether it is that of clinician–client or investigator–participant, are based on the way risks and benefits are distributed. Does posttrial access to research results promote reciprocity or avoid exploitation? It might if access were suggested or permitted, but according to the Declaration of Helsinki it is required. The requirement stipulates that fairness or proportionality cannot occur unless posttrial access is ensured. The requirement does not rule out reciprocity, but does not account for the studies that do not yield posttrial benefits. Suggesting or permitting posttrial access would allow for the research that we do in CSD and other fields that do not yield tangible benefits. The research may be educational, in that we learn more about the condition, or diagnostic, in that we establish baseline measures of functioning and eligibility for other studies. Of course, these studies require that risk be minimized. The educational nature of the research should properly be stated on the consent form.

Rule 5: Risk Payment

The basis of risk payment is that money is not a benefit. The argument is that risks to participants can be offset by the benefit of social value, but money prevents participants from consenting voluntarily. The argument seems to be more of degree than of substance. Money is completely accepted as a compensation for inconvenience (e.g., time, transportation), but IRBs are sensitive to any indication that participants are paid in proportion to the risk involved (i.e., more money for more risk). Why does money have the potential to undermine voluntariness in one condition but not in the other?

Rule 6: Undue Inducement

The undue inducement rule is intended to prevent participants from acting against their better judgment because they are being paid a great deal or receiving a great many services. The argument that money is coercive is false because coercion reduces the number of reasonable options and money increases them. Remember that money is a promise made by governments that it can be exchanged for all goods and services of equal value. Even if money is not coercive, it can be persuasive and affect an individual's autonomy in making decisions. Many of us have taken jobs we didn't like and even had an element of risk because we needed the money. In a review of studies on voluntariness, Applebaum, Lidz, and Klitzman (2009) found that an increase in monetary incentives influenced but did not distort decision making. Sachs (2011) suggests that deferring or portioning payments for participation in research might reduce the allure of a single large payment that can result in impulsive consent. We also need to be aware that certain vulnerable populations, such as those people who are incarcerated or are specifically recruited from a low socioeconomic background, are likely to be more susceptible to high financial incentives.

Rule 7: Right of Withdrawal

The last rule is the right of withdrawal without penalty or loss of benefits to which the participant might otherwise have been entitled. There is also an issue here of protection against harm. For example, if participants in a stress study cannot complete the stressor, they should still be partially compensated and not be forced to finish the study or else forfeit all reward. In a clinical setting, they must not be denied other treatment services based on their inability to finish an experiment. The argument that a participant loses some autonomy by agreeing to participate in a study is the same as saying that you lose some freedom whenever you make a choice. When you choose one option (e.g., marriage), you forfeit other choices (a billion other eligible people to marry). Later in this book (Chapter 6) we will discuss degrees of freedom as a statistical concept.

UNINTENDED CONSEQUENCES OF RESEARCH

Participants in a study may experience effects that last beyond the period of the experiment. Problems that arise later on, but may be prompted by the research experience, need to be considered. What might happen is discussed in the following text. What the researcher's ethical responsibility should be is the subject of the present chapter. The consumer and producer of research needs a strong foundation in ethics before undertaking either endeavor. Earning a certificate from the Collaborative Institutional Training Initiative (CITI) based on successful completion of the online course on the protection of human research participants and studying the Belmont Report are good ways to start.

In medical research and practice, more care may lead to harm (Fisher & Welch, 1999). More diagnosis and more treatment may lead to identification of pseudodisease and a lower treatment threshold. The harms these can create increased worry and disability, unnecessary treatment, mistakes, and adverse effects. It is not a logical leap to suggest that similar outcomes can occur in speech-language and audiological intervention. Below are examples of both negative and positive unintended consequences of behavioral and social studies (Box 3–2).

Negative: Rapist Roosters

The celebrated animal behavioral scientist and autism advocate Temple Grandin wrote about an unintended consequence of selective breeding in the poultry industry (Grandin, 2006). In its zeal to create chickens with larger breasts and more white meat (that sells for a higher price than dark meat), the industry appeared

Box 3–2. Unintended Consequences of Research

Effects on participants may last beyond the period of the experiment.

More care may lead to harm.

Manipulating variables experimentally may lead to unanticipated effects.

Unintended consequences may be positive or negative.

to have neglected the mating behavior of chickens and roosters. It seems that roosters initiate a wiggle dance to mate with hens, and the hens return the wiggle dance to acknowledge their willingness to mate. Hens with bigger breasts could not return the courtship behavior, and the enraged roosters raped and killed the hens.

In a subsequent book, Grandin and Johnson (2010) suggested that rapist roosters might have resulted from a different poultry industry experiment. The industry is obviously continuing to selectively breed for more white meat because breast size is still getting larger. In fact, some big-breasted male turkeys are unable to mate at all, and turkey hens have to be artificially inseminated. The authors cite the work of Duncan (1981), who claimed that the broiler industry may have misdiagnosed the problem. Large-breasted male chickens that had decreased fertility were seen to have low sex drive. The roosters were bred for increased aggressive behavior that the experimenters equated with higher libido, resulting in a cohort of rapist roosters.

We may never know what specifically caused the roosters to act in the destructive way they did, but there were negative, unintended consequences of the poultry experiments regardless of whether hyperaggression and bad courtship behavior were the same problem or two problems occurring at the same time. Industry breeding programs are trade secrets, and they aren't telling.

Positive: Curb Cuts

A new consideration for people with disabilities, similar to a social experiment, resulted in curb cuts or curb ramps; that is, a dip in a sidewalk to make it flush with the gutter. Curb cuts were first used in metropolitan areas to allow returning World War II veterans who used a wheelchair access to cross streets, and these cuts or ramps were codified in 1990. The Americans with Disabilities Act (ADA) was signed into law on July 26, 1990, by President George H. W. Bush. ADA is an extension of the equal opportunity rights provided to people without regard to race, color, religion, sex, or national origin (the Civil Rights Act of 1964) and Section 504 of the Rehabilitation Act of 1973, but this time it applies to people with disabilities.

An unintended positive consequence of curb cuts is the benefit it provides to people pushing babies and toddlers in carriages and strollers. Indeed, in some places curb cuts are called pram cuts. Of course, curb cuts also provide a benefit for people pushing shopping carts and luggage from one street to another.

NIH/CITI ONLINE TRAINING COURSE

Some of the most important and prestigious funding of research in speech-language pathology and audiology comes from the National Institutes of Health (NIH). From trainee stipends to early-career grants covering three-year (RO3) to five-year awards to established researchers at the top of their fields (RO1), the numbers of these NIH grants and their awardees often appear in the acknowledgments section of the most impactful journals (e.g., *Journal of Speech, Language, and Hearing Research*). Effective in 2000, anyone submitting a grant proposal to the NIH must show evidence of successful completion of the computer-based training course on the protection of human research participants. This certificate that comes in printable form with a pretty blue border must be renewed every three or four years. At present, the minimum passing score is 80% correct, and individual quizzes in the course may be retaken until the score is achieved. Subject to change, the CITI online training course has replaced the NIH training course. Many universities have their own links to the review course, and some have a CD version that is available on request. The link through Adelphi University is https://research-grants.adelphi.edu/irb/policy/. Most people complete the course in 2 to 3 hours (Box 3–3 and Figure 3–1).

According to the NIH website (https://phrp.nihtraining.com/introduction/02_intro.php), anyone designing or conducting NIH-funded human participants research must complete the review course. Investigators are obliged to protect the rights and welfare of participants in research. The policy of required education in the protection of human research participants was established on June 5, 2000, and revised on August 25, 2000 (https://grants.nih.gov/grants/guide/notice-files/not-od-00-039.html), and all key personnel working on the grant-funded project must complete the CITI course or one of many similar training courses to meet the policy requirement. The announcement also reminded institutions that they are required to oversee their Institutional Review Boards and clinical investigators to assure compliance.

Box 3–3. CITI Online Training Course

Required since 2000 for submission of grants or IRB proposals

Passing score is 80% correct; individual quizzes may be retaken

Printable certificate, good for three or four years, is awarded to those who pass

Includes an introduction, history, codes and regulations

Reviews material in the Belmont Report

The content of the CITI review course includes an introduction, history, codes and regulations, as well as the material covered in the Belmont report (National Commission for the Protection of Human Subjects of Biomedical and Behavioral Research, 1979; see the following section): respect for persons, beneficence, and justice. Some historical events include the Nazi medical war crimes committed from 1939 to 1945, the Nuremburg Code of 1947, the Tuskegee syphilis study in the early 1950s, and the cold war human radiation experiments from 1944 to 1974. The hope is that these or similar atrocities will not be repeated if researchers as well as individuals reviewing proposed experimental designs are aware of past horrors masquerading as research.

THE BELMONT REPORT

Introduction

The CITI training course has devoted much of its content to the Belmont Report (1979). The goal is for investigators to comply with regulations of the Department of

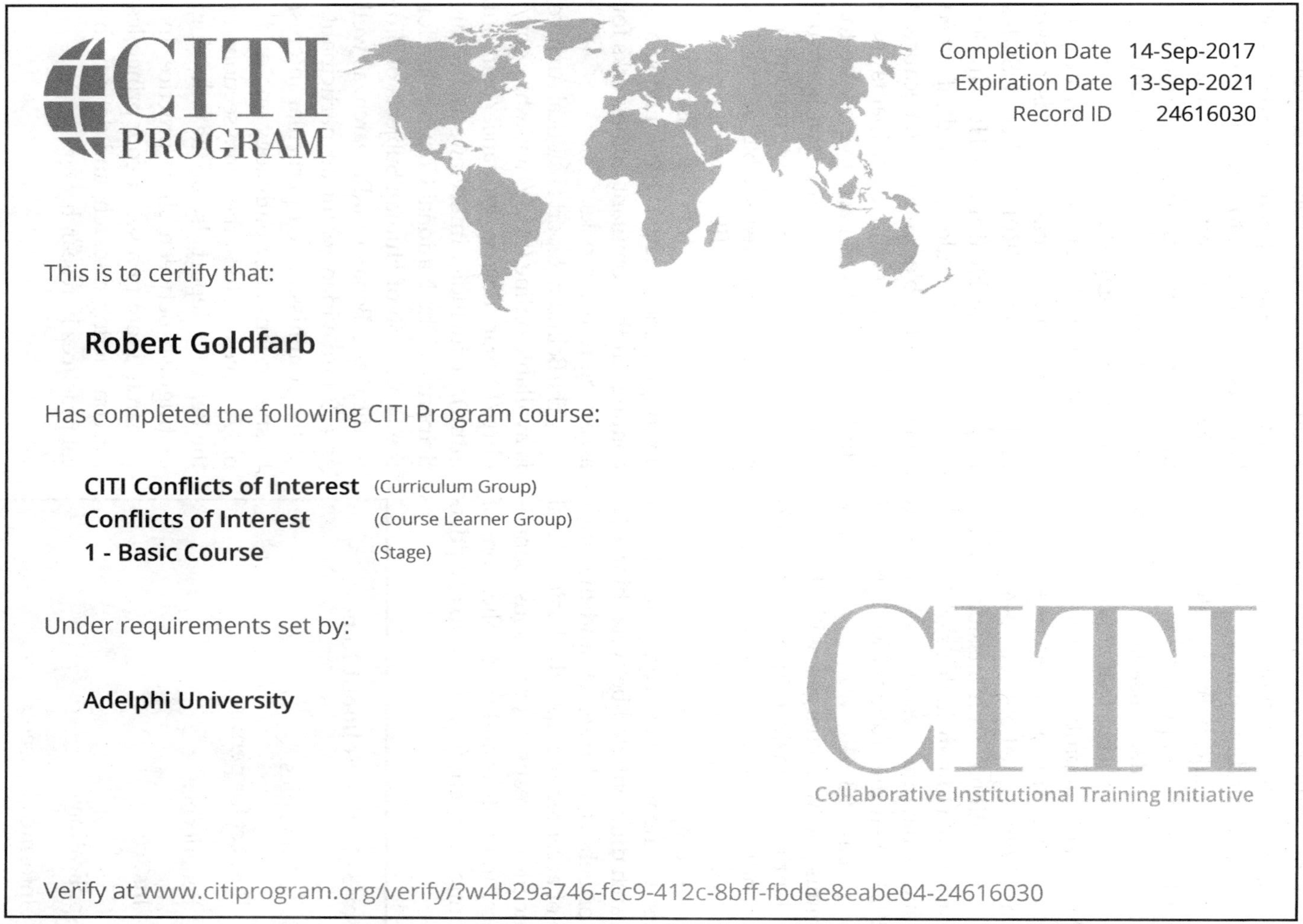

CITI PROGRAM

Completion Date 14-Sep-2017
Expiration Date 13-Sep-2021
Record ID 24616030

This is to certify that:

Robert Goldfarb

Has completed the following CITI Program course:

CITI Conflicts of Interest (Curriculum Group)
Conflicts of Interest (Course Learner Group)
1 - Basic Course (Stage)

Under requirements set by:

Adelphi University

CITI
Collaborative Institutional Training Initiative

Verify at www.citiprogram.org/verify/?w4b29a746-fcc9-412c-8bff-fbdee8eabe04-24616030

***Figure 3–1.** The author's CITI certificate.*

Health and Human Services by demonstrating comprehension of the following: the risks assumed by humans participating in research and how to protect them against these risks; populations, such as children, the mentally disabled, and those incarcerated in prisons that are vulnerable and need special protections; and circumstances where human subject research is exempt from regulations (Box 3–4).

The National Commission for the Protection of Human Subjects of Biomedical and Behavioral Research was created in 1974 when the National Research Act (Public Law 93-348) was enacted. The Commission was charged with the task of identifying basic ethical principles for conducting biomedical and behavioral research with human participants. The resulting Belmont Report had three parts: boundaries between practice and research differentiated between biomedical or behavioral research and the practice of accepted therapy; the basic ethical principles of respect for persons, beneficence, and justice; and the applications of informed consent (divided into consideration of information, comprehension, and voluntariness), assessment of risks and benefits (divided into consideration of nature and scope and systematic assessment of risks and benefits), and selection of subjects (now called "participants" by community-engaged researchers).

Box 3–4. The Belmont Report

Basic Principles

- Respect for persons
- Beneficence
- Justice

Applications

- Informed consent
- Assessment of risks and benefits
- Recruitment and selection of participants

The federal regulation governing research with human participants is known as the "Common Rule" (United States Department of Health and Human Services, 2009). The rule preceded informed consent and subject selection, because it is unethical to recruit participants for a study if the risks of participation are too great. The IRB is charged with ensuring that risks to subjects are minimized and that risks are reasonable in relation to anticipated benefits. This requires an adequate process for risk assessment, although London (2017) has found shortcomings in the dominant frameworks for assessing research risks.

The Belmont Report Historical Archive is available online (http://www.hhs.gov/ohrp/humansubjects/guidance/belmont.html). It includes interviews with participants of the National Commission for the Protection of Human Subjects of Biomedical and Behavioral Research, as well as a 9-min video featuring participants of the commission. Of particular interest to speech-language pathology and audiology investigators, the three sections of the Belmont Report also do the following: distinguish between clinic practice and research, identify a set of core principles for conducting research, and define ethical practices in research.

Respect for Persons

Respect for persons requires that researchers treat participants as autonomous agents, and those with diminished autonomy must be protected. For example, parents are required to give consent for their minor children to participate in research. The capacity for self-determination may change during a person's life because of maturation, illness, mental disability, or circumstances that restrict liberty. Accordingly, some protected classes include children, those who are imprisoned, who are physically sick or mentally ill, and who are pregnant. As will be discussed in the following text, belonging to a protected class does not mean that these individuals cannot or should not participate in research. Failure to include certain populations in research may limit their ability to benefit from experimental findings. For example, without prior research on the protected class of children on the autism spectrum, SLPs would not know if applied behavior analysis was the only option for therapy.

Regarding the application of informed consent, information must be provided to a person who is competent to comprehend the information in order to make a decision. In Goldfarb, Fromson, Gorrindo, and Birnbaum (2012), participants viewed a video of a standardized psychiatrist obtaining informed consent for treatment with atypical antipsychotic medication from a simulated patient. Two groups rated the doctor's performance on the elements of informed consent, what they believed should have been discussed, and to assess comprehension to indicate the time and dosage of the medication prescribed. Although both groups rated the doctor's performance highly, they had different priorities regarding what should be addressed in an informed consent process, and demonstrated inconsistent retention for the information presented by the doctor. Best practices were not "best" with regard to the desired outcomes.

The difference between what is legal and what is ethical becomes clearer when considering voluntariness. A decision is considered to be voluntary, in a legal sense, if there is no evidence that someone has coerced or unduly influenced the person deciding. Consent is not legal if it is given under duress. The legal definition of voluntariness does not take into account the circumstances, such as those who are financially needy, or participant groups, such as children, prisoners, pregnant women, mentally disabled people, or economically or educationally disadvantaged people that need special protections. Applebaum et al. (2009) suggest a modified form of the MacArthur Perceived Coercion Scale (Gardner et al., 1993), a five-item questionnaire, to determine which decisions participants believe are not their own. Respondents answer, "True," "False," or "Don't Know" to questions such as "I had enough of a chance to say whether I wanted to come into the hospital" or "People tried to force me to come into the hospital." Even voluntary decisions may be unwise or uninformed, that is, not optimal. It is important to continue to study how behavior by researchers may compromise voluntary consent.

Beneficence

The second ethical principle of the Belmont Report raises the following question: Are beneficent acts morally obligatory or are they optional ideals (Beauchamp, 2013)? Beneficence as an ethical concept includes any action intended to benefit or promote the good of another person. It is different from benevolence, a character trait that disposes a person to benefit another. Some moral philosophers argue that beneficence is obligatory, but all embrace obligations of nonmalfeasance. That is, rules that prohibit causing harm are moral imperatives. However, as noted previously, participant consent can overrule the moral imperative against causing harm if the perceived benefit is large and the perceived risk is small.

The Belmont Report, in its first beneficence framework enjoining researchers to minimize potential risks and maximize potential benefits, offers no guidance on how to balance these relevant moral concerns. Here are two questions where the Belmont Report does not guide us.

1. How do we measure the importance or value of knowledge that may be gained? Often the importance of research findings becomes clear only in the passage of time. Decades of research had shown that adults with aphasia could only improve in their language abilities, but the discovery of primary progressive aphasia revealed that language gets worse in this condition. It has been said that the questions stay the same, but the answers change. If, for example, research findings reveal how a personal listening device can cause noise-induced hearing loss and then a completely new technology replaces the devices about which the data were collected, are the original findings still important?
2. How do we balance the weight or trade-off of that potential benefit against the interests of the research participants? Here we depend on the IRB, rather than the Belmont Report to guide us.

The second framework, exemplified as the Duty of Personal Care Approach, is a therapeutic obligation (Marquis, 1983) that requires physicians and others to advance the interests of their patients to the best of their ability. The patient or participant can enter into clinical trials only if there is substantial uncertainty or equipoise about the efficacy of the trial treatments. Limitations of the rule of equipoise were discussed at the beginning of this chapter.

Justice

The last part of the Belmont Report deals with justice in selection of human research subjects. The standard view of fair human subject selection addresses who will be included in a research study, according to the following: inclusion and exclusion criteria; and strategies for recruiting subjects, including which communities will be included as study sites and which groups will be approached. If the primary motivation of research is to do good science, with risks minimized and benefits emphasized, then fair subject selection requires that the groups that assume the risks should reap the benefits and those who are likely to benefit assume the risks and burdens. On the other hand, if, as has historically been the case, most research continues to be done with men, then we don't learn enough about women.

Regarding justice in subject selection, MacKay (2016) claims that potential subjects *do not have a right* to participate in research (p. 674, emphasis added). If research represents something good, then to whom should it be allocated, considering that persons should be treated as moral equals? Inclusion and exclusion criteria must respect this moral equality and exclude potential participants only for legitimate reasons. MacKay's (2016) paper deals with the challenges of distinguishing between legitimate and illegitimate reasons by saying that researchers have a legitimate reason to treat people differently if it is the only way to realize the legitimate purposes of their studies. For example, if the research goal is to learn more about developmental stuttering, then it is ethical to exclude individuals with acquired stuttering secondary to brain injury. It would be illegitimate to exclude individuals with acquired stuttering if the goal of the research is to find out how many people have ever stuttered.

Additional problems with justice in research are seen in international clinical research, where there are discrepancies in health care and health research systems (Pratt & Loff, 2011). Ethical guidelines are mostly silent in indicating what is owed to communities in developing countries when the health care research is sponsored externally. Fairness requires that the community that bears the burdens of research should gain a similar quantity of benefits. Collective benefits to research participants and host communities might include better public health facilities, development of research and health care capacity, and continuing collaboration with the external sponsors and research institutions (Pratt & Loff, 2011, p. 78).

ETHICAL BLINDNESS AND SOCIETY'S RESPONSES

The next section deals with research horrors that occurred because they took place before the adoption of the Belmont Report and, in some cases, ignored ethical and moral imperatives entirely.

The Dachau Hypothermia "Study" and Other Unethical Research

In a *New York Times* editorial, Wade (1990) asked if data obtained unethically could be permitted in science. He reviewed some of the Nazi experimental atrocities, such as those performed on twins by Mengele in concentration camps, and found them to be "brutish and demented." However, one study to assess the possibility of reviving people from icy waters has been cited in scientific literature. The purpose was to find a way to help Nazi pilots who were shot down over the North Sea. Wade wondered if the results were too tainted to be trusted. The ethical argument in favor of citation is that the data are permissible only if they can be used to save lives and similar results are not available from medical records or animal data. Subsequent examination of the hypothermia data has revealed them to be grossly flawed, and there are no other Nazi concentration camp data that meet the criteria of uniqueness and life-saving value. Wade concluded that unethical studies are likely to be flawed in other ways as well (Box 3–5).

Box 3–5. Unethical Research

Unethical studies may be flawed in other ways as well

Nuremburg Code defined basic human research protections

Declaration of Helsinki provided rules for human subject research

Children and those who are incapacitated or incompetent need special protections

The Nuremburg Code

The Nuremburg Code resulted from trials of war crimes against Nazi leaders and organizations in Nuremburg, Germany from 1945 to 1946. All subsequent efforts to codify and define basic human research protections are based on this code. The most important principle in the code is voluntary consent by human subjects to experimentation. That is, people have the right to decide whether or not to participate in a research study. Other principles that are also described in the Belmont Report are beneficence, defined at Nuremburg as a reasonable expectation that the results of research will be meaningful and beneficial. Risk to human research participants should be minimized, and never have the possibility of leading to death or disabling injury; and there must be an offsetting benefit to the research.

Although the Nazi experiments are unique in their malignancy, the following studies are unquestionably unethical. In 1928, a study on African-American men in Macon, Georgia was begun with private financial support. The study aimed to test and treat African-American men in the southern United States for syphilis. However, the Great Depression occurred and the private donor was no longer able to finance the study. The U.S. Public Health Service decided to continue the study without treatment to observe the natural progression of syphilis. The Tuskegee Institute, because of its ties to the community, received some funding from the Public Health Service to recruit volunteers for the study. The participants received free medical checkups, transportation, and meals, but were not told that they had syphilis and were not treated for the disease. The study continued until 1972, even though penicillin was discovered to treat syphilis in 1943. The national outrage over the blatant disregard for the lives and health of the participants in the Tuskegee study led Congress to enact legislation to ensure protections for human participants in publicly funded medical research. The Tuskegee experiment violated the Nuremburg Code in two ways: there was no informed consent, because the participants were not told that they had syphilis and would not receive treatment for the disease (even when such treatment was readily available); and the participants assumed risk with no corresponding benefit.

The Declaration of Helsinki

The Declaration of Helsinki followed a World Medical Assembly in Finland in 1964, and has undergone several revisions through 1996. The declaration expanded the principles of the Nuremburg Code and provided rules for the conduct of researchers engaged in human subject research. The declaration specified that information must be provided before asking for consent to participate in research, and that the information must include a description of risks and benefits. Further, the participant must have a complete description of the research protocol, and would be free to withdraw from participation at any time. The declaration addressed unintended coercion, as when the participant's own physician is also the researcher. It also established procedures for potential participants who need special protections, including children and those who are incapacitated or incompetent.

Sadly, there are many more instances of unethical research that are described in the CITI online training course. Next, we focus on a study in our own field, sometimes referred to with the hyperbolic term, "The Monster Study."

THE TUDOR STUDY

Media attention to a 1939 master's thesis that has become known as the Tudor Study prompted Goldfarb (2006) and others to revisit the ethical consideration of this study in order to explore ethical issues in current clinical and research practices. "The Monster Study," as it was described more than 60 years later (Reynolds, 2003; reprinted in Goldfarb, 2006), included the following experimenters and participants: Wendell Johnson, a professor at the University of Iowa and one of the founders of the science of speech-language pathology who said he became a speech pathologist because he needed one (he spent his career trying to understand the stuttering that affected him all his life); Mary Tudor, a graduate student who completed her master's thesis at the University of Iowa in 1939; and the participants, 22 children (10 identified as stuttering) from the Iowa Soldiers and Sailors Orphans' Home in Davenport, Iowa. Johnson and Tudor's findings that they were allegedly able to induce stuttering in normally fluent children supported their hypothesis, but have also raised serious ethical concerns.

The study was designed to assess Johnson's (1942) diagnosogenic theory of stuttering. The theory may be described as follows: the kind of speech shown by individuals who stutter at the onset of stuttering is not distinguishable from normal disfluency; the diagnosis of stuttering is made by a lay person, usually a parent, which explains why stuttering runs in families; once the diagnosis is made, the child experiences disfluencies as speech failures, and begins avoidance and escape behaviors characteristic of stuttering.

The experiment included four groups. In Group 1A, five children identified as stuttering were told, "You do not stutter. Your speech is fine." In Group 1B, five children identified as individuals who stutter were told, "Yes, your speech is as bad as people say." In Group IIA, six children, ages 5 to 15, who did not stutter, were told that their speech was not normal at all, that they were beginning to stutter, and that they must correct this immediately. This is the group that would lead to the lawsuit against the University of Iowa. In Group IIB, six fluent children, similar in age to those above, were complimented on their nice enunciation.

What was unethical about the Tudor Study (Box 3–6)? The participants were treated unethically in two ways. First, their status as children would have required special consideration by today's ethical

> **Box 3–6. What Ethical Principles Were Violated in the Tudor Study?**
>
> The children, given their status as orphans, were exceptionally vulnerable.
>
> The study involved deception.
>
> If the theoretical assumptions were correct, some children were put at risk for emotional stress and communication disorder.
>
> The study may have reflected acceptable ethical principles of its time.

standards. Second, as orphans, the children did not have a competent adult advocating for them. The study also involved deception of the children in Groups IA, where children who stuttered were told that they did not, and IIA, where children who were fluent were told that they stuttered. The fact that, contrary to what Johnson and Tudor had claimed, there was no effect of verbal labeling and that the diagnosogenic theory was not confirmed (Ambrose & Yairi, 2002) is irrelevant in terms of the ethical conduct of the study. The best defense to be made for the treatment of the children in Group IA is that there was equipoise between the standard treatment for stuttering and verbal labeling of fluency, in which case either treatment could be assessed experimentally. However, there was no benefit to the children in Group IIA; rather, a clear potential for the harm of inducing stuttering, a harm that Johnson knew intimately. Even if, as Johnson and Tudor claimed, the children whose stuttering was induced would regain fluency following speech therapy, there were other psychological harms that the litigants claimed in their lawsuit decades later. Finally, there was the possibility of coercion of Tudor, a student, by Johnson, her mentor. Johnson was committed to the diagnosogenic theory and to gathering evidence to support it, and he may have used his authority to sway Tudor in her choice of a master's thesis topic. There is a substantial power differential between mentor and student (see Chapter 9), and the mentor must exercise care to avoid even the appearance of coercion. In his impassioned defense of his father, Nicolas Johnson (2006), a former law professor at the University of Iowa (and Wendell Johnson's son), noted that the design of the Tudor Study was consistent with research practices of the time and put the study in the perspective of occurring before the Nuremburg Code, the Declaration of Helsinki, and other guidelines for the ethical conduct of research.

AAA AND ASHA CODES OF ETHICS

To guide professional practitioners and researchers in speech-language pathology and audiology, the American Speech-Language-Hearing Association (ASHA) has promulgated and updated a Code of Ethics, with the most recent revision in 2016 (available at http://www.asha.org/Practice/ethics/Code-of-Ethics-2016-Revision-Summary/). Another Code of Ethics for audiologists, also revised in 2016, is available from the American Academy of Audiology (AAA) (https://www.audiology.org/publications-resources/document-library/code-ethics).

Principle 6 of the AAA Code of Ethics deals with ethical standards of research, including deception or misrepresentation in public statements or publications. Rule 6a addresses misrepresentation of credentials and competence, including training and academic degrees. It is not unusual for consumers to confuse audiologists with medical doctors, and the AuD, a doctoral degree, is the minimum degree for safe practice. While staff can certainly refer to the audiologist as "Dr. Smith," they should not refer to the audiologist as "the doctor." Rule 6b forbids misrepresentation of research results, including claims that are false, misleading, or deceptive (Box 3–7).

The ASHA Board of Ethics began revising the Code of Ethics in August

> **Box 3–7. AAA and ASHA Codes of Ethics**
>
> AAA
>
> No deception or misrepresentation in public statements or publications
>
> No misrepresentation of credentials or research results
>
> ASHA
>
> Principle I: Researchers hold the welfare of participants to be of paramount importance.
>
> Principle II: ASHA members must not permit misrepresentation of professional competency.
>
> Principle III: Rules for accurate and honest information about an individual's contributions to research activities.

2000, with a focus on ethics in research and professional practice. The revised Code of Ethics took effect in January 2003. The Code of Ethics was revised again and the new version took effect in 2016. Before being revised, the code contained four specific references to research in only two areas: rights and welfare of participants in research, and public statements about research results.

The revisions in Principle of Ethics I add humane treatment of animals to the section on welfare of participants, and also address issues of nondiscrimination, informed consent, confidentiality, and security of research data. Principle of Ethics II refers to professional competency. Finally, Principle of Ethics III requires accurate and honest information about an investigator's contributions to research activities.

According to the ASHA (2014) update on ethics in research and scholarly activity, in 2006, nearly 1,700 ASHA members considered research to be their primary or secondary employment activity. In addition, students and professionals in CSD regularly read the peer-reviewed ASHA journals and attend conventions to stay current with the research in our field. Accordingly, the ASHA Code of Ethics was first revised in 2010 to recognize research and scholarship, with a full revision completed in 2016. The three main themes in the revised Code's focus on research and scholarship are ethical treatment of research participants, competence, and honesty.

Specifically, Principle I of the Code of Ethics requires that researchers hold the welfare of participants to be of paramount importance. The three major areas of the Belmont Report (1979)—respect for persons, beneficence, and justice—are also reflected in the Code of Ethics. Principle I, Rule C requires that we do not discriminate in subject selection. Researchers may not exclude certain groups because they are not readily available or it is not convenient to include them. Principle I, Rule H requires that participants give informed consent and researchers inform participants about the possible effects of the study; Rule I requires researchers to ensure that participation is voluntary. Principle I, Rule O requires that researchers maintain confidentiality about participants' records, and in Rule P, that professional and personal information regarding participants is kept confidential. Lack of confidentiality is a potential source of harm to participants. They may have preexisting conditions that they do not want revealed to someone who might be in a position to deny or charge more for their health insurance.

Research and scholarly activity are also included in the rules (Principle I, Rule A and Principle II) indicating that we must perform our duties competently, and that we maintain the highest levels of competence and performance. Principle I, Rule J requires that the intended purpose of a research endeavor is accurately represented. Principle II, Rule C requires that researchers abide by federal, state, and institutional requirements, even if they are not specified in the Code of Ethics. Rule E requires that administrators and supervisee engage only in research activities for which they have expertise and education. All these rules are intended to ensure that research will be done only by people qualified to do it, that all laws are obeyed, and that all local policies are followed.

Principle of Ethics III refers to the duties we owe to the public in providing information and advocating for the professions of speech-language pathology and audiology. The focus is on acting honestly. This means that researchers must not misrepresent their credentials, education, competencies, and experience (Rule A); their research activities (Rule C); their grants and contracts for services provided (Rule D; this falls into the category of fraud); their statements to the public about research and scholarly activities (Rule E); and they must complete all materials honestly and without omission (Rule G). These rules that have the central theme of honesty are meant to reassure the public, honor the profession, and protect the practitioner or investigator.

The ASHA (2014) update addresses three challenges to treating human research participants ethically. The first is that while researchers who work in universities or institutions with an Institutional Review Board (IRB) gain approval for a research proposal that includes the ethical treatments of participants, many institutions do not have an IRB. Those researchers will have to provide their own oversight for the ethical conduct of their studies. The Code of Ethics can provide guidelines for protection of human research participants even in the absence of an IRB. A second challenge is to provide accurate representation of data. It is very difficult to get funding or publish an article when the results of a study support a null hypothesis; that is, there is no effect of a treatment or no difference between treatment groups. It may then be tempting to fabricate data, because one's job may depend on grant support or publications. Such conduct is unethical and ultimately likely to be found out. The third ethical challenge has to do with conflicts of interest. These conflicts usually involve money, when there is temptation to manipulate data because it supports the goals of a funding source, the investigator's own proprietary product, or the salary given to the investigator by a public or private party.

Other ethical challenges are likely to arise. Not all can be addressed by the AAA and ASHA codes of ethics explicitly, but there are enough implicit references to research and scholarship to serve as reminders that there is nothing more important than the welfare of the people we serve. A discussion of protecting the confidentiality of health information continues in the next section.

HEALTH INSURANCE PORTABILITY AND ACCOUNTABILITY ACT OF 1996 (HIPAA)

Established by the 104th Congress on August 21, 1996, as Public Law 104-191, HIPAA amended the Internal Revenue Code of 1986 in part to combat waste, fraud, and abuse in health care delivery. One purpose of HIPAA was to establish standards and requirements for electronic transmission of health information and to encourage the development of a health information system while allaying concerns about privacy and confidentiality. The second was to secure health information when workers changed jobs and could be denied employee health insurance coverage because of preexisting conditions.

Many aspects of HIPAA are relevant to practitioners in communication sciences and disorders. The term "health information" includes oral or recorded forms created by a health care provider (such as a speech-language pathologist or audiologist), a school, or a university that refer to the physical or mental health of an individual in the past, present, or future. Information for HIPAA regulations for professionals is available at https://www.hhs.gov/hipaa/for-professionals/index.html

Individually identifiable health information is protected. This includes demographic or other physical or mental health information that can reasonably be believed to identify an individual. Security standards and safeguards are incorporated in the 16-page document, as are monetary and incarceration penalties for failure to comply with requirements and standards (Box 3–8).

A general strategy used to protect health information is called de-identification. Specific strategies may include substituting alpha-numeric codes for a person, a disorder, and a geographic location. The aim is to prevent reidentification, or the ability of an individual not involved with data collection to determine whose health information is being cited in the research. There are legal issues here, especially when looking at illegal drug use or psychiatric conditions that could harm the participants if discovered. Cybersecurity is becoming an important issue for protected health information (PHI). Any unencrypted PHI collected as part of a

Box 3–8. HIPAA

Purposes

- Establish standards and requirements for electronic transfer of health information
- Respect privacy and confidentiality
- Prevent denial of health care coverage because of preexisting conditions

Strategies

- De-identification and reidentification
- Linear programming
- Need strategy to assure confidentiality while providing access to records

research study could be stolen (see http://www.hipaajournal.com/unencrypted-device-theft-continues-to-plague-hipaa-ces-8158/). The individual involved in the study may still be able to decode the numbers, as when the author volunteered to participate in a friend's PhD dissertation on speech respiration and determined he was participant #8 because he knew his own vital capacity.

One model used to de-identify data sets is called linear programming (Jung & El Emam, 2014). It is a sophisticated mathematical model that Jung and El Emam used to de-identify a data set of nearly 12,000 postal codes in the city of Ottawa, Canada. The motivation was compliance with the HIPAA Privacy Rule's Expert Determination method; that is, to reduce the risk of reidentification of data. Sometimes, there is a "legal and ethical tightrope" (Wiener & Gilliland, 2011, p. 15) where librarians in institutions with health science historical collections have a professional obligation to provide access to the records, but are constrained by the requirement to protect the confidentiality of those whose health information is included in the records. In an extensive review, the Wiener and Gilliland (2011) did not find an accepted strategy.

CONCLUSION

Our codes of ethics in speech-language pathology and audiology ensure that clients' rights are protected above that which is required by law. However, ethical dilemmas arise in clinical practice in both professions that are not addressed by either codes of ethics or laws. For example, the family of a child with gender dysphoria who is considering transitioning to a different gender may consider it immoral to provide voice therapy. As another example, members of the Deaf community may perceive deaf parents seeking a cochlear implant for their deaf child as an affront to their culture.

Many of the potential ethical conflicts noted in this chapter were reported in a paper on ethical dilemmas in audiology (Callahan et al., 2011). The authors concluded that practicing audiologists need ethics training that focuses on clarification of laws and guidelines regarding confidentiality of patient information, disclosure of information, release of information, and ownership of client records. Ethical dilemmas continue in the areas of pay sources and funding, interactions with coworkers and supervisors, compliance with regulations, and interaction with caregivers (Callahan et al., 2011, p. 82). Weinstein (2001) identified four principles that can assist audiologists in ethical decision making: get the relevant facts, identify pertinent values, find options, and test each option against the facts and values. In discussing ethics in speech-language pathology, Eadie and Charland (2005) reviewed the Belmont Report principles of respect for persons, beneficence, and justice, and added the category of nonmalfeasance that had two principles. The speech-language pathologist must not act in a way that takes power away from clients; and the SLP must not act selfishly or deceptively, even if these actions are well intentioned. The authors conclude with a call for an ongoing clinical ethics forum.

Finally, here is an example where informed consent was not obtained. In current times, there are also HIPAA implications. The case of the "immortal" cells of Henrietta Lacks (Skloot, 2010) is required reading on some campuses. Tissue cells were taken from the tumors of an African

American woman without her permission. Even though her cells helped researchers to develop treatments for cancer after Ms. Lacks died, her family had the right to, and did not, consent to their use. That a white scientist obtained the cells only added to the racist connotations of the case.

ADVANCED STUDY

The author proposes that research ethics skills are necessary for an individual to be granted power of professor. With new generations of scholars and researchers needed every 10 years, professors and master clinicians have an obligation to prepare individuals with adequate knowledge and skills to undertake the tasks of scholarship and research, and research ethics is a key component. For evidence of the requisite research ethics skills, complete the following, and have your instructor, academic adviser, mentor, or CSD department chair review that you have completed the requirements and sign and date where indicated.

Student's Name: ______________________________

1. List seven rules or principles that have been defended as essential to protect human research participants. Provide a critique for one of them.
2. Write a paragraph or two indicating a possible positive and a possible negative unintended consequence of research.
3. Present your Certificate of Completion of the CITI online training course for the protection of human research participants.
4. Write a paragraph or two on the Belmont Report, including the basic principles (respect for persons, beneficence, and justice) and applications (informed consent, assessment of risks and benefits, and selection of subjects).
5. Write a paragraph or two about an example of past research that was unethical. You can choose one described in this volume, in the CITI online training course, or elsewhere.
6. Write a paragraph or two explaining what you would do to make the Tudor Study more ethical.
7. Write a paragraph or two explaining how you would comply with one of the ethical rules in the AAA or ASHA codes of ethics.
8. Write a paragraph or two explaining how you, as an audiologist or speech-language pathologist, would comply with HIPAA regulations.

Date of Completion: ______________________________

Faculty/Supervisor Signature: ______________________________

REFERENCES

Ambrose, N. G., & Yairi, E. (2002). The Tudor study: Data and ethics. *American Journal of Speech-Language Pathology, 11*, 190–203.

American Speech-Language-Hearing Association. (2014). *Issues in ethics: Ethics in research and scholarly activity.* Retrieved from http://www.asha.org/Practice/ethics/Ethics-in-Research-and-Scholarly-Activity/

American Speech-Language-Hearing Association. (2016). *Code of ethics.* Retrieved from http://www.asha.org/Code-of-Ethics/

Applebaum, P. S., Lidz, C. W., & Klitzman, R. (2009). Voluntariness of consent to research: A conceptual model. *Hastings Center Report, 39*, 30–39.

Beauchamp, T. (2013). The principle of beneficence in applied ethics. In E. N. Zalta (Ed.), *The Stanford encyclopedia of philosophy.* Stanford, CA: Center for the Study of Language and Information. Retrieved from https://plato.stanford.edu/archives/win2016/entries/principle-beneficence

Bromley, E., Mikesel, L., Jones, F., & Khodyakov, D. (2015). From subject to participant: Ethics and the evolving role of community in health research. *American Journal of Public Health, 105*, 900–908.

Callahan, A. J., Lass, N. J., Richards, K. L., Yost, A. B., Porter, K. S., Schrock, J. J., & Vetica, M. D. (2011). Ethical dilemmas in audiology. *Contemporary Issues in Communication Science and Disorders, 38*, 76–86.

Duncan, I. J. H. (1981). Animal rights—animal welfare: A scientist's assessment. *Poultry Science, 60*, 489–499.

Eadie, T. L., & Charland, L. C. (2005). Ethics in speech-language pathology: Beyond the codes and canons. *Journal of Speech-Language Pathology and Audiology, 29*, 27–36.

Fisher, E. S., & Welch, H. G. (1999). Avoiding the unintended consequences of growth in medical care: How might more be worse? *Journal of the American Medical Association, 281*, 446–453.

Gardner, W., Hoge, S. K., Bennett, N., Roth, L. H., Lidz, C. W., Monahan, J., & Mulvey, E. P. (1993). Two scales for measuring patients' perception of coercion during hospital admission. *Behavioral Sciences and the Law, 20*, 307–321.

Goldfarb, E., Fromson, J. A., Gorrindo, T., & Birnbaum, R. J. (2012). Enhancing informed consent best practices: Gaining patient, family and provider perspectives using reverse simulation. *Journal of Medical Ethics, 38*, 1–6.

Goldfarb, R. (Ed.). (2006). *Ethics: A case study from fluency.* San Diego, CA: Plural Publishing.

Grandin, T. (2006). *Animals in translation.* San Diego, CA: Harcourt.

Grandin, T., & Johnson, C. (2010). *Animals make us human: Creating the best life for animals.* Boston, MA: Houghton Mifflin Harcourt.

Johnson, N. (2006). Retroactive ethical judgments and human subjects research: The 1939 Tudor study in context. In R. Goldfarb (Ed.), *Ethics: A case study from fluency* (pp. 139–199). San Diego, CA: Plural Publishing.

Johnson, W. (1942). A study of the onset and development of stuttering. *Journal of Speech and Hearing Disorders, 7*, 251–257.

Jung, H.-W., & El Emam, K. (2014). A linear programming model for preserving privacy when disclosing patient spatial information for secondary purposes. *International Journal of Health Geographics, 13*, 13–16.

London, A. J. (2017). Equipoise in research integrating ethics and science in human research. *Journal of the American Medical Association, 317*, 525–526.

MacKay, D. (2016). Fair subject selection in clinical research: Formal equality of opportunity. *Journal of Medical Ethics, 42*, 672–677.

Marquis, D. (1983). Leaving therapy to chance. *Hastings Center Report, 13*, 40–47.

Milgram, S. (1963). Behavioral study of obedience. *Journal of Abnormal and Social Psychology, 67*, 371–378.

National Commission for the Protection of Human Subjects of Biomedical and Behavioral Research. (1979). *The Belmont Report: Ethical principles and guidelines for the protections of human subjects of research* (GPO Office 887-890). Washington, DC: Government Printing Office.

Pratt, B., & Loff, B. (2011). Justice in international clinical research. *Developing World Bioethics, 11*, 75–81.

Reynolds, G. (2003, March 16). The stuttering doctor's "monster study." *The New York Times.* Retrieved from https://www.nytimes.com

Sachs, B. (2011). Going from principles to rules in research ethics. *Bioethics, 25*, 9–20.

Skloot, R. (2010). *The immortal life of Henrietta Lacks.* NY: Crown Publishing Group.

Wade, N. (1990, May 27). The editorial notebook: The errors of Nazi science. *The New York Times*. Retrieved from https://www.nytimes.com

Weinstein, B. (2001). Thinking through questions of ethics: Four steps to better decision-making. *Advance for Speech-Language Pathologists and Audiologists, 11*(45), 28-29.

Wiener, J. A., & Gilliland, A. T. (2011). Balancing between two goods: Health Insurance Portability and Accountability Act and ethical compliancy considerations for privacy-sensitive materials in health sciences archival and historical special collections. *Journal of the American Library Association, 99*, 15–22.

4

The Scientific Method

INTRODUCTION

The scientific method is a way to solve problems by thinking and behaving systematically. It is a research plan, rather than a fixed set of rules that all investigators must follow. Many different procedures or approaches may be acceptable as adhering to the scientific method, as long as they control and measure the influence of one variable upon another and try to rule out outside influences that may lead to alternative explanations of the findings.

Research and clinical intervention in the practices of speech-language pathology and audiology, as scientific professions, rely on two assurances to the public (Finn, Bothe, & Bramlett, 2005):

- we derive and base our conclusions about communication disorders on scientific evidence; and
- assessment and treatment are evaluated by empirical methods.

In other words, speech-language pathologists (SLPs) and audiologists (As) assure the public that they are engaging in evidence-based practice (EBP) and developing practice-based evidence (PBE; see Chapter 2 for more information about EBP and PBE).

This chapter begins with a description of the scientific method, followed by comparisons of the scientific method to "common sense" (also known as conventional wisdom) and pseudoscience. Some of the content in this chapter appeared in earlier writing (see, for example, Goldfarb & Serpanos, 2014). It has been updated and expanded for the present volume.

Learning Objectives

After reading this chapter, the student will be able to

- describe the scientific method;
- differentiate the rules of science from "common sense" and pseudoscience; and
- formulate experimental and clinical hypotheses.

THE SCIENTIFIC METHOD

The discussion of the scientific method begins with some definitions of terms. Beginning with the understanding that the scientific method requires testable hypotheses, we need to review "hypothesis" and explain how it is different from a theory. A hypothesis is a proposition (or a premise) for an explanation (or an argument) about the occurrence of a specific group of phenomena. Theories are statements or principles that explain phenomena. Theories tend to result from repeated experimental testing. In other words, a theory results from hypotheses when some of the facts are in.

The hypothesis is created in the mind of a scientist. It can be falsified or confirmed, but never proven. If, for example, we want to test the hypothesis that rate reduction increases fluency in children who stutter, we try to find a representative random sample of children who stutter. Because we cannot test everyone in the world who stutters, we hope that we can avoid a sampling or other systematic error, and we hope the participants we select represent the larger population of all children who stutter. The experimental design may be wrong, the analysis may be inappropriate, or the sample may not accurately represent the population, so it is incorrect to claim that an experiment proves the research hypothesis. Chapter 6 on statistics will develop this reasoning more broadly; and see Chapter 11 on writing clinical hypotheses.

The scientific method also guards against describing coincidence or correlation as causation. An outrageous example is the following: blue eyes cause potato crops to fail. After all, one of history's worst potato famines occurred in Ireland, where most of the population had blue eyes. Just because B follows A, we cannot form a conclusion based on the two variables. There may be causation, a correlation, or only a coincidence. A coincidence simply means that two or more things occurred at the same time or in nature. There is no apparent cause–effect relationship. If blue-eyed people live in a country where there was a potato famine, there is no reason to accept that having blue eyes leads to potato crop failure. Similarly, a stock market rally on your birthday this year is no indication that you will make money on your birthday in subsequent years. Maxwell and Satake (1997) compared correlation to causation. A correlation indexes an association between variables, but not evidence that one variable causes the other to happen. Snyder et al. (2018) reported that nursing your baby for more than six months is associated with smaller waist size 10 years after delivery in the mothers studied. At present, this finding represents a correlation; it will take much more evidence before researchers can claim a causal relationship. Once we understand what underlies variables A and B, we can then create models, mechanisms, or hypotheses that connect the two. The data that we collect then gives us an indication about the relationship between A and B, as well as the confidence we should have in that relationship.

What do researchers mean by the term *variable*? A good place to start is to consider a variable as the relationship between an object and an event. A clinical researcher may vary objects with the goal of having a child produce the same (invariant) response. The objects may be a picture of a ball, a physical ball, or your lips pressed together while you say /b/, but the goal is the production of "ball" by the child. Similarly, you may hold the object invariant and have variable goals. The same set of cards (objects) may be used for the goals (events) of sorting, matching, or naming. More often, both objects and events will be variable and these quantities will change as circumstances change.

Variables may be independent or dependent. Think of independent variables as setting the stage and dependent variables as the Broadway show. In behavioral terminology, using the example above, the independent variables, called antecedent events (S^D), are the script for the play and the stage design; the dependent variables are the lines spoken by the actors and their interaction with the scenery, called the performance (R); and the reaction by the audience is the payoff or consequent event that may be applause (S^{r+}) or booing (S^{r-}). An independent variable is presumed to cause the dependent variable to occur, and the dependent variable is presumed to be the effect of the independent variable. That is, if the stage design includes a table set with a coffee pot and cups, it is presumed that an actor will pour coffee into a cup, and the pouring behavior is presumed to be the effect of the table setting.

We can also think of independent and dependent variables mathematically, where variable B is said to be a *function* of variable A. You learned about the functional relationship of pressure and volume in the lungs (Boyle's law) in respiration. The pressure (P) of a gas in the lungs (variable B) tends to increase as the volume (V) of the lungs (variable A) decreases in exhalation, and the reverse occurs in inhalation. We can write the equation as $PV = K$, where K is some kind of a constant. In other words, there is an inverse relationship between pressure and volume: $P\uparrow V\downarrow$ or $P\downarrow V\uparrow$. Mathematically, as V increases for inhalation and decreases for exhalation, P, as a function of V, decreases for inhalation and increases for exhalation.

In the speech and hearing center, what the clinician does is the independent variable and what the client does is the dependent variable. The audiologist controls the volume on an audiometer, and when the tone is loud enough, the client's hand goes up. The client's hand-raising behavior *depends* on the volume of the signal presented by the audiologist.

The realization of the scientific method in clinical speech-language pathology and audiology is evidence-based practice (EBP). An early example of a critical evaluation of EBP in our disciplines was the systematic review (see Chapter 2 for many other examples of systematic reviews and meta-analyses) provided by the Academy of Neurologic Communication Disorders and Sciences (ANCDS) writing committee on dysarthria (Yorkston et al., 2001) that established practice guidelines in speech-language pathology based on evidence-based medicine. The authors considered *evidence-based practice* to be an approach to decision making that the clinician uses, in consultation with the client, that is based on the best evidence available and that suits the client best. The explicit statements called *practice guidelines* help clinicians and clients make these decisions. These guidelines should be rigorous and scientific, include input from both clinician and client, cover a range of conditions and problems, and be practical working documents (Yorkston et al., 2001, p. 248). Zippoli and Kennedy (2005) reported the results of a survey of SLPs that indicated generally positive attitudes about EBP, but that a lack of time, access to computerized databases, and a lack of access to appropriate resources limited clinicians' use of EBP.

All of the above that can be called the received wisdom about the scientific method may soon be obsolete in light of the advent of big data. In this case, "big" means massive amounts of data, and in some fields, petabytes of data. In communication sciences and disorders, there has been substantial progress in assembling large data sets for disfluency and other disorders. The author recently received an e-mail from the high-impact journal *Brain and Language* with a request to submit the raw data from previously published articles in the journal to be made available to other researchers. The *Journal of Speech, Language, and Hearing Research* started a Figshare data portal in late 2017. This portal allows the journal to display and archive supplemental data and multimedia associated with the articles that it publishes. These materials are citable as publications and have digital object identifiers (DOIs). Big data has already had a profound effect on the bench sciences, where gigantic computing clusters reveal patterns that the scientific method could not uncover. We do not yet know if correlation will replace theory, but for those of us who are interested in big data, for example in neuroscience, the scientific method of the future may be very different from our present understanding of it.

One goal of science is to uncover some kind of natural truth. Natural truth is probably better seen as a metaphysical concept that refers to the purpose of nature. Truisms in nature may be no more than the slogans, aphorisms, or clichés that appear in the artwork of Jenny Holzer. A second and perhaps more important goal is to extend laboratory findings beyond the laboratory, that is, to generalize verifiable statements. In clinical practice, this type of "bench-to-bedside" work is called translational research that will be discussed in detail in later parts of this book. For those who deal with speakers and listeners identified as having a clinical communication disorder, the job of explaining theories entails an extra responsibility. Bernstein and Weismer (2000), in a special issue of the *Journal of Phonetics*, proposed that any evidence that has been gleaned from research on clinical disorders must also increase our understanding of typical speaking and listening behavior. The experiments described in the special issue covered deafness, hearing loss, dysarthria, aphasia, and voice disorders.

It is unfortunate, but not surprising to report that, in recent years, there has been what may be called a science confidence gap (Achterberg, De Koster, & Van der Waal, 2016). Science has become politicized and characterized by declining public trust. However, trust in scientific methods and principles has declined more than trust in current scientific institutions. The gap seems to be inversely related to level of education. That is, more years of education are associated with a smaller gap in confidence about scientific findings.

THE RULES OF SCIENCE

The Max Planck Society (2000) adopted 10 rules of good scientific practice in 2000. Some of these rules, similar to those in the Belmont Report, apply to research ethics and have been noted in Chapter 3. In general, the rules are based on scientific honesty, and violations can result from lack of care in applying scientific methods to outright fraud and deceit.

One especially noteworthy rule that does not appear in international law is the rule of systematic skepticism. That is, the scientist must be open to doubt, even about the researcher's own results. Reproducibility or replication of results is essential to any scientific claim. Some other regulations in the Max Planck report prohibit hindering the scientific work of others and actively promoting the science of junior colleagues, as well as being open to criticism expressed by other scientists.

A former director of the Max Planck Institute of Neurobiology in Martinsried, Germany (Kreutzberg, 2004) elaborated on the rules of good scientific practice. He noted that the respect and trust of the public depends on the scientist's honesty and adherence to the rules of good scientific practice. These rules govern the following four main principles in scientific research: day-to-day scientific practice, relations and cooperation with colleagues, publication of results, and the appointment of ombuds officers at every institute (Kreutzberg, 2004, p. 332). An ombuds officer is essentially a fair hearer who should be contacted regarding unprofessional conduct, as well as in cases of allegations of harassment, retaliation, or discrimination.

The rules of science describe and explain phenomena, and are different from those of magic, the pseudosciences, and common sense or conventional wisdom. Anderson (1971) proposed five rules of empirical verification, four for description and one for explanation, unique to the scientific method. They have been adapted and expanded for relevance to communication sciences and disorders (CSD).

Empirical Verification

Descriptive statements must correspond with observed reality. We define *observed reality* as sense data or information that we receive through sight, hearing, touch, taste, and smell (this rules out intuition and divine revelation) on which different observers agree (this rules out hallucinations). As others may do the observing for us, there are rules for reporting:

- specific operations are required for making the observations;
- observations are reported;
- there is clear reasoning that leads from observations to statements;
- the process is described clearly and in sufficient detail for us to evaluate it; and
- the authority of the person making the statement should be irrelevant.

There are three other rules for description that are specific procedures for empirical verification.

Operational Definition

All terms in a descriptive statement are defined by the operations involved in manipulating or observing their referents. Here is a descriptive statement with the term needing an operational definition written in italics.

> Patients who *benefit* most from group treatment have been assessed as having
>
> _____ mild aphasia
>
> _____ moderate aphasia
>
> _____ severe aphasia

Adults with aphasia may be fluent or nonfluent; they may also have a mild, moderate, severe, or profound communication impairment, and we set different goals according to type and severity of aphasia. If "benefit" refers to improved naming and word finding, the answer might be "mild aphasia." If "benefit" refers to improved social interactions and quality of life, the answer might be "severe aphasia."

An operational definition is like a recipe: it is a set of instructions. The truth of the statement, "Julia Child liked Boston cream pie" depended on the recipe. An operational definition requires that we specify what we are talking about in the following ways:

- We use only sense data in descriptive statements.
- Our meaning is clear enough that different observers can agree on the sense data.

If we have succeeded, our operational definition is a testable statement. That means it can be falsified or strengthened, but not proven.

Controlled Observation

If a change in condition or event A causes a change in condition or event B, then

- B must be observed when there are different values of A; and
- all variables other than A are discounted as causes of the change observed in B.

Compare the above with the post hoc fallacy described in the following section "Uncontrolled Observation."

Consider this advertisement: "The next time you service your hearing aids, replace your present batteries with Bob's batteries, and you'll be amazed at the difference." It would be amazing if there were not a difference. The kind of battery is not the only variable that could produce a change in performance. Others include:

- condition of the present batteries;
- condition of the hearing aids before servicing;
- switching to Bob's batteries; and
- some combination of these factors.

In the following examples, assume that variable A refers to hearing aid batteries with two values, Bob's and Brand X. Assume also that variable B refers to spondee reception threshold (SRT). If one type of hearing aid is better than the other, then the superior brand should result in lower SRTs. There are five bases for discounting one variable as a possible cause of an observed change on another, as the following sections explain.

Experimental Control

Keep variables constant so that the same value occurs at each value on variable A. By using only new hearing aids and only new batteries, perfect running order (the same value of this variable) will occur at each of the two values of variable A, Bob's and Brand X batteries. Variables that do not change cannot produce changes on any other variable.

Statistical Control

Estimate the magnitude of the effect the variable will have on variable B and subtract this from the change that is observed.

If removing cerumen lowers threshold by 10 dB, then we add 10 dB to thresholds after both removing cerumen and installing Bob's batteries. Whatever difference remains can be attributed to the change caused by Bob's batteries.

Assuming Invariance

You neither control nor measure the variable in question, but assume that it does not vary appreciably. Humidity affects comfort level, possibly reducing performance. If hearing aid batteries are tested one right after the other, then any change in humidity would probably be so slight as to be negligible.

Assuming Irrelevance

You don't care at all whether the same value of the variable occurs at each value of variable A. You assume that the variable has no effect on variable B. The color of the hearing aid is such a variable; you wouldn't bother to match the aids on color, because color is irrelevant to performance.

Randomization

Manipulate the variable in a strictly random fashion with respect to variable A, so that the same average value will be likely to occur at each value on variable A. Test a large number of hearing aid users and toss a coin to decide whether to install Bob's or Brand X batteries. When there is a subset of a variable that is larger than two, coin tossing will not work, and it may become advisable to consult a table of random numbers. The experimenter may also choose to order presentation of batteries pseudorandomly, where, for example, there are never three consecutive occurrences where Bob's batteries are presented first. The purpose of randomization is to control for the threat to internal validity called the order of presentation effect (see Chapters 7 and 8 for information about controlling order of presentation in experimental research and diagnostic testing, respectively).

Statistical Generalization

It is impossible to observe every individual or condition representing the communication disorder we wish to study. For example, there may be a child with autism spectrum disorder who lives on a forgotten street in New Delhi and communicates in a way nobody thought of before. One way we use statistics (see Chapter 6) is to test a random sample of individuals with a certain condition (say, 30 adults with Broca's aphasia) and generalize the findings to a larger population (all adults with Broca's aphasia). We may also want to generalize an observation to other conditions, an important part of carryover exercises in therapy. For example, it is important to generalize children's language gains made in the clinic to home and school environments.

The way to accomplish these goals is to obtain random samples from the set of conditions or set of individuals. Statistical inference is the procedure for deciding if the size of the effect and the number of participants justify generalizing the result from the sample to the population. For many of the analyses we do in research, the statistical difference between about 30 samples and infinity samples is trivial. Obtaining about 30 samples is usually sufficient to limit the adverse effect of low statistical power.

The power of a test refers to the likelihood that we will make a certain kind of mistake when making statistical inferences. These mistakes are called Type I and Type II errors, and they refer to acceptance or rejection of the null hypothesis. A possible hypothesis is that Treatment X will reduce stuttering, and the null hypothesis is that Treatment X will not reduce stuttering. In a Type I error, the experimenter rejects the null hypothesis when it is true. In a Type II error, the experimenter accepts or retains the null hypothesis when it is false. Statistical power refers to the probability of rejecting a false null hypothesis. In other words, we ask if the sample size is adequate to increase the probability that the experimenter will reject the null hypothesis when the null hypothesis is actually false. In previously mentioned example, the null hypothesis that Treatment X will not reduce stuttering is false; Treatment X will be shown to reduce stuttering if you treat enough people who stutter. There are formulas for calculating the number of participants needed to assure adequate statistical power in a given experiment (see Chapter 6 for statistical treatments of differences between experimental and control groups).

Empirical Confirmation

Empirical confirmation means that beliefs or explanatory statements must be evaluated by outside independent tests. An explanatory statement is more likely to be true when it is consistent with:

- verified descriptive statements; and
- confirmed explanatory statements.

Inconsistency between a descriptive statement and an explanatory statement leads to rejection of the explanatory statement. Using the principle of controlled observation, we may propose the following:

> If A, then B
>
> Not B
>
> Therefore, not A
>
> Or,
>
> If Mary is deaf (A), she will fail the audiology screening (B).
>
> Mary did not fail the audiology screening (not B).
>
> Therefore, Mary is not deaf (not A).

However, one successful prediction is not sufficient to prove the explanatory statement that logically implies it, nor are two, nor, in most cases, are 100. Based on the fact that Mary failed the audiology screening, we cannot be certain that she is deaf (she could be distracted, her ear canals could be occluded with cerumen, or she could be hard of hearing, among other possibilities). Successful predictions confirm the explanatory statement, or increase the probability of its being correct.

Empirical confirmation requires that the scientist or clinician always regard explanatory statements as tentative, seek new ways to test them against observations and other explanations, and never accept them as final truths.

THE SCIENTIFIC METHOD VERSUS COMMON SENSE OR CONVENTIONAL WISDOM

This section uses Anderson's (1971) model, with changes to make it relevant to communication sciences and disorders. By *common sense* or *conventional wisdom,* we mean patterns of thoughts that are both widespread and unscientific. They may be widely held beliefs that are unsubstantiated by evidence. This is also referred to as *fallacious reasoning* or what *not* to do according to the scientific method. Accordingly, all information in the following topics from "psychological verification" to "bolstering" represents examples of what *is not done* in good research.

Consideration of the value of common sense goes back at least as far as Aristotle, who considered *sensus communis* to be the ability to integrate stimuli to derive commonalities in them. Scientists who shun common sense run the risk of pursuing only a specific and narrow field of study, blocking promising research avenues, or failing to follow unexpected paths or improbable directions. The common sense reported by nonscientists results from evolutionary steps or refinements by large groups and across generations (Erren, Koch, & Meyer-Rochow, 2013).

Earlier in this chapter, I noted that the scientific method relies on controlled observations, and that divine intervention and hallucinations cannot be cited as causes for the observed phenomena. But is it possible that religion, common sense, and the scientific method can coexist in the same person's mind just as many languages can be mastered without confusion in the polyglot speaker? The cognitive notion of *polyphasia* is based on the proposal that science, religion, and other forms of knowledge can coexist as modes of thought shared as common sense (Falade & Bauer, 2017, p. 4).

It is unlikely that many of us will conduct scientific experiments to inform the daily decisions we make. Sometimes, according to Garin and DeVoogd (2008, p. 341), common sense just makes sense. Although the authors focused their report on scientifically based reading research (Garin & DeVoogd, 2008, p. 336), they generalized their claims to consumers of research of any instructional method. By claiming that an experimental model may not be appropriate to educational research because classrooms are not laboratories, the authors are, in essence, challenging the integrity of some high-quality journals, such as *Language, Speech, and Hearing Services in Schools.* Research results do not confer certainty, and hypotheses are never proven. However, common sense, as demonstrated in the following section, is often nonsense or, at least, at odds with the scientific method.

Psychological Verification

Descriptive studies use the weakest of research designs to explain causal relations among variables. They try to clarify specific features of research variables through classification or illustration. A descriptive statement is considered to be true if it is authoritative, comforting, or familiar. Empirical verification requires that we observe, but the principle of psychological verification tells us not to observe. The corollaries suggest ways to avoid observation. In empirical observation, we try to find consistencies among explanatory statements and between explanatory and descriptive statements, but in psychological verification, we are instructed not to think logically (better yet, not to think at all) about relationships among statements.

The essential point is to avoid the test of observation, because it is difficult, cumbersome, and time consuming to apply. We may be forced to discard some fine thoughts merely because they are not supported by facts. Common-sense reasoning, therefore, is to avoid any test that might not support the desired outcome.

The Test of Authority

Focus on the authority figure, rather than statements or evidence. In this way, we can accept each authoritative statement without being concerned about truth or falsity. We can decide in advance to accept or reject future statements based on our evaluation of the authority figure. Evaluation criteria might include prestige, power, wealth, and personal confidence. If the authority is a group, the criterion might be the size of the group. For example, you should believe what you just read, because the author is an expert in his field.

The Test of Comfort

This is also known as *wishful thinking*, in that we accept pleasant statements and reject those that are unpleasant. For example, global warming might be a good thing because it reduces the harshness of winters. Feelings of hate, anger, or fear are justified as the responses of righteous people to wrongdoing by others. As an example, children with Down syndrome may be thought to be docile and sweet, whereas children with autism may be considered distant and difficult.

The Test of Familiarity

We accept familiar statements and reject those that are unfamiliar. Advertisements are repeated so often that they must contain at least a germ of truth. People with brain damage are "vegetables" and those who are deaf are also "dumb," according to the test of familiarity.

Verbal Definition

Anderson (1971) suggested the following principles as ways of avoiding the test of observations, in other words, avoiding the scientific method. If terms in a descriptive statement are undefined or defined in strictly verbal terms, then they avoid testability. The scientific method requires explanatory statements that are observable and empirically testable, but the other ways of explaining phenomena, as described in the following sections, do not adhere to the scientific method.

Use Vague Terms

Terms that are sufficiently vague in their reference to observations will not be useful in determining truth or falsity of statements in which they are used. For example, it is impossible to insult elderly individuals with Alzheimer disease because they don't care if you do.

Use Verbal Definitions

When required to define terms, substitute one set of operationally vague terms for another. Explain that the child who does not attend to a task must lack focus.

Use Circular Statements

For example, stuttering is everything you do to stop stuttering. An individual who continues to stutter didn't stop trying to stop stuttering.

Attach a "Nonobservability" Clause

The phenomenon will not appear if it is being looked at. For example, write in your diagnostic report that the only time the child hears normally is when it is absolutely quiet.

Uncontrolled Observation

When the test of observation must be applied, it can be made more flexible by inferring causality from natural co-occurrences or naturally occurring correlations. The definition of *post hoc ergo propter hoc* reasoning (after this therefore because of this) is, If B follows A, then A is the cause of B. The child with hyperfunctional voice disorder became hoarse after attending a baseball game, so the parents are counseled to discontinue taking the child to any more games.

Overgeneralization

Once you have arrived at a conclusion, generalize it as broadly as possible. Don't burden your conclusions with restrictions and qualifications. If you state the conclusion simply enough, then there will be no need for further observations.

Generalize to Unexamined Values of Independent Variables

For example, ASHA membership is growing at an astounding rate. The number of ASHA members quadrupled from 1980 to 2000. If the number keeps quadrupling every 20 years, there should be nearly a half million ASHA members by 2020 and more ASHA members than people in about 150 years.

Generalize to Unexamined Values of Sampled Variables

This is a method for extending conclusions. If you prepare an individualized educational plan (IEP) for a child with a language disorder, the same IEP should be useful for all other children with language disorders (see, for example, the "gray book" for preparing an IEP).

Generalize to Unexamined Values of Controlled Variables

This is reasoning by analogy. For example, M&Ms have been used as effective reinforcers in behavior modification studies with children on the autism spectrum. Extend this conclusion to use chocolate in dysphagia management treatments.

Generalize to Different Operational Definitions of Variables

Many bilingual Spanish–English tests have been standardized using Spanish-speaking children living in Mexico. If you are testing a child who learned Spanish in any of the other 21 countries where Spanish is spoken, you should not be concerned about this.

Psychological Confirmation

Once you accept an explanatory statement, you never need to reject it. You can deal with inconsistencies found in other statements by discarding or altering the competing statements or by ignoring or modifying the relationships between them. Because your awareness of inconsistency is the result of thinking, not of observation, then the solution is either

- do not think; or
- if you must, think very carefully.

Do Not Think

Ignore One of the Ideas or the Relationship Between Them. Repression is a well-known and time-tested way of dealing with conflicting ideas. If deaf children are convinced by their elders that cochlear implants represent a betrayal of their Deaf community, then they will be less likely to think about the consequences of being able to hear.

Logic-Tight Compartmentalization. Keep ideas from coming into contact, so you can think about them both. For example, you support special education services for all children with communication disorders in your community but vote against any tax increase to expand school budgets.

Think Carefully (If You Must Think)

Produce an Appearance of Compatibility. Modify one of the ideas or the relationship between them. Psychologists call this thinking *rationalization*; another term is *whitewash thinking*. There are two ways to modify one of two conflicting ideas to make it appear compatible with the other:

- *Differentiating:* Split the idea into two. If the caregiver's report does not correspond with your findings on a diagnostic test, then indicate that the caregiver is not a reliable informant.
- *Bolstering:* Change your attitude toward one idea so that it seems more congruent with the other. In "sour grapes" thinking, we emphasize undesirable aspects of the issue. If a client is hard to test, say he couldn't be conditioned. In "sweet lemon" thinking, we emphasize the desirable aspects. If you use facilitated communication, you have a heightened interest in articles that extol its virtues.

THE SCIENTIFIC METHOD AND PSEUDOSCIENCE

An emphasis on evidence-based practice (EBP) based on the scientific method started with the medical profession in the 1990s and was adopted in audiology and speech-language pathology, as well as other health care professions, around the year 2000. The motivation was the need to move away from craft-based or intuition-based treatments to treatments whose efficacy was supported by evidence (Lof, 2011). However, there are still questionable treatments that may be marketed as alternative, with no substantial evidence that they work. We refer to these treatment rationales as pseudoscience or quackery. One reason for their appeal is that our treatments are not always completely effective. Another is that EBP may be hard to do, involving data collection, perusal of current research, and commitment in time and effort for both clinician and client. Pseudoscientific approaches, on the other hand, often promise quick and easy results.

Herreid (2016) noted that an overwhelming majority of Americans do not understand the scientific process, and those with more scientific knowledge are no more or less skeptical of pseudoscientific claims than students who scored poorly on science knowledge tests. One solution is to provide everyone with a Baloney Detection Kit (Herreid, 2016, p. 62). The individual confronting possible pseudoscience should ask four questions:

- What is the consumer of research asked to accept?
- What evidence supports the claim?
- What, if any, are the alternative explanations or hypotheses?
- What evidence supports these alternatives?

Finn et al. (2005) provide warning signs that alert a consumer or student that a claim may only appear to be scientific. The more such signs are in evidence, the greater the likelihood that the assertion, belief, or treatment approach is pseudoscientific. The article highlights 10 criteria that differentiate between science and pseudoscience. Described in the following text are the six that refer to the quality of evidence used to support a treatment claim or a research finding.

One device that Finn et al. (2005) criticized is the SpeechEasy, prompting a reply by Kalinowski, Saltuklaroglu, Stuart, and Guntupalli (2007). In the disclosure statement on the first page of the article, Kalinowski and Stuart indicate that they are coinventors of the SpeechEasy and have a financial interest in the product. That the evidence for using the SpeechEasy was thought to be based on pseudoscience on 8 of 10 criteria (Finn et al., 2005), prompted Kalinowski et al. (2007) to claim that the evaluators were biased in differentiating science from pseudoscience in research on the SpeechEasy, that the term "pseudoscience" has a history of being misused, and that the metaphors and analogies they (Kalinowski et al., 2007) used were appropriate, because the theoretical underpinning for the neural basis of stuttering is lacking. The authors Kalinowski et al. (2007) presented a detailed rebuttal of Finn et al.'s (2005) claims of pseudoscience. They indicated that they would adjust their orientation in light of new, persuasive data, and challenged Finn et al. (2005) to do the same.

Untestable

Finn et al. (2005) ask if the treatment is not able to be tested or falsified. There are legitimate academic pursuits, such as theoretical linguistics, where models are never exposed to real-world tests. For example, assume the model called TPWSGWTAU (or *the place where sentences go when they are understood*). Theoretical linguists are comfortable developing what we might call an "armchair hypothesis" that is not testable. There is no intent to subject this model to empirical observation. Rather, the model serves as a stimulus for empirical sciences to examine it further. Neurologists may study the brain structure of TPWSGWTAU; psychologists may consider processes leading to TPWSGWTAU. It is up to other disciplines, such as CSD, to develop specific testable hypotheses that explain how TPWSGWTAU is affected by communication disorders.

Pseudoscience is exposed when there are claims of a research finding or treatment's benefits, but the claim is not testable or capable of being disproved. For example, all three judges found that efficacy of facilitated communication, a treatment sometimes used for autism, is not testable (Finn et al., 2005). Recall that an essential part of a hypothesis is that it must be testable.

Remember that these assertions or hypotheses may never be proven, because the treatments are applied to a sample rather than to the entire population. Theories may be strengthened if the results of empirical testing support the hypothetical construct and they may be falsified or disproved if the treatment does not work as claimed. Other pseudoscientific claims are testable in principle, but are never tested in practice. Empirical tests that refute the claims are ignored or explained away with such generalities as, "No treatment works on everyone and everything."

Unchanged

Finn et al. (2005) ask if the treatment approach remains unchanged even if there is contradictory evidence. It is possible for a good treatment to have errors, misconceptions, or inaccuracies.

For example, Melodic Intonation Therapy (MIT) is a well-known means of treating moderate nonfluent aphasia, based on the premise that the musical abilities of the undamaged right cerebral hemisphere can facilitate word retrieval after a stroke in the left hemisphere of the brain. However, Albert, Sparks, and Helm (1973) erred in the original protocol that required their patients to shift from intoned forms of utterances to normal speech prosody. They recognized their error and instituted a transitional stage called *sprechgesang* (speech-song) that bridged the gap between speaking and singing, resulting in an effective treatment.

Because pseudoscientific claims are not typically exposed to empirical testing, the errors are seldom self-corrected. The treatment of stuttering offers many examples of this type of pseudoscience. Relating the problem of stuttering to the structure of the individual's tongue is at least as old as Aristotle, and the claim found its avatar in the 1800s in Diefenbach, who performed partial glossectomies to "cure" stuttering. Removing the tongue would remove the stuttering. (It is fortunate that a similar claim was not made for headaches.)

Confirming Evidence

Finn et al. (2005) ask if the rationale for the treatment approach was based only on confirming evidence, so that disconfirming evidence was ignored or minimized. Even a pseudoscientific treatment may garner some corroborating or confirming evidence. However, there are different levels of evidence, ranging from the weakest level of expert opinion (Level IV) to the strongest level of randomized controlled trials (Level I) (see Chapter 2). Positive results from a single therapy session with an individual client may be meaningful, but lack the force of results from randomized, double-blinded, placebo-controlled clinical trials replicated by independent investigators. It is a human frailty that we tend to assign greater credibility to evidence that confirms rather than disconfirms our beliefs.

Pseudoscience is not the practice of only ignoring disconfirming evidence; rather than being receptive, even if evidence is disconfirming, pseudoscientists explain away the differences, and save the original idea by adding some ad hoc hypotheses that incorporate the new evidence.

The tendency to overemphasize confirming evidence is most apparent in studies where the researchers have a financial interest in the outcome. That is, there is a monetary reward for confirming one's findings and a penalty for disconfirming them. Many scientific journals (ASHA's publications among them) require a disclosure statement from prospective contributors regarding a possible conflict of interest. It is important for consumers to know if they are reading reports of independent research versus research and development undertaken to bring a product to market.

Anecdotal Evidence

Finn et al. (2005) ask if the evidence supporting the treatment relies on personal experience and anecdotal accounts. Case study research is designed to examine in-depth specific individuals or situations in order to illustrate important principles that might be overlooked in examining group data. For example, the relatively new syndrome of primary progressive aphasia was identified after a case study in Canada was followed by a decade of similar reports of cases around the world. Useful as they are, scientists recognize that case studies provide a weak foundation for making valid inferences about treatment. Proper examination of treatment efficacy or evidence for clinical practice requires experimental controls that are not found in case studies.

Pseudoscience uses case studies, testimonials, and personal experiences as its bread and butter. The claim of repressed and recovered memories, popular a generation ago, resulted in well-meaning individuals testifying in court about events from decades earlier that they just recovered in memory. These testimonials threatened to result in the incarceration of innocent people, until the claims of repressed and recovered memories fell out of fashion.

There are many threats to the validity (generalizability of the data) of an experiment, including practice effects and the placebo effect. We need to eliminate alternative explanations that might account for the treatment effects: the fewer the alternative explanations, the greater the internal validity of the experiment.

Inadequate Evidence

Finn et al. (2005) ask if treatment claims are not commensurate with the level of evidence required to support those claims. There is an old saying that extraordinary claims require extraordinary evidence. The purpose of research is no more or less than a search for a piece of truth. Note that the word *truth* includes a lowercase *t*. Outcome research follows phases, which address different questions using different methods. Eventually, it is possible that the pieces of lowercase *t* truths that are revealed are collected into a capital-*T* Truth.

Pseudoscience often jumps right into the upper case. Asserting a fundamental right to the Truth, pseudoscientists turn the process of discovery on its head, claiming that it is the responsibility of their critics to prove them wrong. The argument from this position of ignorance that a claim must be correct represents fallacious reasoning.

Avoiding Peer Review

Finn et al. (2005) ask if treatment gains are unsupported by evidence that has been evaluated critically. The gold standard that evidence has undergone critical evaluation is publication in a peer-reviewed journal. The ASHA journals, including *Journal of Speech, Language, and Hearing Research; American Journal of Speech-Language Pathology; American Journal of Audiology;* and *Language, Speech, and Hearing Services in Schools,* are all peer-reviewed publications. In 2018, the publications called *SIG Perspectives* of ASHA's Special Interests Groups (SIGs) became peer reviewed. (Note that the *ASHA Leader* invites articles and is not considered peer reviewed.) Authors submit unsolicited articles to the editor of the journal who forwards the material to an associate editor with expertise in the area of study. The associate editor requests usually three experts in the field to serve as ad hoc reviewers (selected from volunteers who have previously been appointed to a review panel) to write a detailed critique of the paper. Recommendations for or against publication are generally in the four categories of accept, accept with minor revisions, accept with major revisions, and reject. The journal editor makes the final determination, and forwards the critical evaluations to the authors.

The peer-review process may be subverted by reviewers who wish to promote a particular agenda, style, or method of research. Even when the peer review is putatively blind, with reviewers and authors remaining anonymous, it is not uncommon for reviewers to recognize the work of scholars from laboratories that may be competing with the reviewers' labs for funding and recognition. On the other hand, authors whose work has been rejected from journals with the most rigorous review process can often find a home for their work, even if it is in an online journal where authors are responsible for submitting their own external peer reviews (presumably from sympathetic friends).

Papers that are self-published, either in hard copy or on the Internet, have not undergone peer review. Pseudoscientific approaches to treatment may be promoted directly to the public, often very effectively, through advertisements or stories that emphasize emotional rather than intellectual content. The scientific process of peer review should include challenges to claims that may be one-sided or biased, whereas the pseudoscientific approach is less likely to do so.

CONCLUSION

How does the student or professional clinician avoid implementing treatments that are based on pseudoscience or quackery? First, be skeptical. Be open to new ideas, but be ruthless in your scrutiny of all ideas, both new and old (Lof, 2011). Understand that a principal goal of the scientific method is raising questions for the sake of discovery. Second, pay attention to the disclosures required in journal articles and presentations at professional conventions. See if the author has a financial interest in or is being paid to promote a particular treatment. Understand the difference between objective research and research and development that is used to market a product. Finally, engage in practice-based evidence (PBE), that is, the way that practitioners contribute to EBP by using research methodologies to examine the quality of clinical intervention. Better EBP depends on more PBE.

ADVANCED STUDY

The author proposes that skills in the scientific method are necessary for an individual to be granted power of professor. With new generations of scholars and researchers needed every 10 years, professors and master clinicians have an obligation to prepare individuals with adequate knowledge and skills to undertake the tasks of scholarship and research, and the scientific method is a key component. For evidence of the requisite scientific method skills, complete the following, and have your instructor, academic adviser, mentor, or CSD department chair review that you have completed the requirements and sign and date where indicated.

Student's Name: ______________________________

1. Explain the difference between a hypothesis and a theory.
2. Explain the difference between coincidence and correlation.
3. Give five examples of systematic skepticism using the rules of science.
4. Give five examples of common sense that do not conform to the scientific method.
5. Give five examples of pseudoscience.

Date of Completion: ______________________________

Faculty/Supervisor Signature: ______________________________

REFERENCES

Achterberg, P., De Koster, W., & Van der Waal, J. (2016). A science confidence gap: Education, trust in scientific methods, and trust in scientific institutions in the United States, 2014. *Public Understanding of Science, 26*, 704–720.

Albert, M., Sparks, R., & Helm, N. (1973). Melodic intonation therapy for aphasia. *Archives of Neurology, 29*, 130–131.

Anderson, B. F. (1971). *The psychology experiment*. Belmont, CA: Brooks/Cole.

Bernstein, L. E., & Weismer, G. (2000). Basic science at the intersection of speech science and communication disorders. *Journal of Phonetics, 28*, 225–232.

Edelstein, W., & Hofschneider, P. H. (Eds.). (2000). *Verantwortliches handeln in der wissenschaft* (p. 139). Munich, Germany: Max-Planck-Gesellschaft.

Erren, T. C., Koch, M. S., & Meyer-Rochow, V. B. (2013). Common sense: Folk wisdom that ethnobiological and ethnomedical research cannot afford to ignore. *Journal of Ethnobiology and Ethnomedicine, 9*, 1–12.

Falade, B. A., & Bauer, M. W. (2017). 'I have faith in science and in God': Common sense, cognitive *polyphasia* and attitudes to science in Nigeria. *Public Understanding of Science, 1*, 1–18.

Finn, P., Bothe, A. K., & Bramlett, R. E. (2005). Science and pseudoscience in communication disorders: Criteria and applications. *American Journal of Speech-Language Pathology, 14*, 172–186.

Garin, E. M., & DeVoogd, G. (2008). The benefits of sustained silent reading: Scientific research and common sense converge. *The Reading Teacher, 62*, 336–344.

Goldfarb, R., & Serpanos, Y. (2014). *Professional writing in speech-language pathology and audiology* (2nd ed.). San Diego, CA: Plural Publishing.

Herreid, C. F. (2016). Science, pseudoscience, and nonsense. *Journal of College Science Teaching, 45*, 61–65.

Kalinowski, J., Saltuklaroglu, T., Stuart, A., & Guntupalli, V. K. (2007). On the importance of scientific rhetoric in stuttering: A reply to Finn, Bothe, and Bramlett (2005). *American Journal of Speech-Language Pathology, 16*, 69–76.

Kreutzberg, G. W. (2004). The rules of good science. *European Molecular Biology Organization, 5*, 330–332.

Lof, G. L. (2011). Science-based practice and the speech-language pathologist. *International Journal of Speech-Language Pathology, 13*, 189–196.

Max-Planck-Gesellschaft. (2000). *Rules of good scientific practice; rules of procedure in cases of suspected scientific misconduct* (p. 22). Munich, Germany: Author.

Maxwell, D. L., & Satake, E. (1997). *Research and statistical methods in communication disorders.* Baltimore, MD: Williams & Wilkins.

Snyder, G. G., Holzman, C., Sun, T., Bullen, B., Bertolet, M., & Catov, J. M. (2018). Breastfeeding greater than 6 months is associated with smaller maternal waist circumference up to one decade after delivery. *Journal of Women's Health.* Advance online publication. doi:10.1089/jwh.2018.7393

Yorkston, K. M., Spencer, K., Duffy, J., Beukelman, D., Golper, L. A., Miller, R., . . . Sullivan, M. (2001). Evidence-based medicine and practice guidelines: Application to the field of speech-language pathology. *Journal of Medical Speech Language Pathology, 9*, 243 –256.

Zippoli, R. P., & Kennedy, M. (2005). Evidence-based practice among speech-language pathologists. Attitudes, utilization, and barriers. *American Journal of Speech-Language Pathology, 14*, 208–220.

5

Types of Research

INTRODUCTION

Now that you understand why professors and students do research; why the researcher must have high moral or ethical standards; how the material you learned in your courses applies to language, speech, and hearing intervention in the clinic; and how basic knowledge of the scientific method can help you to understand the design of most experiments, it is time to learn the types of research that are performed in the communication sciences and disorders (CSD) professions.

Learning Objectives

After reading this chapter, the student will be able to

- evaluate different types of research;
- interpret clinical files and design evidence-based clinical research studies; and
- critically examine survey forms.

EXPERIMENTAL, QUASIEXPERIMENTAL, AND NONEXPERIMENTAL DESIGNS

Recall that an *independent variable* is defined as a phenomenon that is manipulated by the researcher and that is predicted to have an effect on another phenomenon, and *dependent variable* is defined as a phenomenon that is affected by the researcher's. manipulation of another phenomenon. The application to experimental research is the following: for the independent variable, the experimenter presents a stimulus, such as a picture; for the dependent variable, the participant produces an observable behavior, such as naming the picture. The participant's response *depends* on what the experimenter has presented. The experimenter can manipulate the presentation, for example, by blurring it or limiting the length of time of exposure to see if there is an effect on the participant's picture naming ability.

In an award-winning article in the *American Journal of Audiology* (Humes et al., 2017), a study examined efficacy of hearing aids for older adults by controlling three independent variables: audiology best practices, over-the-counter hearing aids selected by the consumer, and placebo devices. The experimenters also manipulated the purchase price of the hearing aids, with half the participants paying the typical price and the other half paying a reduced price. The dependent variable was a 66-item self-report of satisfaction completed by consumers. The report of the study that won the best article award in the same year for the language division of the *Journal of Speech, Language, and Hearing Research* (Van Horne, Fey, & Curran, 2017) assigned children with developmental language disorders to two groups where training targeted grammatical morphemes of verbs. About half of the children were assigned to training where harder forms came first and the other group received training where easier forms came first. There were no differences between groups in number of therapy sessions or trials to criterion for mastery of the forms. The hard-first group made greater gains in accuracy on both trained and untrained verbs than the easy-first group. The independent variable was the treatment protocol and the dependent variable was the number of correct responses produced by the children.

Group Experimental Design

The strongest research design is called a true experiment. The most basic kind involves randomized assignment to one of two groups where only the posttest is measured. One group gets the experimental treatment and the other group gets the standard treatment or no treatment. There is no need for a pretest to assure comparable groups, because assignment to groups is random (called probabilistic equivalence). However, the most common true experimental design is called the pretest–posttest control group design, as well as by its other names, the classical experimental design or the randomized before and after control group design. The experiment typically compares the change in Group A with the change in Group B. Statistical analyses are used to rule out the likelihood that differences are due to chance alone. The study of the children who learned either easier-first or harder-first forms of verbs (Van Horne et al., 2017) was a randomized controlled trial. In the study of satisfaction with hearing aids (Humes et al., 2017) cited previously, there were three groups that participated in a randomized, placebo-controlled, double-blinded clinical trial.

Group characteristics must be carefully considered. Ideally, groups will be identical except for the variable under study. For example, uncontrolled variables, such as age, gender, education, and socioeconomic status, can confound your results, and the researcher must answer the question of why these variables were controlled, but not others (e.g., handedness, premorbid history, medications). There may be pairwise matching (one participant in Group A matched to one participant in Group B) or group matching (all participants in Group A matched to all participants in Group B).

Quasiexperimental Designs

Sometimes, usually because of time or financial constraints or ethical concerns about no-treatment control groups, researchers will opt to use quasiexperimental designs to rule out some alternative explanations that threaten internal validity (truthfulness and generalizability) of the experiment.

Nonequivalent Control Group Design

In this quasiexperimental design, the comparison group is as similar as possible to the experimental treatment group, but there is no random assignment into the groups. There may be pairwise or group matching but, once the matches are made, the participants are deliberately assigned to one group or the other. This strategy saves the time and expense, as well as the need for many more participants, to achieve the same balance randomly. The same design can be used to replicate an existing study, using that completed study as the comparison group.

Time-Series Design

The second type of quasiexperimental design is called the time-series design. These designs use repeated measurements of the dependent variable over an extended period of time with a single subject or a small number of participants. There is no control or comparison group. The design allows participants to act as their own controls in order to reduce bias. There are at least three observations taken before and after the intervention (sometimes called an interrupted time series design). For example, a multicenter study of heat and moisture exchangers (HME) on the pulmonary function of individuals who had undergone total laryngectomy (Parrilla, Minni, & Bogaardt, 2015) had a 2-week initial baseline period, followed by 12 weeks of HME use. Baseline measurements included a questionnaire regarding quality of life, as well as initial measurements of coughing and forced expectorations. Measurements were repeated after 2, 6, and 12 weeks of HME use. This design is also useful in behavior modification research. In the following design, "O" refers to observation and measurement of the dependent variable; "A" is the baseline; and "B" is the experimental segment, beginning with the "X" marker. Simplest is the A–B design (Box 5–1).

An example of the A–B design is the finding in both single-subject (Ingham, Martin, & Kuhl, 1974) and group studies (Kalinowski, Armson, & Stewart, 1995) that stuttering does not consistently increase with increased speech rate.

The Nonexperimental One-Group Pretest–Posttest Design

This is more commonly used in studies of efficacy of CSD treatments. There is no comparison group and pretest measures are not repeated. All members of the group receive the experimental treatment with the pretest and posttest providing the basis for comparison.

The most common type of nonexperimental design is the one-group pretest–posttest design that mirrors in a group what the clinician does with an individual in therapy. How do you know if there is an effect of intervention if you don't have some form of baseline measurement (pretest) before you start treatment? What is

Box 5–1. The A–B Design

A segment		B segment
O_1, O_2, O_3, O_4	X	O_5, O_6, O_7, O_8

true for the therapy you do in your speech and hearing center is also true for group experiments of efficacy of clinical intervention. In other words, research using the one-group pretest–posttest design that is published in a peer-reviewed journal follows the same evidence-based practice model that good clinicians use daily in their treatment of communication disorders.

Recall from Chapter 2 that it is not only unethical but illegal for an individual who may want treatment to be randomly assigned to a no-treatment control group. Therefore, a typical study of two groups will include one group receiving an experimental treatment and the other receiving the standard treatment, or one group receiving individual therapy and the other receiving group therapy, as long as there is equipoise—an equivalent expectation of outcome—in the two intervention types. Of course, there must be proper randomization that clarifies how participants are assigned to groups; a sample size that ensures adequate statistical power; and allowance for attrition or mortality, because not everyone who starts the experiment completes it.

AB is a randomized control group design (Box 5–2), where participants are randomly assigned to two groups, for example, experimental and control. There are now within-subjects and between-subjects components. The dependent variable A is measured repeatedly before intervention B is initiated. A change in A indicates that B has had an effect. By measuring A repeatedly before initiating B, then the clinician can make a reasonable claim that any change is more likely to be the result of intervention and not maturation (if working with children) or spontaneous recovery (if working with neurologically-impaired adults).

ABA or "Reverse" Design

ABA or "reverse" design (Box 5–3) means that there is a reversal to baseline after completion of the experimental segment. This design is considered to be more powerful than an AB study, but it is more useful in assessing drug interventions than speech, language, or hearing interventions. In pharmacological studies, the dependent variable A, let's say environmental allergies, decreases following intervention B of, say, allergy medication, and allergies return to baseline when medication B is withdrawn. In speech and language interventions, we hope that improvements following treatment cannot be reversed or unlearned. In audiology, there is little to be gained, other than satisfying a clinician's curiosity, from withdrawing an effective hearing aid.

Box 5–2. The AB Randomized Control Group Design

	A segment		B segment
Experimental Group	O_1, O_2, O_3, O_4	X	O_5, O_6, O_7, O_8
Control Group	$O_9, O_{10}, O_{11}, O_{12}$	X	$O_{13}, O_{14}, O_{15}, O_{16}$

Trials O_{13}–O_{16} represent a "pseudo-B segment" with no experimental treatment applied.

Box 5–3. The ABA or "Reverse" Design

A segment	B segment	(X removed)	A segment
O_1, O_2, O_3, O_4	O_5, O_6, O_7, O_8		$O_9, O_{10}, O_{11}, O_{12}$

SINGLE-SUBJECT AND CASE STUDIES

Controlled Single-Subject Experiments

The single-subject design is more rigorous and can provide a stronger level of evidence than case studies. Publication of research using the single-subject design for assessing therapy usually depends on large effect sizes. Effect size is a measure of the existence of a phenomenon of interest in a population. For example, if preoperative counseling by an SLP for an individual undergoing a laryngectomy shows a large effect size in improving a patient's ability to develop esophageal voice postsurgically, then this counseling should be part of preoperative protocol. Another way of looking at effect size is to relate it to the power of a test to result in a significant finding when the hypothesis is true.

Strengths

Single-subject research designs (SSRDs), sometimes called single-subject experimental designs (SSEDs) are self-controlling. That means that there is no need for a control group to compare to the research group. The individual participant responds to the experimental factor, compared to the same person's response to a control factor. For example, an individual who stutters (IWS) can read aloud in unison with the experimenter (experimental factor), and this factor is compared to that same IWS who reads aloud alone (control factor). A second strength of the SSRD is that it is usually faster and cheaper to find a single participant than a group of participants. Finally, the SSRD may be ideal for assessing the viability of a speech, language, or hearing intervention in everyday practice, generating evidence-based practice (EBP) (Byiers, Reichle, & Symons, 2012). SSRDs can also provide practice-based evidence (PBE) for scaling up, or justifying randomized clinical trials.

Here are some examples of SSRDs in speech, language, and hearing. Nordgren (2016) tracked changes in fundamental frequency of two Swedish boys with autism spectrum disorder following a yearlong intervention of phonological segmentation. At the end of the study, the boys developed prosody similar to typically developing peers. A nonlinear approach to target selection was used for a 6-year-old girl with speech sound disorders in an A-B-A-B (see description of this design later in this chapter) single-subject experimental design (Shoaf, Iyer, & Bothe, 2009). Nonlinear phonological analysis describes and explains phonological patterns. The 18-session treatment, conducted at a public school, showed that clinicians who were not associated with the development of this approach could apply it successfully. Finally, Plant, Gnosspileus, and Levitt (2000) used tactile supplements to improve lipreading in a deaf adult using speech tracking testing.

Weaknesses

Single-subject research designs (SSRDs) used to study efficacy of CSD therapy may have low internal validity (truthfulness and generalizability) because of weaknesses in design, assessment, and observational measurements. That means that the empirical value, or the ability to generalize the findings of the SSRD experiment to a larger population, will not be a strong as the value of results from a larger group study. In a review of 25 SSRDs dealing with language therapy for aphasia, Fukkink (1996) suggested that internal validity can be increased by applying A-B-A-B designs, multiple-baseline designs, control tests, objective tests, and a blind procedure with objective measurement. Multiple baseline measurements, before and after intervention, motivate a conclusion that the therapy did or did not have an effect. We refer to the measure of a behavior before treatment as the initial baseline, and the measure after treatment as baseline recovery.

Case Study Research

This research is designed to examine specific individuals or situations in depth in order to illustrate important principles that might be overlooked in examining group data. These studies are used to evaluate phenomena that occur rarely and that can provide important information. They are also valuable in examining exceptions to generally accepted rules. If case studies aim to evaluate efficacy of clinical interventions, they must move beyond descriptive analysis and use rigorous research methodology, including a clinical hypothesis or research question (Vance & Clegg, 2012). These studies in language, speech, and hearing can show gains in communicative abilities over time.

Strengths

The ethical proscription of random assignment of some participants in a group study to a no-treatment control group (see Chapter 2) that is both immoral and illegal is avoided. The factors that threaten internal validity (truthfulness and generalizability) in experimental research may be the substance of the case study approach, especially history and maturation. Research designs typically exclude external factors that can serve as alternative explanations for the findings; this is the threat of history. For example, if a child receives speech-language therapy in a university clinic and in school, any improvements in language may be attributable to the work done in the clinic, in school, or in both places. Maturation refers to changes in the participants themselves that can serve as alternative explanations for the findings. For example, did a child acquire a new speech sound because of clinical intervention or because it was a normal consequence of getting older?

Weaknesses

Case studies allow little generalization. They are also more likely to be contaminated by subjective biases on the part of the investigator.

Case studies and case study series can contribute to the evidence base for intervention in communication disorders if they include some element of experimental control. Within the framework of types of research, as noted in Chapter 2, evidence that follows single participant research is of lower value than evidence gleaned from group studies using randomized controlled trials, as well as systematic reviews and meta-analyses of randomized controlled trials. However, the strength of evidence based on $N = 1$ research is higher than that of observation and expert opinion. Vance and Clegg (2012) make a case for case study research as a methodology that practitioners should use to show effectiveness of their interventions.

In her article on single-subject controlled experiments in aphasia, Thompson (2006) presents a history of $N = 1$ experimental designs over more than 200 years. Probably the best known CSD case is that of Leborgne (called "Tan" because that was all he could say), described by Broca in 1861. As we have noted elsewhere (Halpern & Goldfarb, 2013), it is somewhat ironic that the patient who inspired the common understanding of Broca's aphasia and Broca's area did not have Broca's aphasia (Broca described the disorder as "aphemie" or aphemia, but Tan probably had global aphasia), and the lesion was not restricted to Broca's area (it included much of the zone of language or the perisylvian region, according to Damasio, 2008). Thompson (2006) noted that case study research in aphasia was important for establishing a starting point for evaluating the efficacy of speech-language therapy, but that the single-subject experimental design was better at controlling extraneous variables. In other words, the researcher could isolate the treatment as the independent variable responsible for the experimental effects. The single-subject experimental analysis is different from the case study (or $N = 1$) design in that the former can be replicated within and across multiple study participants.

Descriptive case studies explain an aspect of a client's communication difficulties. When a condition is rare, such as the young child with a suspected in utero stroke described in Chapter 1, the case report adds to the literature on this disorder. In describing my own brainstem stroke (Goldfarb, 2016), I hoped to foster a better understanding of the nature of my speech and swallowing difficulties. However, shining a light on communication disorders that follow a stroke from the perspective of an aphasiologist does not serve to evaluate interventions, nor is it designed to.

The A-B-A-B Design

The treatment effect is studied twice (the B segment) for all participants in the single-subject design experiment.

Strengths

The A-B-A-B design is well suited to show conditions under which stuttering is reduced or absent. For example, one or more individuals who stutter are asked to read a phonemically balanced story (such as the "Grandfather Passage" or the "Rainbow Passage"). There is no intervention in the first or second A phase and delayed auditory feedback (DAF) is set at 200 msec in the first and second B phase. The number of instances of stuttering will be higher in both A phases and lower in both B phases, indicating that DAF can reduce overt symptoms of stuttering. Replication may be calculated as $N \times 2$, so that five participants allow observation of the treatment effect 10 times. Yairi (personal communication, 2016) has demonstrated the DAF effect in unpublished videos. Box 5–4 provides an example of how to record this kind of data.

Weaknesses

The A-B-A-B design may be ill suited to clinical research in language intervention, as shown in the following example: A behavior, such as a word-finding deficit, is observed in the initial A phase; a treatment, such as a cue of the initial phoneme of the target word, is applied during the first B phase; the treatment is withdrawn during the second A phase, and the behavior (word retrieval) is observed; and lastly, the treatment (phonemic cue) is reapplied in the second B phase (Box 5–5).

Thompson (2006) indicates that the A-B-A-B design is not recommended for aphasia therapy because withdrawal of treatment must result in unlearning to

Box 5–4. The A-B-A-B Design to Study Disfluencies per Minute (DPM) under Delayed Auditory Feedback (DAF)

Participant	No DAF (A)	DAF (B)	No DAF (A)	DAF (B)
1	18	3	21	4
2	15	2	16	1
3	8	0	7	0
4	12	4	11	1
5	17	3	17	0

Box 5–5. Example of the A-B-A-B Design in a Language Task for Adult Aphasia

Stimuli include highly associative open-ended sentences with or without initial phonemic cues.

First A: Wash your hands with soap and _____ ("water" is not produced).

First B: Someone is knocking at the front d_____ ("door" is produced).

Second A: The American flag is red, white, and _____ ("blue" is not produced).

Second B: Every morning I brush my t_____ ("teeth" is produced).

demonstrate experimental control. That is, the second A observation should *not* show that the first B phase has generalized to the second A phase. Successful therapy should not result in reversal, and reversal to the initial A phase may not even be possible.

Multiple-Baseline Design

This is a within-subjects design because all subjects participate in the two conditions—baseline and experimental segments. Compare a participant's performance in the baseline with performance in the experimental segment to see the effect of the experimental treatment on the dependent variable. Multiple-baseline designs can be used in two ways. In a staggered-start design, different participants start the intervention at different times, but the same dependent variable or behavior is measured. For a single individual, there are two or more dependent variables or different behaviors that are measured as a result of intervention.

Strengths

The following are strengths of the multiple-baseline design: Repeated measurements of the dependent variable in the baseline provide control over the threats to internal validity posed by maturation, pretesting, regression, and instrumentation (see Chapter 8). Participants act as their own controls because the repeated measurements involve an experimental intervention.

Weakness

A weakness is the threat to internal validity of the experiment by history. History refers to an event that does not occur during baseline but that does occur during the experimental segment; this event may compete with the experimental treatment in affecting the dependent variable. For example, improvement in speechreading/lipreading may follow therapy in the university clinic, but the child with hearing loss may also have received aural rehabilitation in school at the same time. How do you know which treatment resulted in improvement in speech discrimination?

PROOF-OF-CONCEPT AND PILOT STUDIES; PHASE O, I, II, III, AND IV TRIALS

Pilot Study or Pilot Experiment

This is often carried out before conducting a large-scale research project. Pilots are small-scale studies that may be used to predict the sample size needed for a randomized clinical trial (RCT), the so-called gold standard of research. RCTs are rare in CSD research (although they are becoming more prevalent), partly because they take a great deal of time and money to carry out. Another explanation for the rarity of RCTs is the ethical and legal proscriptions against random assignment to a no-treatment or placebo control group. However, it is possible to use the RCT design with a stagger-start control group where one group (perhaps individuals on a waiting list) starts the intervention at a later time (see the multiple-baseline design above). Pilot studies are used for the following three reasons:

- *Assessing feasibility:* Examine the key steps of the main study such as recruitment of participants, eligibility criteria, and retention or drop-out rates.

- *Assessing problems with time and resources:* These may occur in the main study, including time to complete forms of evaluation, and types of equipment or instrumentation.
- *Assessing management problems:* These include data collection and storage. At the conclusion of a pilot study, the investigator typically reports one of four outcomes (Box 5–6).

Some Examples of Published Pilot Studies in CSD

Some examples of published pilot studies in CSD include an examination of alternative and augmentative (AAC) devices used to support conversation in chronic aphasia (Brock, Koul, Corwin, & Schlosser, 2017); using a computerized false–belief understanding task in children with autism (Carlsson, Miniscalco, Gillberg, & Johnels, 2018); using objective measurements of voice in older people with or without Parkinson disease in their natural environments (Donovan, Boudreaux, & Savage, 2015); and measuring off-topic speech in the discourse of healthy middle-aged and older adults (Wills, Capilouto, & Wright, 2012). These studies generally concluded with a section on future research where the authors recommended a greater number of participants, different types of measures, and better control for interaction of variables.

Box 5–6. The Four Possible Outcomes of Pilot Studies

- The main study is feasible without changes to the protocol.
- The main study is not feasible.
- The main study is feasible with changes to the protocol (with proposed changes clearly outlined).
- The main study is feasible with close monitoring.

Proof-of-Concept Studies

Proof-of-concept evidence demonstrates the feasibility of an experimental design. It is sometimes used as a synonym for a pilot study, but it is not the same as a prototype. For example, a recent paper (Mazerolle & Marchand, 2015) presented preliminary data about TypingSuite, a prototype software that may be able to identify users based on keystroke dynamics. The authors noted that the results of their study were necessary before undertaking the more challenging proof-of-concept task to determine if TypingSuite was useful in collecting biometric data. In other words, a prototype allows innovators to visualize how a product will function, and proof-of-concept verifies or strengthens a theory that can be achieved in development.

The proof-of-concept study described previously is designed to lead to Phase I, II, and III clinical trials in medical research. Although Phase I trials are the earliest ones done on people, it may be possible to join a Phase 0 study to find out if a drug works in the way that researchers expect it to. Phase I trials are usually small, recruiting only a few participants. Not all Phase I trials make it to Phase II, where there may be up to 100 people taking part and where a placebo is often used. Phase III trials involve many more participants and compare the new treatment with the best currently available treatments. Finally, Phase IV trials are done after a drug has been shown to work and has been granted a license.

While typically used by physicians testing new drugs, the various phase trials have also been used in CSD research. In a Phase I trial, an electromagnetic driver coupled with a target magnet was temporarily affixed to the malleus of six hearing aid users with sensorineural hearing losses. Resultant benefits in gain and output characteristics led to Phase II of the project with the magnet surgically implanted in an ossicular prosthesis (McGee et al., 1991). In an SLP example, I consulted on a Phase I trial (Perkins et al., 2007) to determine if a drug (modafinil, a generic form of Provigil, a treatment for narcolepsy) that promotes wakefulness without the side effects of caffeine would be helpful for patients with nonfluent aphasia secondary to acute stroke when they undertake speech-language therapy.

GROUP DESIGNS

There are three broad categories of research: quantitative, qualitative, and mixed-methods designs.

Quantitative Designs

The experimenter has maximum control over independent variables, and the predicted (in the study's hypotheses) dependent variables are carefully measured. Quantitative research is used to generate numerical data and to generalize results from a larger sample population. Data collection methods are much more structured than in qualitative research. Statistical analyses are performed to test the hypotheses of the study. The quantitative design is well suited to research done in laboratories where maximal control is possible. The statistical methods described in Chapter 6 may be appropriate in quantitative research.

Qualitative Designs

The experimenter has less control over independent variables, and participant behaviors are observed in a more natural setting. This research is used primarily to understand underlying reasons, opinions, and motivations. The insights gained from qualitative research can lead to hypotheses that are tested in quantitative research. Rather than using sophisticated statistics, qualitative research often reports trends, using broad measures of central tendency and dispersion. The qualitative design is well suited to preliminary research done in schools. Qualitative designs often stipulate triangulation of data, such as data collected from group discussions, individual interviews, and participant observations. The Council on Academic Accreditation (CAA), in evaluating graduate programs to award or continue accreditation, visits master's programs in SLP as well as audiology (AuD) programs to examine compliance with the CAA standards for accreditation. In our site visits we triangulate the data by looking for three places where there is evidence of compliance. For example, there may be evidence of compliance with curricular requirements in the graduate handbook, the PowerPoint presentation given to students at a mandatory orientation meeting, and in the minutes of a departmental meeting.

Mixed-Methods Designs

These have both quantitative and qualitative components, and are well suited to survey studies. The questionnaire part of the survey is the quantitative part, subject to statistical analyses of both the questions and the responses. Responses to follow-up, open-ended questions are evaluated in the qualitative portion of the survey study. For example, a study on coping with stuttering (Swartz, Irani, & Gabel, 2015) used a mixed-methods approach of a forced-choice questionnaire and open-ended questions to conclude that adults whose stuttering was not severe managed their stuttering with no negative impact.

RETROSPECTIVE RESEARCH

Retrospective studies are designed to examine data already on file before the formulation of the research problem. The availability of the data makes it enticing to think about all the potential studies housed in speech and hearing center cabinets. However, the researcher may have had no control over the quality of the data or the individuals who performed the assessments in the files. There are still many reasons why retrospective studies are reasonable and even desirable forms of research. In low-incidence populations or unusual cases, the retrospective design may be used to determine if there is a pattern of development of the disorder. For example, spousal reports on file that described the first indications of primary progressive aphasia (PPA) across the three PPA variants (nonfluent and logopenic progressive aphasia and semantic dementia) depended on caregivers' recollections of the earliest emerging signs (Pozzebon, Douglas, & Ames, 2018). Retrospective research has strengths and weaknesses.

Strengths

This type of research can offer support for existing hypotheses. For example, the Linguistic Coding Differences Hypothesis predicts that weakness in one native language component will have an adverse effect on learning a foreign language (Sparks, Patton, Ganschow, Humbach, & Javorsky, 2006). In a retrospective and cross-sectional analysis over 10 years, the authors concluded that native language aptitude is the best predictor for foreign language proficiency, but that these predictors change over time. Similarly, the symptomatic, familial, and cognitive overlaps between reading disability and phonological disorders were supported in prospective and retrospective studies (Tunick, 2002). Retrospective studies may also help resolve differences between competing hypotheses. For example, should bilingual children with hearing loss receive therapy for both languages or only for the language of the majority culture? Retrospective analyses of language measures indicated that dual-language support resulted in better expressive language than support in English alone (Bunta, Douglas, Dickson, Cantu, Wickesberg, & Gifford, 2016).

Weaknesses

In retrospective studies, subject classifications and criterion variable measurements may have been performed at a different time and possibly by a different person. The investigator may not know the reliability (consistency) and validity (truthfulness) of these file data. For example, audiograms may have been obtained by a new graduate student who committed procedural errors; in addition, the equipment may have been out of calibration. DaParma, Geffner, and Martin (2011) examined the files of 100 children who had received diagnoses of attention deficit/hyperactivity disorder (ADHD). The authors reviewed five years of files from a university speech and hearing center. The children with ADHD had also received audiological evaluations and subtests of a language assessment. The conclusion that children with ADHD had receptive language impairments to a greater degree than typical children was reasonable, but may have been tainted by test results over which the authors had limited or no control. A retrospective study of 34 postsurgical patients with glottal insufficiency concluded that thyroplasty improved acoustic parameters of voice regardless of whether the tumor was benign or malignant (Ng, Wong, Wei, Wong, & Lam, 2008). While palliative thyroplasty is likely to improve voice production, the uncontrolled variables inherent in this retrospective study limit generalization of the findings. Similarly, chart reviews of the audiograms of 144 adults with sensorineural hearing loss formed the basis of a study (Robertson, Kelly-Campbell, & Wark, 2012) of hearing-aid ownership and use. The data seemed to support the authors' claim that speech-in-noise tests could differentiate patients who would be likely to use hearing aids from those who would not. Commendably, the authors included a section on study limitations where they recognized that, as the study was based on chart review, they could not know how participants were counseled regarding speech-in-noise test results.

Because of the uncontrolled variables that have been identified in retrospective studies, it may be best to conduct retrospective research only when the researcher has had administrative control over data collection and when it would be difficult to collect new data because of financial or other administrative considerations.

SURVEY RESEARCH

Survey research is designed to provide a detailed inspection of the prevalence of conditions, practices, or attitudes in a given environment. The old method of stopping random people on the street and asking them questions has been replaced by surveys that use advanced technology, such as random dialing (the dreaded "robo-calls"), questions on the TV in your hotel room that you must answer before checking out electronically, or a request to please stay on the line to answer a few brief questions for quality assurance. Surveys are different from other ways of answering research questions because they remotely ask people about the questions instead of observing participants directly. Surveys are most frequently used academically as a means of measurement in applied social research. They use questionnaires, interviews, or both. However, researchers, businesses, and governments use questionnaires for collecting information from a wide range of persons, and use interviews for more detailed information from a more restricted sample. Sometimes a broadly distributed questionnaire (such as filing your income tax form) is followed by a smaller-sample follow-up interview (as in an income tax audit). In this example, the Internal Revenue Service (IRS) is using a mixed-methods design where the IRS Form 1040 generates quantitative data, but the auditor may make a qualitative judgment to disallow your deduction for a home office. One current problem is that survey information may be gleaned from people who did not choose to participate, but their data resides in storage that is accessible, often in an unrestricted manner. A U.S. Supreme Court ruling in June 2018 in favor of privacy of phone data may indicate a trend toward consumer privacy protections.

Strengths

Researchers can use surveys to correlate attitudes and beliefs with actual abilities or knowledge. Surveys are often indirect measures that can yield some initial evidence quickly and at relative low cost. Results of surveys can serve as the basis for future, more-detailed direct investigations. Some survey topics in our professions include knowledge of aging and attitudes toward older people by CSD students (Darling, 2016); abilities versus attitudes and beliefs of CSD students regarding information literacy (Swartz, Ratcliffe, & Ivanitskaya, 2015); and knowledge and use of complementary and alternative practices in SLP (Marshall & Basilakos, 2014). Results of these surveys and similar ones can be used to motivate changes in graduate or continuing education in CSD.

Weaknesses

Survey research reflects group data and may not apply to an individual. Assume you are an undergraduate student or advising an undergraduate student about potential graduate programs in communication sciences and disorders (CSD). Based on survey research (see, for example, Pavelko, Malani, Lieberman, & Hans-Vaughn, 2015), the most important consideration was the cost of the graduate program. Other influential factors were accreditation, opportunity to engage in research and conference presentations, and availability of specialty clinics. Factors ranked unimportant in a student's decision about which CSD program to attend included family affiliation (so-called "legacy" schools), religious and cultural diversity, and flexibility for family responsibilities. Graduate students, on the other hand, listed family obligations as the top reason they would not pursue a PhD in CSD (Davidson, Weismer, Alt, & Hogan, 2013). It is likely, or at least possible, that an individual undergraduate applicant would find what were identified as unimportant factors to be more salient than factors deemed influential. For example, Adelphi University has accelerated master's-degree programs in CSD on two campuses where all academic courses are offered on Sundays. These classes are filled with students for whom flexibility for family responsibilities is of major importance.

Not all survey questionnaires are returned, so the ones returned may not be an unbiased representation of the problem. There are also problems in determining the accuracy and honesty of respondents' answers to various questions. Following are some threats we need to consider in evaluating survey research.

Adequate Sample

Was the survey sent to an adequate sample? Some techniques to assure this, addressed in Chapter 6, include random sampling (where every possible sample has a predetermined probability of being chosen), stratified sampling (where the population is divided into smaller groups according to common characteristics), cluster sampling (where the whole population is divided into groups and a group is sampled randomly), and systematic sampling (similar to cluster sampling, but the researcher uses pseudorandom sampling, such as looking at every 10th data point to get 100 data points in a population of 1,000).

Adequate Response Rate

Was the response rate adequate? A response rate of 50% is adequate; 60% is good; 70% is very good. A mortality threat (see Chapter 8) refers to the number of people who failed to respond.

Adequate Survey Construction

Was the survey constructed adequately? An instrumentation threat (see Chapter 8) is related to the adequacy of the survey instrument, questionnaire, or interview. In constructing a survey, make sure the questions are clear and unambiguous; that they are objective and nonthreatening; and that they lead to nonbiased responses.

Appropriate and Consistent Design

Is the research design appropriate to and consistent with the purpose of the study? As an example, consider the following evaluation of a course evaluation form. Table 5–1 is an example of a course evaluation that I received from students in a graduate course in Research Methods.

As a class assignment, we critique the course evaluation form as an example of a survey with shortcomings that limit its usefulness. For example, it seems odd that Question #1 that asks if I know the subject matter is given the same statistical weight as Question #5 that asks if I return tests and assignments quickly. Students complete the survey using a 5-point Likert scale where a score of 3 indicates neutral; 1 and 5 indicate strongly disagree or strongly agree, respectively; and 2 and 4 indicate disagree or agree, respectively. A related tool is the 7-point semantic differential that I have used (Goldfarb, 1987) to evaluate connotative as opposed to denotative meanings of words used by adults with aphasia. The quantitative data derived from either scale is calculated by adding the score for each question and dividing by the number of scorers, yielding a mean score for each question. The sum of all means may then be divided by the total number of questions, but then there is (I think false) equivalence between such questions as whether your instructor knows what he's talking about and his speedy return of tests and assignments.

At the conclusion of the last contract negotiated by the American Association of University Professors on behalf of the faculty, the administration at Adelphi University agreed not to include scores on the course evaluation form in making decisions about retention, promotion, and

Table 5–1. *Example of Survey Research*

Instructor Evaluation	Valid Answers	Strongly Agree (5)	Agree (4)	Neutral (3)	Disagree (2)	Strongly Disagree (1)	Not Applicable	Mean
1. The instructor presents the subject matter in a clear and understandable way	10	40.0%	60.0%	0.0%	0.0%	0.0%	0	4.4
2 The instructor uses class time effectively and efficiently	10	60.0%	30.0%	10.0%	0.0%	0.0%	0	4.5
3 The instructor stimulated my interest in the subject	10	50.0%	50.0%	0.0%	0.0%	0.0%	0	4.5
4 The instructor creates an atmosphere that encourages questions and discussion	10	70.0%	30.0%	0.0%	0.0%	0.0%	0	4.7
5 The instructor returns examinations and assignments in a timely manner	10	90.0%	10.0%	0.0%	0.0%	0.0%	0	4.9
6 The instructor provides useful feedback on coursework	10	70.0%	30.0%	0.0%	0.0%	0.0%	0	4.7
7 The instructor clearly explains what is expected of the students	10	40.0%	50.0%	10.0%	0.0%	0.0%	0	4.3
8 The instructor treats students with respect	10	60.0%	40.0%	0.0%	0.0%	0.0%	0	4.6
9 The instructor is available for help/consultation outside of class	10	60.0%	40.0%	0.0%	0.0%	0.0%	0	4.6

10 Given the choice, or opportunity, I would take another course with this instructor	10	50.0%	50.0%	0.0%	0.0%	0.0%	0	4.5
Course Evaluation	***Valid Answers***	***Strongly Agree (5)***	***Agree (4)***	***Neutral (3)***	***Disagree (2)***	***Strongly Disagree (1)***	***Not Applicable***	***Mean***
11 Exams and/or assignments are well connected to course objectives	10	80.0%	10.0%	10.0%	0.0%	0.0%	0	4.7
12 I find this course intellectually challenging	10	50.0%	30.0%	10.0%	10.0%	0.0%	0	4.2
13 Textbook and other assigned material are relevant to class	10	70.0%	30.0%	0.0%	0.0%	0.0%	0	4.7
14 The technology used (Moodle, websites, or other resources) enhances the class experience	10	70.0%	30.0%	0.0%	0.0%	0.0%	0	4.7
15 I would recommend this course to other students	10	60.0%	40.0%	0.0%	0.0%	0.0%	0	4.6
Student Learning	***Valid Answers***	***Excellent Progress (5)***	***Good Progress (4)***	***Adequate Progress (3)***	***Little Progress (2)***	***No Progress (1)***	***Not Applicable***	***Mean***
16 In gaining knowledge of this subject	10	40.0%	60.0%	0.0%	0.0%	0.0%	0	4.4
17 In improving my writing	10	70.0%	20.0%	10.0%	0.0%	0.0%	0	4.6

continues

Table 5–1. *continued*

Student Learning	Valid Answers	Excellent Progress (5)	Good Progress (4)	Adequate Progress (3)	Little Progress (2)	No Progress (1)	Not Applicable	Mean
18 In improving my critical thinking skills	10	30.0%	60.0%	10.0%	0.0%	0.0%	0	4.2
19 In using information resources to research topics	10	70.0%	20.0%	10.0%	0.0%	0.0%	0	4.6
20 In preparing for a career	10	50.0%	30.0%	20.0%	0.0%	0.0%	0	4.3
21 In increasing my awareness of community and global issues	9	33.3%	55.6%	11.1%	0.0%	0.0%	1	4.2
22 In improving my quantitative reasoning skills	6	33.3%	33.3%	33.3%	0.0%	0.0%	4	4.0
23 In improving my artistic expression and understanding	6	33.3%	0.0%	66.7%	0.0%	0.0%	4	3.7
	Valid Answers	**Less than one (5)**	**1–3 (4)**	**4–6 (3)**	**7–9 (2)**	**10 or more (1)**		**Mean**
24 On average, how many hours per week do you study/prepare for this class?	10	0.0%	10.0%	40.0%	30.0%	20.0%		2.4

Note. Respondent to enrolled completion rate: 38%.

tenure. One striking limitation in the survey is identified as respondent to enrolled completion rate, showing that only 38% of eligible students (a poor response rate) completed the course evaluation. There are ways to improve compliance with completion of surveys. Some institutions (e.g., Yale University) will not allow students to have access to their course grades unless they have completed the course evaluation.

LONGITUDINAL STUDIES (DEVELOPMENTAL RESEARCH)

Longitudinal studies may be experimental or nonexperimental research. In these studies, researchers collect repeated measures of the same variables from the same participants at two or more points in time. These studies are designed to follow participants as they mature or age and to observe changes over time. There are multiple waves of data collection. They refer to studies with repeated observations or measures from the same participants on the same outcome variables over time. Researchers hope to describe changes within and among individuals over time with the goal of explaining the changes in terms of certain other variables. Developmental milestones and typical speech sound acquisition in children are two examples of longitudinal research that speech-language pathologists (SLPs) and audiologists (As) use routinely.

In some considerations, an investigator who uses the longitudinal design is interested in comparing antecedent and consequent relationships through extended tracking of phenomena in context, rather than employing experimental controls or comparisons. However, this design may not be appropriate when the goal of the experiment is to examine the effects of a particular intervention on individual change over time.

Strengths

They show directly how participants mature or develop certain characteristics or behaviors in real time (while participants are actually aging). They provide a better basis for making claims about causality than cross-sectional research because longitudinal data can provide information about the temporal order of the designated cause and effect variables. A major advantage is that the researcher can investigate and explain change over time. As opposed to cross-sectional research, longitudinal studies permit examination of *intra*individual change (whether and how individuals change over time) and *inter*individual change (if individuals change in the same or different ways), as well as the causes and predictors of these changes.

Some fields of research depend on longitudinal study. Second language learning takes a long time, so we need to study it for a long time to understand it. This longitudinal approach permits examination of the following questions regarding second language learning (Ortega & Iberri-Shea, 2005):

- How long does it take second-language learners to gain proficiency in second language (L2)?
- How and when do L2 abilities develop over time?
- What is the pace and pattern of L2 development over time?

- What are the effects of L2 instruction on the nature and durability of L2 learning?

Barkaoui (2014) summarized quantitative analytic methods used in second language research. The L2 studies often used repeated measure designs that are also used for research that is not longitudinal (see Chapter 6 for an example of repeated measures analysis using SPSS). Some of the traditional analyses include the paired *t*-test, repeated measures for univariate and multivariate analysis of variance (ANOVA, MANOVA), analysis of covariance (ANCOVA), and regression analysis. Decisions for research design included the variables and measures that were examined; the participants who were selected; the definition and measurement of time; and the timing, number, and spacing of measurement intervals (Barkaoui, 2014, p. 68).

Weaknesses

They are expensive, time-consuming, and suffer from subject attrition. There are four conditions that make a study longitudinal (Ortega & Iberri-Shea, 2005): the length of the study; data collection at multiple points in time; capturing change as a conceptual focus of the design; and prolonged tracking of the phenomenon in context, rather than through experimental controls or comparisons. Longitudinal research literature in CSD supports only the second and third conditions. The first condition lacks a specific definition, and the last condition does not allow examination of the effects of intervention.

TRANSLATIONAL RESEARCH

Translational research (TR) does not refer to foreign languages. As the concept began in medical fields, the motivation was a faster translation of new laboratory findings to improved standards of care. In our professions, translational SLP/A expands on the "bench-to-bedside" and "bedside-to-community" models to include discovery as a two-way street; that is, both evidence-based practice (EBP) and practice-based evidence (PBE), so that clinical findings can inform scientific exploration. TR also includes the science of dissemination to hasten findings to and from laboratory to practice and practice to community and public health policy.

The following was sent to prospective contributors to a book I edited (Goldfarb, 2012):

> *Translational SLP/A* will include investigations in the broad fields of laboratory, clinical, and public health research. Interdisciplinary and cross-disciplinary papers are encouraged. Aiming to expedite the translation of scientific discovery into new or improved standards of care, the book is intended to promote a wide-ranging exchange among basic, preclinical, clinical, epidemiologic, and health outcomes topics. Also encouraged will be essays describing public health research with potential for application to the clinic, disease prevention, or health care policy. Our professions are somewhat behind the curve, compared to medicine, in not addressing this issue directly, although there certainly have been efforts in this direction by individuals.

Kent (2012) distilled the essence of translational research (TR) into the phrase *discovery to delivery*. The discovery part is the knowledge gained from the basic sciences, and the delivery part is the application of the knowledge to clinical practice and community settings. The types of translation are sometimes called *T-phases*. TR has also been described as "bench-to-bedside" (T1) and "bedside-to-community" (T2) research. However, this description may be oversimplified. Kent (2012) advises us to expand our notion of TR to include bidirectional, even multidirectional influences, such as bench to bedside and back again. We can also think of TR as outcomes research or clinical research.

There are different models of TR, some more appropriate to drug research than to the bio-behavioral studies required for CSD. In one three-part model, T1 speeds the movement between basic scientific research and patient-oriented standards of care; T2 expedites the movement between patient-oriented and population-based research; and T3 promotes interaction between laboratory-based and population-based research. In a four-phase model (Papir-Bernstein, 2012), T1 applies the scientific discovery to a health field; T2 uses the health application to develop evidence-based guidelines (evidence-based practice, or EBP); T3 uses dissemination research to move the guidelines into clinical practice; and in T4, the most problematical phase, the health practice moves into the public sector. According to Mendel, Meredith, Schoenbaum, Sherbourne, and Wells (2008), behavioral change should be the result of *dissemination*, or the spread of knowledge and information. Adoption of strategies for implementation in treatment centers or communities is the result of *implementation*, and the study of factors that result in adoption is called *diffusion*. CSD research focuses mainly on T1 and T2, with dissemination of research (Rosenbek, 2012; see Part III of this book) representing a major challenge. EBP can also become bidirectional as PBE (Papir-Bernstein, 2012), where assessment and intervention techniques that make sense motivate research in these areas.

An example of translational research in CSD shows how the study of brain damage in the zebra finch can inform our therapy for aphasia in adults (LaPointe, Johnson, McNeil, & Pratt, 2012). The authors ask if acquiring birdsong is similar to learning human speech and language. They also ask if destabilized birdsong through brain injury can teach us anything about speech and language recovery in humans after a stroke. Birdsong is not human speech and language and knowing that the bird brain makes new neurons (and recovers its song) after being damaged represents promising but limited information about human brain plasticity.

TR may require skills beyond those needed for basic and applied research in CSD. While educational programs have yet to identify a definitive skill set needed for TR, or develop a curriculum geared to TR, it seems that interdisciplinary study and interprofessional practice will be required.

ADVANCED STUDY

The author proposes that skills in types of research are necessary for an individual to be granted power of professor. With new generations of scholars and researchers needed every 10 years, professors and master clinicians have an obligation to prepare individuals with adequate knowledge and skills to undertake the tasks of scholarship and research, and types of research is a key component. For evidence of the requisite skills in understanding types of research, complete the following and have your instructor, academic adviser, mentor, or CSD department chair review that you have completed the requirements and sign and date where indicated.

Student's Name: ______________________________

1. Explain three similarities and/or differences between single-subject and case studies.
2. Explain four ways that proof-of-concept or pilot studies are used.
3. Give one example each of quantitative, qualitative, and mixed-methods designs.
4. Give one example each of experimental, quasiexperimental, and nonexperimental designs.
5. Cite one strength and one limitation of retrospective research.
6. Cite one strength and one limitation of survey research.
7. Cite one strength and one limitation of longitudinal research.
8. Using any translational research model, explain how to speed the movement between basic scientific research and patient-oriented standards of care

Date of Completion: ______________________________

Faculty/Supervisor Signature: ______________________________

REFERENCES

Barkaoui, K. (2014). Quantitative approaches for analyzing longitudinal data in second language research. *Annual Review of Applied Linguistics, 34,* 65–101.

Brock, K., Koul, R., Corwin, M., & Schlosser, R. (2017). A comparison of visual scene and grid displays for people with chronic aphasia: A pilot study to improve communication using AAC. *Aphasiology, 31,* 1282–1306.

Bunta, F., Douglas, M., Dickson, H., Cantu, A., Wickesberg, J., & Gifford, R. H. (2016). Dual language versus English-only support for bilingual children with hearing loss who use cochlear implants and hearing aids. *International Journal of Language & Communication Disorders, 51,* 460–472.

Byiers, B. J., Reichle, J., & Symons, F. J. (2012). Single-subject experimental design for evidence-based practice. *American Journal of Speech-Language Pathology, 21,* 397–414.

Carlsson, E., Miniscalco, C., Gillberg, C., & Johnels, J. A. (2018). Assessing false-belief understanding in children with autism using a computer application: A pilot study. *Journal of Psycholinguistic Research, 47(5),* 1085–1099.

Damasio, H. (2008). Neural basis of language disorders. In R. Chapey (Ed.), *Language intervention strategies in aphasia and related neurogenic communication disorders* (5th ed., pp. 20–41). Baltimore, MD: Lippincott Williams & Wilkins.

DaParma, A., Gefner, D., & Martin, N. (2011). Prevalence and nature of language impairment in children with attention deficit/hyperactivity disorder. *Contemporary Issues in Communication Science and Disorders, 38,* 119–125.

Darling, R. M. (2016). Knowledge of aging and attitudes toward older people by communication sciences and disorders students. *Contemporary Issues in Communication Science and Disorders, 43,* 50–63.

Davidson, M. M., Weismer, S. E., Alt, M., & Hogan, T. P. (2013). Survey on perspectives of pursuing a PhD in communication sciences and disorders. *Contemporary Issues in Communication Science and Disorders, 40,* 98–115.

Donovan, N. J., Boudreaux, D. M., & Savage, M. C. (2015). Objective measurement of vocal parameters in older people with and without Parkinson's disease in their natural environments: A pilot study. *Contemporary Issues in Communication Science and Disorders, 42,* 100–109.

Fukkink, R. (1996). The internal validity of aphasiological single-subject studies. *Aphasiology, 10,* 741–754.

Goldfarb, R. (1987). The Pollyanna hypothesis in adult aphasia. *Aphasiology, 1,* 361–367.

Goldfarb, R. (Ed.). (2012). *Translational speech-language pathology and audiology.* San Diego, CA: Plural Publishing.

Goldfarb, R. (2016). An aphasiologist has a stroke. *Aphasiology, 30,* 1151–1162.

Halpern, H., & Goldfarb, R. (2013). *Language and motor speech disorders in adults* (3rd ed.). Burlington, MA: Jones & Bartlett Learning.

Humes, L. E., Rogers, S. E., Quigley, T. M., Main, A. K., Kinney, D. L., & Herring, C. (2017). The effects of service-delivery model and purchase price on hearing-aid outcomes in older adults: A randomized double-blind placebo-controlled clinical trial. *American Journal of Audiology, 26,* 53–79.

Ingham, R. J., Martin, R. R., & Kuhl, P. (1974). Modification and control of rate of speaking by stutterers. *Journal of Speech and Hearing Research, 17,* 189–196.

Kalinowski, J., Armson, J., & Stuart, A. (1995). Effect of normal and fast articulatory rates on stuttering frequency. *Journal of Fluency Disorders, 20,* 293–302.

Kent, R. D. (2012). Models and concepts of translational research. In R. Goldfarb (Ed.), *Translational speech-language pathology and audiology* (pp. 27–36). San Diego, CA: Plural Publishing.

LaPointe, L. L., Johnson, F., McNeil, M. R., & Pratt, S. (2012). Birdsong and human speech and language: What the zebra finch uses, loses, and regains. In R. Goldfarb (Ed.), *Translational speech-language pathology and audiology* (pp. 283–300). San Diego, CA: Plural Publishing.

Marshall, R. S., & Basilakos, A. (2014). Hot or not?: A survey regarding knowledge and use of complementary and alternative practices in speech-language pathology. *Contemporary Issues in Communication Science and Disorders, 41,* 235–251.

Mazerolle, E. L., & Marchand, Y. (2015). TypingSuite: Integrated software for presenting stimuli, and collecting and analyzing typing data. *Journal of Psycholinguistic Research, 44,* 127–139.

McGee, T. M., Kartush, J. M., Heide, J. C., Bojrab, D. I., Clemis, J. D., & Kulick, K. C. (1991). Electromagnetic semi-implantable hearing device: phase I. Clinical trials. *Laryngoscope, 101,* 355–360.

Mendel, P., Meredith, L. S., Schoenbaum, M., Sherbourne, C. D., & Wells, K. B. (2008). Interventions in organizational and community context: A framework for building evidence on dissemination and implementation in health services research. *Administrative Policy on Mental Health, 35,* 21–37.

Ng, M. L., Wong, R. K., Wei, W. I., Wong, Y. H., & Lam, P. K. Y. (2008). Acoustic changes in Chinese patients with cancer-related unilateral vocal fold paralysis after medialization thyroplasty. *Contemporary Issues in Communication Science and Disorders, 35,* 17–24.

Nordgren, P. M. (2016). F0, F0 range and duration of utterances: Longitudinal single-subject studies of prosody in two Swedish children with ASC. *Clinical Linguistics & Phonetics, 30,* 29–48.

Ortega, L., & Iberri-Shea, G. (2005). Longitudinal research in second language acquisition: Recent trends and future directions. *Annual Review of Applied Linguistics, 25,* 26–45.

Papir-Bernstein, W. (2012). The artistry of practice-based evidence (PBE): One practitioner's path —Part I. In R. Goldfarb (Ed.), *Translational speech-language pathology and audiology* (pp. 51–58). San Diego, CA: Plural Publishing.

Parrilla, C., Minni, A., & Bogaardt, K. (2015). Pulmonary rehabilitation after total laryngectomy. *Annals of Otology, Rhinology & Laryngology, 124*(9), 706–713.

Pavelko, S. L., Malani, M. D., Lieberman, R. J., & Hans-Vaughn, D. L. (2015). Factors influencing undergraduates' choices in graduate school programs in communication sciences and disorders. *Contemporary Issues in Communication Science and Disorders, 42,* 155–172.

Perkins, C. J., Korgaonkar, M. S., Fiore, S. M., Squires N., Goldfarb R., McCloskey K. M., & Wagshul, M. E. (2007, May). *Functional evaluation of aphasia recovery in stroke patients using fMRI and ERP.* Paper presented at the American Academy of Neurology, Boston, MA; also presented to the American Speech-Language-Hearing Association, Boston, MA (2007, November).

Plant, G., Gnosspileus, J., & Levitt, H. (2000). The use of tactile supplements in lipreading Swedish and English: A single-subject study. *Journal of Speech, Language, and Hearing Research, 43,* 172–183.

Pozzebon, M., Douglas, J., & Ames, D. (2018). Spousal recollections of early signs of primary progressive aphasia. *International Journal of Language & Communication Disorders, 53,* 282–293.

Robertson, M. A., Kelly-Campbell, R. J., & Wark, D. J. (2012). Use of audiometric variables to differentiate groups of adults based on hearing aid ownership and use. *Contemporary Issues in Communication Science and Disorders, 39,* 114–120.

Rosenbek, J. C. (2012). The science of dissemination. In R. Goldfarb (Ed.), *Translational speech-language pathology and audiology* (pp. 37–42). San Diego, CA: Plural Publishing.

Shoaf, K. O., Iyer, S. N., & Bothe, A. K. (2009). Using a single-subject experimental design to implement a nonlinear phonology approach to target selection. *Contemporary Issues in Communication Science and Disorders, 36,* 77–88.

Sparks, R. L., Patton, J., Ganschow, L., Humbach, N., & Javorsky, J. (2008). Early first-language reading and spelling skills predict later second-language reading and spelling skills. *Journal of Educational Psychology, 100*(1), 162–174.

Swartz, B., Ratcliffe, A., & Ivanitskaya, L. (2015). Correlation of attitudes and beliefs with actual abilities of speech-language pathology students regarding aspects of information literacy. *Contemporary Issues in Communication Science and Disorders, 42,* 215–225.

Swartz, E., Irani, F., & Gabel, R. (2015). Coping with stuttering. *SIG4 Perspectives, 24,* 58–68.

Thompson, C. K. (2006). Single subject controlled experiments in aphasia: The science and the state of the science. *Journal of Communication Disorders, 39,* 266–291.

Tunick, R. (2002). The etiological relationship between reading disability and phonological disorder. *Annals of Dyslexia, 52,* 75–97.

Van Horne, A. J. O., Fey, M., & Curran, M. (2017). Do the hard things first: A randomized controlled trial testing the effects of exemplar selection on generalization following therapy for grammatical morphology. *Journal of Speech, Language, and Hearing Research, 60,* 2569–2588.

Vance, M., & Clegg, J. (2012). Editorial: Use of single case study research in child speech, language and communication impairments. *Child Language Teaching & Therapy, 28*, 255–258.

Wills, C. L., Capilouto, G. J., & Wright, H. H. (2012). Attention and off-topic speech in the recounts of middle-age and elderly adults: A pilot investigation. *Contemporary Issues in Communication Science and Disorders, 39*, 105–113.

6

Really Basic Statistics

INTRODUCTION

Why do you skip the Results section when you read a journal article? Why do practicing clinicians shy away from conducting clinical research? One of the main reasons must be the certainty of encountering statistics as a consumer or producer of research. It may also be that you do not think your math skills are sharp enough to understand statistics. Individuals who would never countenance being called illiterate all too cheerfully (and inaccurately) claim to be innumerate. However, the majority of statistical treatments used in communication sciences and disorders (CSD) involve nothing more complex than elementary algebra, a subject most of us learned in 9th grade.

Statistics may be viewed (McElreath, 2015) neither as mathematics nor as a science; it is more akin to a branch of engineering. Introductory statistics courses are likely to be confusing to students because of the diversity of applications. Instead of learning a single method for building, refining, and critiquing statistical models, you are required to learn a variety of tests where each has a particular purpose. In other words, rather than learning how to design a zoo, you are taught about how each animal in it must be treated.

Some statistical problems are worked out in this chapter to bolster the reader's confidence in having the required skills for calculation. The larger questions are what statistics, in its singular form, is for, and how we determine what statistical treatment to use for a given research problem. The purpose of this chapter is to begin to answer these larger questions.

A basic chord progression will enable you to accompany yourself on guitar while singing folk and rock songs. The four chords of C major, A minor, F major, and G7 are all you need to play along with thousands of songs. Learning to transpose to different keys, to play more sophisticated chords, and to shred may come later. In this chapter, you will learn the statistical equivalent of a C progression.

We begin with measures of central tendency (how things come together) and dispersion (how things separate) that are probably a review of old lessons. Learning about sums of squares represents the basic "fingering" for the statistical chords that follow. The four statistical "chords" that appear in this chapter are the parametric measures for comparison of mean differences in calculations of t and F, the correlation coefficient r, and, the last chord, the nonparametric calculation of χ^2.

In the last part of this chapter, you will have a recipe for entering data for a repeated measures design using the general linear model of the Statistical Package for the Social Sciences (SPSS) (George & Mallery, 2007).

Learning Objectives

After reading this chapter, the student will be able to

- reject innumeracy and feel confident about basic math skills;
- interpret the Results section of a journal article; and
- select appropriate measures of statistical analysis to answer some clinical or academic research questions.

SOME STATISTICAL CONCEPTS

Many terms and concepts are defined and described in an alphabetical list at the end of this chapter. Some concepts will benefit from more description and appear below.

Statistics

As indicated in the definition at the end of this chapter, *statistics* in its singular form is a branch of applied mathematics that refers to the practice of collecting, presenting, analyzing, and using numerical data to make inferences about behavioral, social, and physical sciences. Statistics may be descriptive in summarizing and describing a body of data, and inferential in reaching generalizations about entire populations by examining a sample or a portion of the whole population. As noted in the following text, samples must represent populations and data must be obtained in specific ways. The probability that there might be an error in the sampling process must also be specified.

Parametric and Nonparametric Statistics

A parameter is a characteristic of a population. We use parametric statistics to estimate the probability that our findings in a small world (for example, a sample of children who have conductive hearing loss) can generalize to a larger world or population (all children who have conductive hearing loss). In most parametric CSD research that assesses efficacy (effectiveness and efficiency) of a clinical treatment, two or more groups are compared. The two groups may be people with a disorder (an experimental group) and people without a disorder (a control group, matched in many demographic and physical characteristics to the experimental group). The control group as a whole may be matched to the experimental group as a whole (overall matching), or individuals in each group may be matched (paired or pairwise matching). Ideal matching in both groups would include the same individual characteristics (e.g., age, gender, handedness, language spoken, socioeconomic status, educational level, race), with the only difference being presence or absence of a communication disorder. The two groups may also be only people with a disorder, with the goal of comparing efficacy of a standard treatment or diagnostic procedure (e.g., videofluoroscopy for evidence of dysphagia) to that of an alternative treatment or diagnostic procedure (e.g., bedside evaluation for evidence of dysphagia).

Some of the most frequent questions we ask about data are answered by parameters. What is the average difference between treatment groups (or treatment–no treatment groups)? How strong is the association between the treatment and the outcome? How much variation is there between or among groups?

Nonparametric statistics deal with data, not populations. We are not concerned with parameters if our statistical analyses do not make assumptions about population distributions. Nonparametric statistics are used to determine significance of characteristics of sampled data. A *sample* is a portion of the population or data set that we choose to analyze, and *significance* refers to the probability of making a Type I error (rejecting the null hypothesis when it is true). This type of analysis is useful for determining demographic trends, such as incidence of multiple sclerosis or conductive hearing loss in a particular geographic area. The findings will not determine individuals who are at risk for the disorder, nor will they reveal why a particular region is associated with a communication problem.

Some studies have few participants but a large amount of data, such as in speech science research, where hooked-wire electrode placement in various muscles of the speech effector system yields information about muscle function in people with typical or disordered communication. In these cases, the data are treated as the participants in the experiment, and parametric statistical analysis is appropriate. In the example noted previously, the population may be the intrinsic muscles of the larynx.

Random Sampling and Random Assignment

The clinician–researcher who is interested in finding some piece of truth about a clinical population cannot possibly test a hypothesis on every individual with the communication disorder of interest. Even if there were unlimited resources, it would be impossible to identify and test, say, every preschool child with specific language impairment. We use statistical analyses and the method of random sampling in an unrestricted manner to address the limitation of not being able to test, for example, a preschool child in Ulan Ude, Siberia, who has a specific language impairment. Ideally, random sampling will give everyone in the target population an equal probability of being included in the study. We can apply random sampling not only to populations but also to values of the independent variable, order of presentation of stimulus variables, and time of measurement, to mention a few. Note that colloquial use of *random* (e.g., "Some random kid in my class") is quite different from the scientific method criteria used for randomization. We can also randomize *assignments* to comparison groups. When extraneous demographic and physical factors (e.g., socioeconomic status, primary language, gender, intelligence) are equivalent in experimental and control groups, there will not be systematic bias in favor of one group over the other and they will be considered equivalent when the experiment starts. We can then use random assignment to experimental and control groups without worrying, for example, that one group might perform better than the other because of age differences.

Other Sampling Procedures

Other Random Sampling Procedures. *Systematic sampling* is useful where the researcher has access to a membership. For example, your professional state association, American Speech-Language-Hearing Association (ASHA), or American Academy of Audiology (AAA) may be interested in the number of continuing education hours that members earn outside of convention attendance. To reduce bias, the researcher starts with a name on the membership list (not the first) and then selects every tenth name that appears afterward.

In *stratified sampling*, the experimenter divides the population into subgroups (strata). About three-fourths of the members of ASHA are currently employed full time, and systematic sampling may inadvertently survey too many part-time professionals (only about 1% of ASHA members are seeking employment). Stratified sampling would take two groups (one full time, one part time) and then randomly select three full-time employees for every part-time employee. If the two groups are large, then systematic sampling can be combined with stratified sampling, where, for example, every tenth name on the lists for both types of employees would be selected. The 3:1 ratio of full-time to part-time employment status would still be maintained when the researcher combines systematic and stratified sampling.

Another way a researcher can expedite data collection is through *cluster sampling*, where smaller samples are chosen from larger units called clusters. For example, if ASHA wants to learn the percentage of members that attend state association conventions, it does not have to undertake the expense of analyzing data from all 50 states. Because ASHA is interested in percentage of members and not raw numbers, the size of the state doesn't matter and the sample can be regional rather than statewide (e.g., southeast, central, northwest). Investigators can also use cluster sampling in combination with the other sampling strategies described above.

Nonrandom Sampling Procedures Have Limited Scientific Application, But They May Also Be Used in Research. *Matched samples* allow the investigator to restrict differences in comparison groups by pairing them according to predetermined characteristics (e.g., time post-onset of aphasia or severity rating). Because assignment to groups (such as standard therapy versus experimental therapy) is not random, a matched-sample study is a quasi-experimental design.

In *consecutive sampling*, there are predetermined criteria for inclusion in the study, and then the investigator selects all who agree to participate. For example, we examined noun-verb ambiguity in the language of adults with chronic undifferentiated schizophrenia (Goldfarb & Bekker, 2009). The consulting psychiatrist referred to us all outpatients that he diagnosed as having the disorder, and we tested everyone who agreed to participate in our study.

Purposive sampling was done in the early years of identification of three variants of primary progressive aphasia (PPA;

Gorno-Tempini et al., 2011). This type of sampling is useful in studying phenomena that occurs infrequently. The authors convened on three occasions to operationalize earlier published clinical descriptions for PPA subtypes.

Type I and Type II Errors

It is very difficult to know if a sample is actually random. For example, your hypothesis is that undergraduate students at your university are taller than graduate students, and you schedule height measurements in front of a randomly selected building on campus on a randomly selected date and time. Through no fault of your own, the undergraduate basketball team shows up, confirming your hypothesis. You would be in danger of making a *Type I error*, where you reject the null hypothesis of no height difference between the two groups when it should have been the accepted alternative. In a *Type II error*, you accept the null hypothesis when it should have been the rejected alternative. As an example of the latter, we wrote that there was no evidence for a diagnosis of schizophasia separate from a diagnosis of schizophrenia and aphasia (Goldfarb, Eisenson, Stocker, & DeSanti, 1994), but had to acknowledge the possibility that we might be making a Type II error. As an example of the null hypothesis, consider the following *modus tollens* (Latin for mode that denies by denying): Early Europeans formulated the hypothesis that all swans were white (the null hypothesis of no color differences between swans), because they had seen only swans with white feathers. Once they reached Australia, they encountered swans with black feathers. No number of white swan observations could prove the hypothesis, but one observation of black swans could falsify it.

Degrees of Freedom

Every time you make a choice, you lose some freedom. For example, if you select an entrée at a restaurant, you will likely be too full to try the other choices. If you have committed to a life partner, then you have ruled out perhaps a billion other potential mates. The game of Sudoku is an exercise in logic based on degrees of freedom. By filling in one or more of the nine boxes in each grid, you limit the number of options, as numbers may not be repeated.

In statistics, degree of freedom refers to the number of scores or data points that are free to vary. For example, when you know the total of five scores, then only four of them will be free to vary, because the fifth will be obliged by the known total. If you know that the five scores add up to 100, assume that you have obtained four scores of 25, 15, 20, and 30. Because the total of the four scores is 90, and you know that the total of the five scores is 100, then the fifth score *must* be 10. The statistical representation for this example would be $df = n - 1 = 4$. Critical value tables for the statistical treatments discussed in this chapter (t, ANOVA, r, and χ^2) show that $df = n - 1$ for each group, with some adjustments indicated below. CSD studies that include statistical analyses tend to use a much larger n so that $n - 1$ will not have as much of an effect on significance. Critical value tables, or the computer programs that calculate them, show that the number required for statistical significance is quite different between $n = 4$ and $n = 5$, but not so different between 34 and 35. A larger representation of the *data sample* (for nonparametric statistical analyses) or a larger representation of the *population* (for parametric analyses) means that there are more data points to analyze statistically and a lower likelihood that there will be a sampling error. A larger representation of the sample or population has greater statistical power, up to the point where the difference between the *n* in your sample and infinity samples is statistically trivial.

Lies, Damned Lies, and Statistics (Mark Twain): The *p* Value

The *p* value is a common index that indirectly equates to the strength of evidence. The conventional minimal level of significance $p < 0.05$ indicates that there is less than a 1 in 20 (or 5%) chance that the findings resulted from a sampling error or some other systematic error. However, the *p* value has been shown to be neither as reliable nor as objective as most scientists assume (Nuzzo, 2014). A *p* value measures whether an observed result can be attributed to chance. The researcher's real question regarding the odds that a hypothesis is correct is not answered. Those odds depend on how strong the result was and, most importantly, on how plausible the hypothesis is in the first place (Nuzzo, 2014, p. 151).

The dependence on the *p* value for statistical significance has also been identified as a major reason why most research findings have not been replicated and, indeed, why some claimed research findings may be false (Ioannidis, 2005). The probability that a research finding is true depends on three conditions: the prior probability that it was true (that is, that the finding was true before the study began); the study had adequate statistical power to decrease the likelihood of a sampling error; and the level of statistical significance is sufficiently rigorous (Ioannidis, 2005, p. 696). Recall that for CSD research where we compare an experimental group to a control group, a sample from about 30 participants is usually enough to make the difference between the number of participants tested and infinity participants statistically trivial. For most CSD research, $p < .05$ is used as an acceptably rigorous level for statistical significance. However, for some CSD research, such as identifying safe foods to swallow in the presence of dysphagia, a more rigorous level of statistical significance (perhaps $p < .001$) may be required, because an unsafe food described as "safe" to swallow may have catastrophic consequences for an individual with a swallowing disorder.

The *p* level for statistical significance should always be an ad hoc (meaning for this specific purpose) decision; that is, the level of statistical significance should be determined before the study begins, and the rejection or acceptance of the null hypothesis should be based on this predetermined value. If $p < .05$ has been determined as the significance measure, then the results need only indicate either $p < .05$ or $p > .05$. However, computers now generate exact levels of *p*, and these levels (e.g., $p = .0013$) are reported in the results of many journal articles. I think this current form of reporting dilutes the importance of ad hoc determination of the rigor needed to reject the null hypothesis.

Mark Twain used the phrase at the heading of this section to describe how numbers can be persuasive but wrong, especially when statistics bolster weak arguments. An investigation (Bennett, Miller, & Wolford, 2009) was designed to illustrate Twain's pants-on-fire view of some statistically supported studies. The participant in an fMRI experiment was asked to identify the emotion that an individual in a series of photographs was experiencing. The procedure used the blood oxygen level dependent (BOLD) technique of measuring specific brain regions for signal changes during the photo condition compared to a rest condition. The BOLD technique is considered the gold standard for fMRI neuroimaging. Statistical analysis used a form of a *t*-test (see description of *t*-tests later in the chapter), resulting in statistical significance where $p < 0.001$, indicating that the chances were less than one in one thousand that the findings were the result of a sampling error. What makes the experiment notable is that the participant undergoing fMRI measures was *a frozen salmon*. The point that Bennett et al. (2009) wanted to make was not that a dead fish can make these kinds of cognitive judgments, but that random noise may yield spurious results in fMRI testing, unless adaptive measures are taken to control them. In fact, fMRI testing routinely uses adaptive measures to eliminate the kind of statistical "noise" described above, and fMRI is an exceptionally accurate and useful research tool.

DESCRIPTIVE STATISTICS: MEASURES OF CENTRAL TENDENCY AND DISPERSION

We use descriptive statistics in a study to describe the basic features of the data. These statistics are used to summarize information about the sample and the measures. Dividing data into groups or classes and showing the number of observations in each class yields a frequency distribution. Then, dividing the number of the observations in each class by the total number of observations will yield a fraction. This is a *relative* frequency distribution. The sum of the relative frequencies always equals 1. The sum of all observations is the *cumulative* frequency distribution. Frequency distributions are usually displayed in the form of a bar graph called a histogram or a line graph called a frequency polygon; a symmetrical frequency distribution is called the bell-shaped curve (see Figures 6–2, 6–3, and 6–4 in the section on presenting the data later in this chapter).

Central Tendency

This shows the location of a distribution. The mean, median, and mode are the most important measures of central tendency. The arithmetic *mean*, or average, may be calculated for populations (in parametric statistics) and for samples (in nonparametric statistics). The population mean is sometimes represented by the Greek letter mu (μ), and the sample mean is sometimes represented by $\bar{x}$. For clarity, and in accordance with current research practices in CSD, the means in all the examples in this chapter will be represented by M. Similarly, while N is sometimes used to refer to the number of observations in a population and n is used to refer to the number of observations in a sample, all the examples in this chapter will use n to represent the number of observations in a population or a sample. Accordingly, the formula for calculating mean (population or sample) in a frequency distribution is

$$M = \frac{\Sigma X}{n}$$

where ΣX refers to the sum of all observations and n refers to the number of observations in the population or sample.

The *median* is the midpoint or midscore when ungrouped data are arranged either in ascending or descending order in terms of values. In other words, half the scores are above and half are below the median. The median is preferred to the mean in some instances; for example, for purchasers of a home when real estate values can fluctuate wildly in a given neighborhood. Calculating what you can expect to pay for a typical three-bedroom home will not be represented fairly by the mean, where the outliers skew the price upward. In CSD research, an example would be mean number of words per minute (WPM) spoken by children on the autism spectrum. If the population includes too many very low-functioning children who may be mute, the mean WPM will skew low; if the sample includes too many of those who are high functioning, including children with logorrhea, the mean WPM will skew high. Therefore, the median would be more representative.

The *mode* is the most frequent score or value in a data set. It is not used much in CSD research.

The *mean* is used most often as a measure of central tendency and is also used in the statistical formulas that follow. As noted previously, however, the mean is affected by outliers or extreme scores in the data set, but the median and mode are not.

Dispersion

This refers to the spread or variability in the data. The simplest form of dispersion is the *range*, or the lowest score subtracted from the highest score. For example, in the series of scores 4, 9, 3, 7, 8, 8, 6, the range is 6 because the highest score is 9 and the lowest score is 3 (9 − 3 = 6). The measures of dispersion discussed in the present chapter are the *variance* and the *standard deviation*. CSD students are likely to be familiar with standard deviation measures because they are used in diagnostic tests. Calculation of these measures is based on obtaining sums of squares.

ALL YOU NEED ARE SUMS OF SQUARES

In statistics, researchers use the sum of squares to evaluate the overall variance of a data set from its mean. A large sum of squares indicates a large variance. In other words, individual readings fluctuate widely from the mean. A random sample of words per minute taken from all 6-year-old children diagnosed with autism spectrum disorders (ASD) is likely to yield a large variance because of the wide range of severity of communication impairment in children diagnosed with ASD. Even more useful is the square root of the number representing the variance (or sums of squares); it is the standard deviation. Calculation of the total (sum) of the squared deviances from the mean (sums of squares) represents the difficulty level of the math needed for the measures of dispersion and central tendency that follow.

Calculation of Variance and Standard Deviation

Box 6–1 shows calculation of variance and standard deviation in an example of a clinical experiment. The standard deviation shows how spread out the numbers are from the mean. It is the square root of the variance. As shown in in the alphabetical list of terms at the end of this chapter,

Box 6–1. Calculating Variance and Standard Deviation

SLI				TYPICAL			
n	X	$\lvert X-M \rvert$	$(X-M)^2$	n	X	$\lvert X-M \rvert$	$(X-M)^2$
1	100	15	225	1	100	15	225
2	90	5	25	2	100	15	225
3	85	0	0	3	90	5	25
4	85	0	0	4	90	5	25
5	80	5	25	5	65	20	400
6	70	15	225	6	65	20	400
			500				1300

$$M = \frac{\Sigma X}{n}$$

For SLI group, $M = 510/6 = 85$

Median = 85

Mode = 85

Range = 100 − 70 = 30

For typical group, $M = 510/6 = 85$

Median = 90

There is no mode score

Range = 100 − 65 = 35

$$\text{Variance} = \sigma^2 = \frac{\Sigma(X-M)^2}{n}$$

For SLI group,

$\sigma^2 = 500/6 = 83.3$, $SD = 9.13$

For typical group,

$\sigma^2 = 1300/6 = 216.67$, $SD = 14.72$

variance is defined as the mean of the squared deviation scores about the mean of a distribution, and *standard deviation* is defined as the square root of the mean of the squared deviation scores about the mean of a distribution. This is the first example of, "all you need are sums of squares."

In this experiment, six children with specific language impairment (SLI) and 6 typically developing children have responded to a task where the maximum score is 100. The children are identified only as a number (n), in this case one through six. The next column, X, refers to the score that each child earned on the task. Adding the scores and dividing by the number of children in the group yields the mean (M), represented by the formula:

$$M = \frac{\Sigma X}{n}$$

Note that the means of 85 are the same for both SLI and Typical groups, but the median, mode, and range scores are different for the two groups. The column indicated as $|X - M|$ shows the absolute value of the mean subtracted from the participant's score. We use absolute value because we will square this number, so we don't care about assigning a + or – to the number. If you use + and – symbols in the $X - M$ column, the sum of these scores will always equal zero. The next column, $(X - M)^2$, shows this number squared, and when we add all of these numbers and divide by 6 (n, or the number of children in the group), we have calculated the variance (the sums of squares divided by the number of subjects). The uppercase Greek letter sigma Σ means "summation" and the variance is represented by the square of the lowercase sigma, σ, so:

$$\text{Variance} = \sigma^2 = \frac{\Sigma(X - M)^2}{n}$$

Because the variance can be a large number, we take the square root of the number to calculate σ or SD, which is the standard deviation. So, $SD = \sqrt{83.33} = 9.13$ for the group with SLI and $SD = \sqrt{216.67} = 14.72$ for the typically developing group of children.

Sample CSD Experiment

Some of the analyses that follow will relate to the following sample experiment called, "Preference of Orthographic versus Semantic Distinctions in Aphasia" (Goldfarb, DeMetropolis, & Friedman, 2013; Box 6–2).

The lexical discrimination task requires the participant to choose the word that is most different among a foil, an orthographically related word, and a semantically related word (e. g., leopard, leotard, lion). Neurotypical adults should overselect the word that is orthographically related but not semantically related (e. g., "leotard" in the example above) as most different because of the saliency of the semantic pair. Individuals with aphasia (IWA) will overselect the word that is semantically related but not orthographically related (e. g., "lion" in the example above) as most different because of the letter similarities in the orthographic pairs and the semantic deficit common in aphasia. The hypotheses are that

- neurotypical participants will choose the word that is not semantically related as the most different more often than IWA; and

Box 6–2. Stimuli for Participants in "Preference of Orthographic versus Semantic Distinctions in Aphasia"

WHICH WORD IS THE MOST DIFFERENT?

1. daughter	laughter	son	10. charm	chasm	seduce
2. lion	leotard	leopard	11. fool	trice	trick
3. bough	tough	strong	12. hour	four	second
4. lose	dose	find	13. plain	plaid	simple
5. king	grown	crown	14. breath	inhale	breach
6. fix	bread	break	15. odor	scene	scent
7. thin	this	skinny	16. bridle	tunnel	bridge
8. servant	slave	suave	17. closet	open	closed
9. store	stone	rock	18. peach	apply	apple

Source: Goldfarb, DeMetropolis, & Friedman, 2013.

- participants with aphasia will choose the word that is not orthographically related as the most different more often than neurotypical participants.

Participants include about 30 IWA and about 30 matched controls. That there are 30 participants in each group is not arbitrary, as the difference between 30 and infinity participants is statistically trivial in the critical values for significance in *t*-tests and analyses of variance that will be used. There is one standard normal distribution, the symmetrical bell-shaped curve (see Figure 6–2 later in this chapter), but a different *t* distribution for each sample size, *n*. As *n* becomes larger, the *t* distribution more closely approximates the standard normal distribution. When $n > 30$, the two distributions are about equal.

Stimuli (see Box 6–2) include words that are similar orthographically and semantically. The three categories of orthographic, semantic, and foil words are randomized in presentation to all participants to reduce the threat to internal validity called the practice effect (or learning to learn; see Chapter 7). They are rearranged in category order (Box 6–3) for the purpose of analysis.

Before beginning a discussion about statistical analyses, let's address some areas of interest for consumers of research.

Box 6–3. Data Sheet for the Question, "Which Word Is Most Different?"

	Foil	*Orthographic Similarity*	*Semantic Similarity*
1.	daughter	laughter	son
2.	leopard	leotard	lion
3.	tough	bough	strong
4.	lose	dose	find
5.	crown	grown	king
6.	break	bread	fix
7.	thin	this	skinny
8.	slave	suave	servant
9.	stone	store	rock
10.	charm	chasm	seduce
11.	trick	trice	fool
12.	hour	four	second
13.	plain	plaid	simple
14.	breath	breach	inhale
15.	scent	scene	odor
16.	bridge	bridle	tunnel
17.	closed	closet	open
18.	apple	apply	peach

How To Evaluate Raw Data Descriptively

Forgetting for the moment about statistical significance, what does the data say about the sample? In the present sample CSD experiment, we are testing the hypothesis that adults with aphasia who have acquired a language deficit affecting semantic comprehension and production will respond differently in a judgment task than neurotypical adults who do not have a semantic language deficit. Specifically, given the three words *leopard, leotard,* and *lion*, people with aphasia are more likely to identify *lion* as the word that is most different and people who do not have brain damage will be more likely to identify *leotard* as the word that is most different. That is, people with aphasia will highlight the word with the spelling that is the most different and neurotypical adults will select the word with the meaning that is the most different.

The visual representation of the data, a line graph in the present example (Figure 6–1), shows that the two samples of adults with and without aphasia responded differently in the experiment. The consumer of research can see that adults with aphasia are more likely to identify the word that is most different in spelling more often than the word that is most different in meaning, and that the opposite is true for neurotypical adults. The written and visual descriptions of the data inform the reader about results of the experiment before the statistical analyses are described.

Drawing a Conclusion When a Finding Is or Is Not Statistically Significant

Statistical significance relates to the hypotheses in an experiment. Remember that there is usually a statement of an experimental hypothesis that there will be a difference (between treatments or between groups) and an implied null hypothesis that there is no difference between treatments or groups. A finding that is statistically significant motivates rejection of the null hypothesis (in other words, there is a difference) and a finding that is not statistically significant motivates acceptance of the null hypothesis that there is not a difference.

Evaluating the Magnitude of the Finding

If we assume that the research hypothesis is true, then we also want to know the extent to which the finding exists in the population. This *effect size* relates to the power of a test to yield statistically significant findings. If the unit of analysis is mean scores, then effect size is calculated by dividing the difference between the means by the averaged standard deviations between groups. Effect sizes may be small, where the two groups are separated by 0.2 standard deviations; moderate (0.5 standard deviations); or large (0.8 standard deviations). Meta-analyses combine effect sizes from different studies into an overall average effect size (Maxwell & Satake, 1997).

If the research question refers to the correspondence or correlation between two or more sets (e.g., groups, events, objects, treatments), then the magnitude of the finding is expressed as the *strength of association*. For example, the association between cleft palate and conductive hearing loss in children below 8 years of age is strong because of otitis media with effusion (OME or "glue ear"). However, the association between cleft palate and phonological disorder is weak, even though these children may have imprecise or

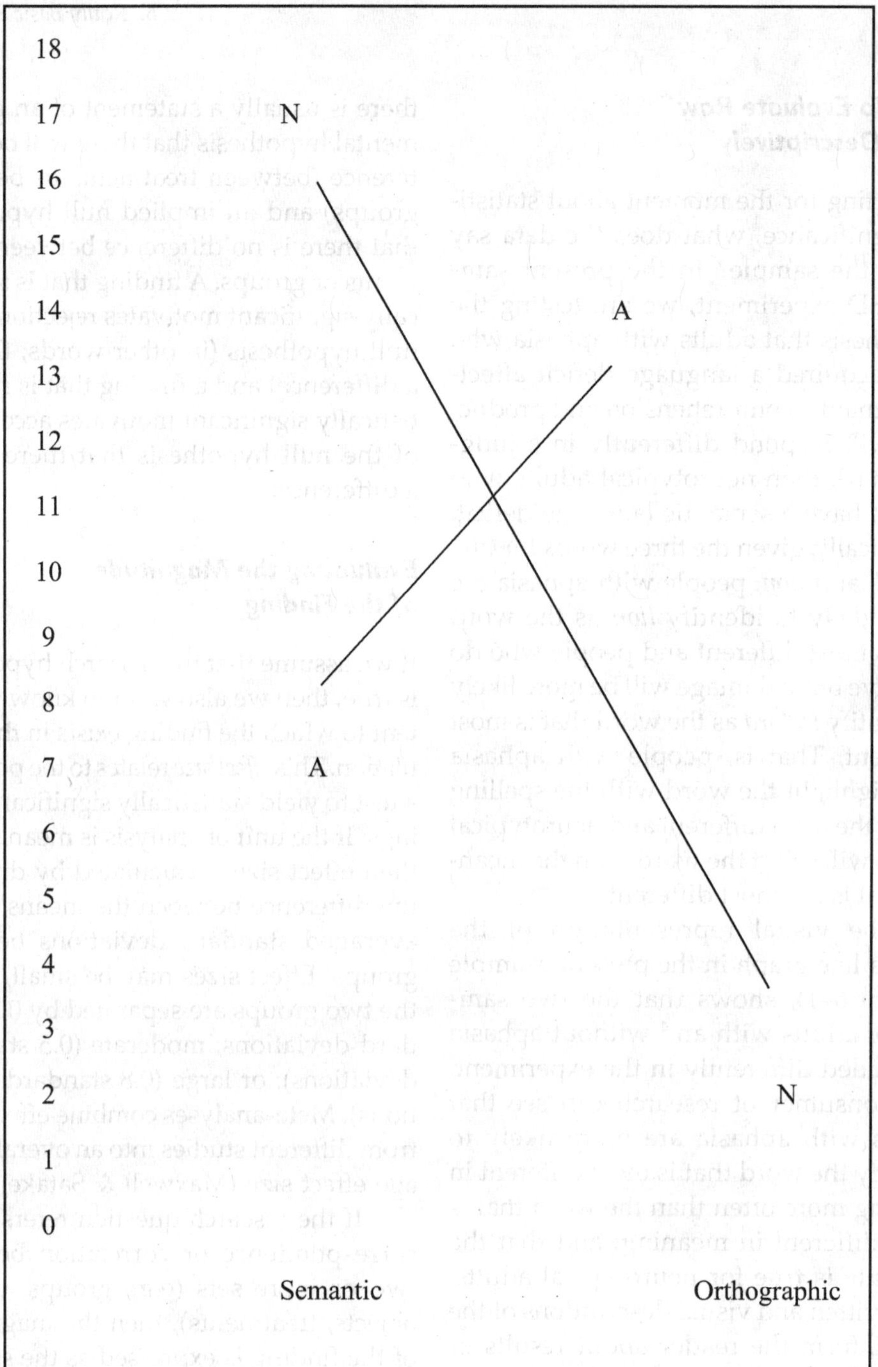

***Figure 6–1.** Mean scores of responses (word that is most different) by adults with and without aphasia.*

distorted speech (the result of an articulation disorder).

Observing Trends

When a relationship exists, a visual display can illustrate the nature or the *trend* of the relationship. Trends are especially useful in developmental studies or experiments that take place over an extended period. For example, deep brain stimulation surgery in the subthalamic nucleus (STN-DBS) for adults with Parkinson disease may improve voice functioning as well as lexical and semantic fluency naming immediately as a result of a microlesion effect, but these gains diminish over time (Crowley, 2018).

Incidence of stuttering (how many have ever stuttered) in the United States (16,000,000) as well as worldwide (362,500,000) is about 5%, while prevalence of stuttering (how many are presently stuttering) in the United States (2,240,000) as well as worldwide (50,400,000) is about 0.7% (Yairi & Seery, 2017). The trend is toward improved fluency, although the data do not indicate how many recover spontaneously and how many improve through clinical intervention.

Calculation of t for Dependent Groups

The *t*-test is a parametric statistical analysis for determining if differences between two related samples or groups are significant. Two groups are dependent—that is, they are related—because they are matched on a number of *parameters* to reduce the effect of extraneous variables. For example, articulation errors are assessed in 10 children, five in Group I and five in Group II (Box 6–4). The children are matched in age, gender, educational level, and monolingual status, but the five children in Group I have low socioeconomic status, while the 5 children in Group II have middle socioeconomic status. The parameters selected for matching depend on the study being conducted. In health care research, diagnosis, type, and severity of the disorder are often studied. The application of "all you need are sums of squares" is seen in the columns for deviations squared (d_I^2 and d_{II}^2).

With $df = 8$ (based on $n - 1$ for each group), the t value needed to reject the null hypothesis at the 0.05 level of significance is 2.306 (this can be found in a table for critical values of t, but any statistical computer program includes these values). Accordingly, because our finding of $t_8 = 2.8$ is greater than the value of t noted above, we are required to reject the null hypothesis that there is no difference between the two groups.

A single group can also be considered to be dependent when the scores used in the analysis come from the same participants, but under different conditions. For example, pretreatment and posttreatment scores are compared to see if, for example, a hearing aid improves spondee reception threshold (SRT) in children with otitis media. In this example, the scores refer to the SRT in dB HL obtained in an audiological evaluation. The weakness of the single-group design is that it is considered quasi-experimental, because it does not include a comparison to a control group. Therefore, it is difficult to support a claim of effectiveness of treatment.

A *t*-test for dependent groups makes four assumptions:

- Dependent variables are measured at interval or ratio levels (interval refers

Box 6–4. Example of the Calculation of *t*

	Grouped data		*Deviations from sample means*		*Deviations squared*	
	I	II	d_I	d_{II}	d_I^2	d_{II}^2
	61	50	4	−2	16	4
	53	48	−4	−4	16	16
	59	56	2	4	4	16
	55	54	−2	2	4	4
	57	52	0	0	0	0
M	57	52			40	40
n	5	5				

Next, calculate variance: divide d_I^2 by n (40/5 = 8) and d_{II}^2 by n (also 40/5 = 8 in this example) to obtain σ_I^2 and σ_{II}^2

$$t = \frac{M_1 - M_2}{\frac{\sqrt{\sigma_I^2 + \sigma_{II}^2}}{N}}$$

When the samples are equal in Groups 1 and 2, then $n_1 = n_2 = N$. So,

$$t = \frac{5}{\frac{\sqrt{16}}{5}} = \frac{5}{\sqrt{3.2}} = \frac{5}{1.78} = \mathbf{2.8}$$

to time, while ratio refers to number of trials; see Chapter 11).

- There is a normal or near-normal distribution of scores.
- The differences between groups are dependent because they are based on matching or because the participants serve as their own controls.
- Differences between paired scores are independent.

In the "Preference of Orthographic versus Semantic Distinctions in Aphasia" (Goldfarb, DeMetropolis, & Friedman, 2013) study, the *t*-test can be used for two analyses: to determine significance of preference (semantic or orthographic difference); and a second *t*-test to determine significance of presence of neuropathology (difference between experimental and control groups).

Sample Calculation for One-Way Analysis of Variance

An analysis of variance (ANOVA) is used to test the hypothesis that the means of more than two groups are the same or different when the populations are normally distributed and have equal variance. For our experiment "Preference of Orthographic versus Semantic Distinctions in Aphasia" (Goldfarb et al., 2013), we can use a 2 × 3 ANOVA to determine if there are significant differences between groups. The independent variable is presence of neuropathology (e.g., in aphasia vs. control groups); the dependent variable is choice of which word is most different (orthographic, semantic, or foil). We could test the hypotheses that people with and without aphasia select orthographic stimuli differently than semantic stimuli or differently than foils (two *t*-tests), that they select semantic stimuli differently than foils (a third *t*-test), or we could use a single ANOVA to address all three hypotheses. For practice in this chapter, we will focus on the simpler one-way ANOVA rather than the more complex multivariate analysis of variance or MANOVA.

A one-way ANOVA is used to test equality of three or more means at one time by using variances. We use this analysis to test the null hypothesis that means from three or more groups are the same. Assuming that we have three means, A, B, and C, then we can use three *t*-tests to compare Groups A and B, B and C, and A and C, or use a single one-way ANOVA. The null hypothesis of a one-way ANOVA is that all population means are equal, and the experimental hypothesis is that at least one mean is different. There are three assumptions made about a one-way ANOVA:

- The samples were obtained from a population that is normally or nearly normally distributed.
- The samples are independent.
- The variances of the populations are equal.

Following is a CSD example of a one-way analysis of variance. Assume that the data refer to the number of disfluencies produced in a 5-min spontaneous speech sample by 4-year-old children who are fluent (Group I), who stutter (Group II), and who clutter (Group III). The application of "all you need are sums of squares" is seen in the columns for deviations squared (d_I^2, d_{II}^2, and d_{III}^2). The summary table is followed by a check.

The null hypothesis for this experiment assumed that all three groups came from the same population. One-way ANOVA is used to estimate how much variability among individual scores would be expected. This variability is shown as the within-group variance. If the *F*-test number (32.64 in this example) is large enough to reject the null hypothesis, then at least one of the means is different. ANOVA does not indicate where the difference is, but a post hoc analysis, such as the Sheffé or Tukey test, can identify where the difference lies.

There are two ways to look at data from fluent individuals compared to those who stutter or clutter. *Between group* differences show how two groups (or more than two groups) are different, and *within group* differences show differences among participants who are in the same group. With $df = 2$ for between groups (based on $n - 1$ for the 3 groups [3 − 1 = 2]) and 12 for within groups (based on $n - 1$ for the 5 scores in each group [5 − 1 = 4], multiplied by the 3 groups [3 × 4 = 12], the $F_{2,12}$ value needed to reject the null hypothesis at the 0.05 level of significance is 19.41 on the table of critical values of *F*. Accordingly, because our finding of $F_{2,12} = 32.64$ is greater than the value of *F* noted above (19.41), we are required to reject the null hypothesis that there are no differences between the three groups.

I	d_I	d_I^2
51	−1	1
53	1	1
49	−3	9
55	3	9
52	0	0
$M_I = 52$		20

II	d_{II}	d_{II}^2
59	−3	9
64	2	4
61	−1	1
63	1	1
63	1	1
$M_{II} = 62$		16

III	d_{III}	d_{III}^2
59	2	4
58	1	1
56	−1	1
57	0	0
55	−2	4
$M_{III} = 57$		10

Grand mean: 52 + 62 + 57, divided by 3 = 57

The grand mean is the total of all the data values divided by the total sample size (15 in the previous example) divided by the number of groups (3 in the previous example). You can find it in two ways. If you have all the sample data, you can add it and divide by the total number of scores. In the previous example, add all 15 scores and divide by 15. If you have the sample means, then find their weighted average, as shown in the previous example.

Within SS = Σd_w^2

Score deviations (d_w^2) from group means: 20 + 16 + 10 = 46

The sum of squares (SS) within groups denotes the variation caused by differences within individual samples. There is no interaction between samples because each sample is considered independently.

Between SS	I	II	III
Group means (*m*)	52	62	57
Group deviation from grand mean (d_b)	−5	5	0
Squared deviation (d_b^2)	25	25	0
Group *n* times d (nd_b^2)	125	125	0

Between SS = Σnd_b^2 : 125 + 125 + 0 = 250

The sum of squares between groups denotes the variation caused by the interaction between the samples. When sample means are close to each other, then they will also be close to the grand mean and the variation will be small (*MS* indicates mean square). Total variation represents the sum of the squares of the differences of each mean with the grand mean. It is not the same as variance. Mean square (*MS*) is the sum of squares (*SS*) divided by its degrees of freedom (*df*), and the *F* value is found by dividing the Between *MS* by the Within *MS*. The degrees of freedom in the *F*-test are indicated in the same order as they appear in the table, as subscripts of *F* (e.g., $F_{2,12}$ in the present example).

$$F = \frac{MS \text{ between}}{MS \text{ within}}$$

The *F* statistic is the ratio of two sample variables. In other words, it is the ratio of two independent chi-square (χ^2) variables divided by their degrees of freedom. See examples of χ^2 computations later in this chapter.

Summary Table

Source	*SS*	*df*	*MS*	*F*
Between	250	2	125	32.64
Within	46	12	3.83	
Total	296	14		

CHECK

Total SS

Score deviations (d_g) from grand mean (57 in this example)

I	d_{gI}	d_{gI}^2
51	−6	36
53	−4	16
49	−8	64
55	−2	4
52	−5	25
		145

II	d_{gII}	d_{gII}^2
59	2	4
64	7	49
61	4	16
63	6	36
63	6	36
		141

III	d_{gIII}	d_{gIII}^2
59	2	4
58	1	1
56	−1	1
57	0	0
55	−2	4
		10

Total SS = 145 + 141 + 10 = 296

Calculation of the Correlation Coefficient *r*

The correlation coefficient measures the degree of association between two or more variables. In the two-variable case, the simple linear correlation coefficient *r* for a set of sample observations is given by the formula below. The closer *r* is to ±1, the greater is the degree of positive or negative linear relationship. A zero correlation means that there exists no linear relationship whatsoever between *X* and *Y* (i.e., they tend to change with no connection with each other). The range of correlation scores is from −1 to 1.

Example I

Suppose that the data from two students scoring a standardized test are

x	6	2	2	−2
y	5	5	−3	−3

The means are:

$M(x) = (6 + 2 + 2 - 2) / 4 = 8 / 4 = 2$

$M(y) = (5 + 5 - 3 - 3) / 4 = 4 / 4 = 1$

Columns (1) and (2) in the following section are the scores provided by the students; columns (3) and (4) are the deviations from the mean for the *x*s and *y*s obtained from columns (1) and (2) by subtracting the proper mean. Note that the sum of each set of deviations is 0 (columns [3] and [4]), as is always the case. Columns (6) and (7) are the squares of these deviations (all you need are sums of squares).

(1) x	(2) y	(3) $x - Mx$	(4) $y - My$
6	5	4	4
2	5	0	4
2	−3	0	−4
−2	−3	−4	−4
		0	0

(5) $(x - Mx)(y - My)$	(6) $(x - Mx)^2$	(7) $(y - My)^2$
16	16	16
0	0	16
0	0	16
16	16	16
32	32	64

If we divide the sums of these columns (6 and 7) by the number of observations, four, the variances of x and y are

$$\sigma_x^2 = 32 / 4 = 8$$

$$\sigma_y^2 = 64 / 4 = 16;$$

and the standard deviations are

$$SD_x = \sqrt{8} = 2.8$$

$$SD_y = \sqrt{16} = 4$$

Column (5) contains the product of each entry in column (3) and the corresponding entry in column (4). Be careful of the signs here. Both positive and negative products may occur. The sum of the entries in column (5) is the sum in the numerator of r. We need only divide by the number of observations $n = 4$ (NOT $n = 8$, because n is the number of bivariate observations). So, finally

$$r = \frac{32/4}{(2.8)(4)} = \frac{8}{(2.8)(4)} = \frac{2}{2.8} = 0.71$$

The purpose of the example above is not to show you how to calculate r; we have computers to do that. This is a recipe for what the correlation coefficient r says. There are five points to be made when we interpret r.

- The correlation coefficient r makes sense as a measure of association; it is positive when the association is positive and negative when the association is negative.
- The correlation coefficient r always has a value between −1 and +1.
- The extreme values $r = -1$ and $r = +1$ indicate perfect straight-line association.
- The correlation coefficient r measures how tightly the points on a scatterplot cluster about a straight line.
- There is a specific way in which r measures straight-line association. The square (r^2) of the correlation coefficient is the proportion of the variance of one variable that can be explained by straight-line dependence on the other

variable. This is sometimes called the strength of association measure. Because r is almost always less than 1 (or more than −1) and r^2 results from multiplying a fraction, then r^2 will be a smaller number than r. As a general rule, r^2 greater than .80 indicates a strong association and r^2 lower than .60 indicates a weaker association. That is, even though a statistical finding may be significant, it may also be weak.

To summarize, the finding above of $r = .71$ sounds pretty good, but r^2 indicates that only half the variance of one variable can be explained by the other variable.

Example 2

There is a similar formula for calculating the Pearson product–moment correlation coefficient, abbreviated as Pearson's r. This formula is used for parametric correlation analysis (for nonparametric correlation analysis, use Spearman's rank correlation). Let x = score assigned by one SLP. Let y = score assigned by the other SLP. This might be a statistical treatment to assess interscorer or interrater reliability (see Chapter 8). Test the null hypothesis that there is no relationship between scores assigned by the two SLPs. Remember that the range for Pearson's r is from −1.0 (for perfect disagreement) to 0 (for no relationship) to 1.0 (for perfect agreement). Sums of squares appear in the last two columns.

$$r = \frac{\Sigma xy}{\sqrt{\Sigma x^2 \, \Sigma y^2}}$$

$$df = n - 2$$

n	x	y	xy	x^2	y^2
1	1.2	0.7	0.84	1.44	0.49
2	0.5	0.5	0.25	0.25	0.25
3	1.1	0.6	0.66	1.21	0.36
4	0.6	0.7	0.42	0.36	0.49
5	3.1	1.0	3.10	9.61	1.00
			5.27	12.87	2.69

$$r = \frac{5.27}{(\sqrt{12.87 \times 2.69}} = \frac{5.27}{5.89} = 0.89$$

With $df = 3$ (we calculate df as $n - 2$, and we have $n = 5$), we need $r = .878$ to reject the null hypothesis at the 0.05 level of significance. Since we have found $r = 0.89$, we reject the null hypothesis, and find that there ***is*** a relationship between the scores obtained from the two SLPs. Squaring the r of 0.89 yields about .80 or four-fifths of the variance of one variable that can be explained by a straight-line dependence on the other variable, a strong association between the scores provided by the two SLPs.

Example 3

In a repeated measures single-subject design (Arroyo, Goldfarb, & Sands, 2012), we wanted to determine how use of an augmentative and alternative communication (AAC) device correlated with three different communication behaviors exhibited by an adult with severe aphasia. While the calculation of r could have been done nearly instantly by a dedicated computer program, it was not very difficult to do it by hand (Box 6–5).

There were four measurements that were subjected to statistical analysis: the

Box 6–5. Correlation of Usage of AAC (U) with Initiations (I), Responses (R), and Verbalizations (V) ($n = 17$)

Initiations (I) $M - I = i$			Responses (R) $M - R = r$			Verbalizations (V) $M - V = v$			Used AAC (U) $M - U = u$		
I	**i**	**i^2**	**R**	**r**	**r^2**	**V**	**v**	**v^2**	**U**	**u**	**u^2**
4	−4.53	20.52	4	−10.82	117.07	1	−15.24	232.26	−4	−10.53	110.88
5	−3.53	12.46	5	−9.82	96.43	2	−14.24	202.78	5	−9.53	90.82
8	−.53	0.28	8	−6.82	46.51	8	−8.24	67.90	8	−6.53	42.64
10	1.47	2.16	10	−4.82	23.23	6	−10.24	104.86	10	4.53	20.52
7	−1.53	2.34	7	−7.82	61.15	2	−14.24	202.78	6	−8.53	72.76
7	−1.53	2.34	7	−7.82	61.15	3	−13.24	175.30	7	−7.53	56.70
4	−4.53	20.52	4	−10.82	117.07	2	−14.24	202.78	4	−10.53	110.88
1	−7.53	56.70	1	−13.82	190.99	1	−15.24	232.26	1	−13.53	183.06
11	2.47	6.10	11	−3.82	14.59	9	−7.24	52.42	11	−3.53	12.46
5	−3.53	12.46	5	−9.82	96.43	4	−12.24	149.82	5	−9.53	90.82
6	−2.53	6.40	6	−8.82	77.79	55	38.76	1502.34	6	−8.53	72.76
3	−5.53	30.58	40	25.18	634.03	40	23.76	564.54	40	25.47	648.72
6	−2.53	6.40	26	11.18	124.99	26	9.76	95.26	22	7.47	55.80
12	3.47	12.04	32	17.18	295.15	32	15.76	248.38	32	17.47	305.20
5	−3.53	12.46	25	10.18	100.36	24	7.76	60.22	25	10.47	109.62
5	−3.53	12.46	15	.18	.03	15	−1.24	1.54	15	.47	.22
46	37.47	1404.00	46	31.18	972.19	46	29.76	885.66	46	31.47	990.36
145 / 17			252 / 17			276 / 17			247 / 17		
$M = 8.53$			$M = 14.82$			$M = 16.24$			$M = 14.53$		

number of uses of the AAC device during a single recording session, which formed the basis of comparison to the other three measurements; the number of initiations of communicative interactions by the participant; the number of responses the participant provided to the caregiver; and the number of independent vocalizations the participant produced. There were a total of 17 different recording sessions where there were data in all of the four measurements.

The research question involved the effect of use of AAC on other means of communication. Accordingly, the Pearson correlation coefficient was deemed to be the appropriate statistical measurement. The correlations were significant for all calculations of r: for correlation between use of AAC and initiations, $r_{15} = 0.610$, $p < .01$; for correlation between use of AAC and responses, $r_{15} = 0.998$, $p < .01$; and for correlation between use of AAC and independent verbalizations, $r_{15} = 0.716$, $p < .01$.

A significant finding in a statistical analysis indicates that a relationship is real, but not that it is strong. Recall that strength of association measures are obtained by squaring the r value, with a weak association indicated at a level below 0.60 and a strong association above 0.80. Accordingly, there are weak associations between use of AAC and initiations ($r^2 = 0.372$) and between use of AAC and independent verbalizations ($r^2 = 0.513$); but a very strong association between use of AAC and responses ($r^2 = 0.996$).

The Chi-Square (χ^2) Test of Independence

We use the nonparametric test chi-square (represented as the 22nd letter of the Greek alphabet, χ^2) when we want to know whether variables are associated or independent of each other. In nonparametric statistics, we do not have to fit the data in a normal distribution. The data can be ranked or ordered without relying on numbers. Finally, nonparametric tests can be easier to calculate than parametric tests.

We ask if the observed frequencies differ significantly from expected frequencies when more than two outcomes are possible. The following example refers to a simulated experiment regarding handedness and fluency. The null hypothesis is that handedness will not influence fluency in individuals who are fluent, who clutter, or who stutter. The research hypothesis is that there will be an influence of handedness on fluency. However, the question of whether left-handed people who clutter are more disfluent than right-handed people who stutter will not be answered in a χ^2 test.

The paired observations of handedness and fluency are displayed in a bivariate frequency table called an χ^2 contingency table (Box 6–6) that is used to study the independence or association of handedness and fluency. Contingency tables allow chi-square to be an appropriate test for independence. The observed frequencies are plotted and the expected frequencies (seen in parentheses in Box 6–6) are calculated, using the formula below.

To Calculate Expected Scores (r Indicates Rows and c Indicates Columns)

$$f_e = \frac{\Sigma r \Sigma c}{n}$$

$$\frac{124 \times 118}{413} = 35.4 \qquad \frac{124 \times 195}{413} = 58.5$$

Box 6–6. χ^2 Contingency Table

Contingency table showing relationship between the fluency for 413 participants and calculation of expected values.

	Cluttering	*Fluent*	*Stuttering*	*Total*
L-handed	34 (35.4)	62 (58.5)	28 (30.0)	124
Ambidextrous	27 (21.4)	28 (35.4)	20 (18.2)	75
R-handed	57 (61.1)	105 (101.0)	52 (51.8)	214
Total	118	195	100	413

$$\frac{124 \times 100}{413} = 30.0 \qquad \frac{75 \times 118}{413} = 21.4$$

$$\frac{75 \times 195}{413} = 35.4 \qquad \frac{75 \times 100}{413} = 18.2$$

$$\frac{214 \times 118}{413} = 61.1 \qquad \frac{214 \times 195}{413} = 101.0$$

$$\frac{214 \times 100}{413} = 51.8$$

So, what is the expected proportion of people who clutter and who are L-handed, or people who stutter and who are ambidextrous, and so on?

To Calculate Degrees of Freedom, df = (r – 1) (c – 1)

There are three rows (r = 3) and three columns (c = 3). Therefore, in this example, $df = (3 - 1) \times (3 - 1) = 4$. That means, you need to do only four of the f_e calculations above, instead of all nine (whew!).

To compute χ^2,

$$\chi^2 = \Sigma\frac{(O - E)^2}{E}$$

Calculation of χ^2 data

O	E	(O – E)	$(O - E)^2$	$\frac{(O - E)^2}{E}$
34	35.4	–1.4	1.96	.055
62	58.5	3.5	12.25	.209
28	30.0	–2.0	4.00	.133
27	21.4	5.6	31.36	1.465
28	35.4	–7.4	54.76	1.547
20	18.2	1.8	3.24	.178
57	61.1	–4.1	16.81	.275
105	101.0	4.0	16.00	.158
52	51.8	.2	.04	.001
413	412.8	0		$\chi^2 = 4.021$

The value of χ^2 required for significance at the 5% ($p < 0.05$) level is 9.488. Therefore, we have no grounds for rejecting the hypothesis of independence between fluency and hand laterality.

Are We Playing with Loaded Dice?

Box 6–7 shows another example of observed and expected frequencies. A die (one of a pair of dice) is a cube with six sides, each side having one through six dots. If you roll the die 300 times, you would expect each of the six options to occur 50 times, even though that is extremely unlikely for a fair die. With "loaded dice," the observed frequencies would favor a particular throw (let's say "snake eyes" or one on each die) beyond a reasonable variation from the expected frequency. In Box 6–7, the die is found to be fair, even though none of the observed frequencies matches the expected 50, because χ^2 is not sufficient to reject the null hypothesis of reasonable variation from the expected frequencies.

PRESENTING THE DATA: FREQUENCY DISTRIBUTIONS, HISTOGRAMS, LINE GRAPHS

The shape of a frequency distribution has two features of interest: skewness (whether or not it is symmetrical) and kurtosis (the shape of the peak).

The Bell-Shaped Curve

In a symmetrical bell-shaped curve (Figure 6–2), the mean, median, and mode are equal, as seen in the vertical line in the center of the curve. A distribution may also be positively skewed, where the right tail is longer, and then mean > median > mode; or negatively skewed, where the

Box 6–7. Using Chi-Square to Test If a Die Is Fair

Value of Die	Observed Frequency	Expected Frequency	O – E	$(O-E)^2$	$\frac{(O-E)^2}{E}$
1	43	50	–7	49	.98
2	55	50	5	25	.50
3	39	50	–11	121	2.42
4	56	50	6	36	.72
5	63	50	13	169	3.38
6	44	50	–6	36	.72
Total	300	300	0		$\chi^2 = 8.72$

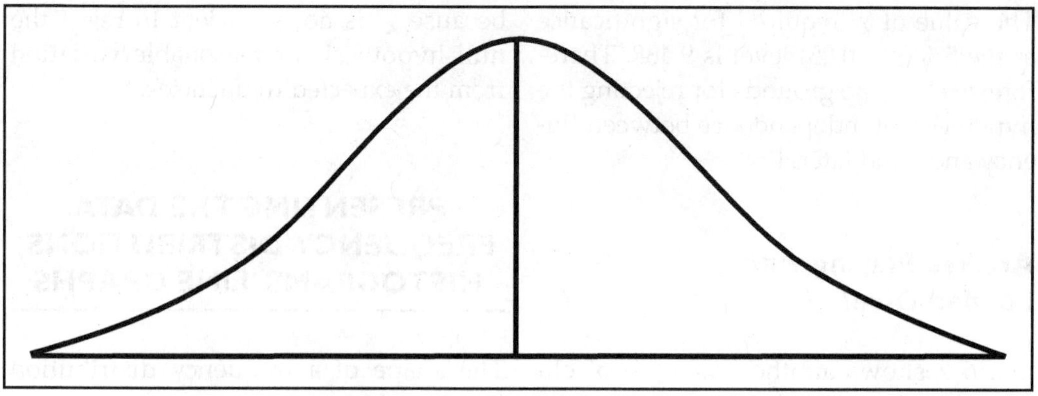

Figure 6–2. *A symmetrical frequency distribution.*

left tail is longer, and then mode > median > mean. When the curve is peaked, it is called leptokurtic, and when it flattens, it is called platykurtic; a curve with a peak between the two is called mesokurtic. Peakedness refers to the concentration about the mean, with platykurtic being least concentrated and leptokurtic being most concentrated.

Note that the curve tails off in both left and right directions. If we consider the vertical line in the middle of the curve to be the historical mean, then any analysis of statistical significance that has to consider data that are above or below the historical mean is called a two-tailed test. An experiment that considers statistical significance in only one direction—either above the historical mean only or below the historical mean only—is using a one-tailed test. An experimenter who uses a one-tailed test has an easier time showing statistical significance, and a new researcher may be tempted to use such a test. But remember the words of Mark Twain about statistics! The consumer of research should be skeptical about research using one-tailed tests, and the author of such research is obliged to demonstrate why it was used appropriately.

The Histogram

Figure 6–3 shows a histogram, a form of a bar graph (technically, a bar graph has spaces between the bars) of a frequency distribution. Classes are measured along the abscissa, or horizontal axis, and frequencies along the ordinate, or vertical axis.

The Frequency Polygon

Figure 6–4 shows a frequency polygon, or a line graph of a frequency distribution that results from joining the frequency of each class that is plotted at the class midpoint. In this simulated study, Figures 6–2 and 6–3 represent baseline data of the effectiveness of botulinum toxin on the ability of patients with spasmodic dysphonia to sustain phonation over time.

RECIPE FOR REPEATED MEASURE ANALYSIS ON SPSS

A research design that contains more than one independent variable is called

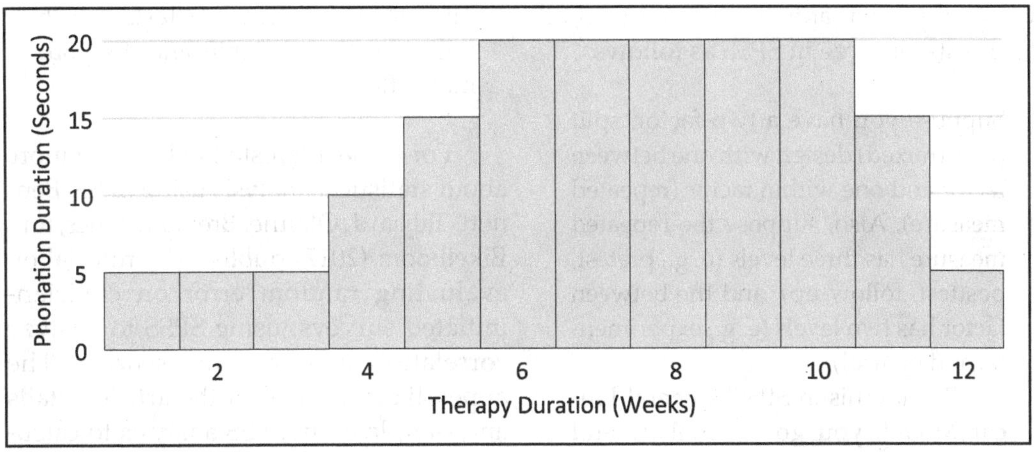

Figure 6–3. *Example of a histogram.*

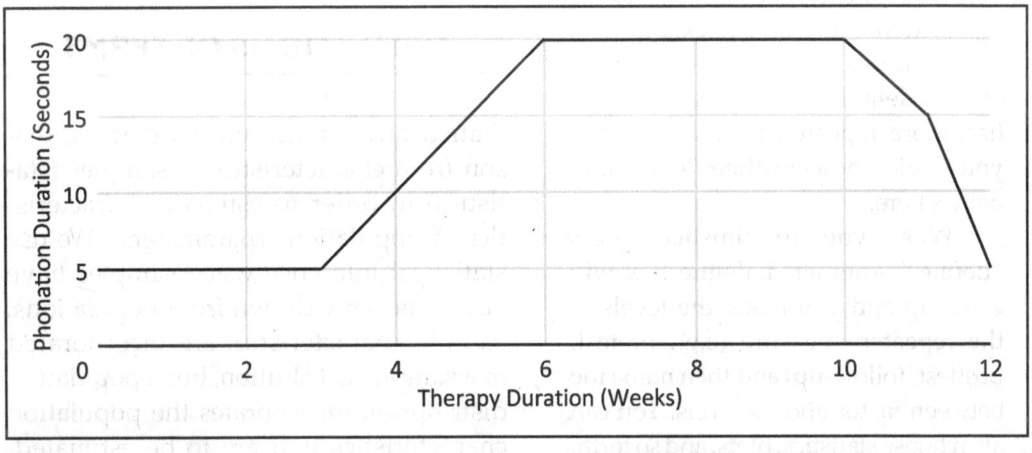

Figure 6–4. *Example of a frequency polygon (line graph) showing the same data as in the histogram.*

a factorial design. Time-Altered Word Association Tests (Goldfarb & Halpern, 2013; available for free on my Adelphi University website at http://home.adelphi.edu/~go18170/tawat/newtest/test7.html) is given at two speeds of stimulus presentation (one independent variable) and through the auditory or visual modality (another independent variable). There are two equivalent word lists of 36 words each (List A and List B). Participants are randomly assigned to slow or fast speed, auditory or visual modality, and List A or List B. For example, Participant 1 gets fast, visual, List B first and slow, visual, List A second. Four testing sessions will be needed to get information about both modalities at both presentation speeds with the alternating word lists used to prevent the practice effect (see Chapter 7 for information about controlling the practice effect, a threat to internal validity).

Once all participants have completed all four tests, analyze in SPSS as follows:

> Suppose you have a two-factor, split plots (mixed) design with one between factor and one within factor (repeated measure). Also, suppose the repeated measure has three levels (e. g., pretest, posttest, follow-up), and the between factor has two levels (e. g., experimental and control).
>
> To run this in SPSS' General Linear Model, you go to Analyze and pick General Linear Model and choose "repeated measures."
>
> In the repeated measures dialogue box, name the number of levels of the repeated measure (in this example, 3), and name the repeated measure (SPSS gives a default name, factor1). If you had more repeated measure factors, you could indicate their levels and names here.
>
> When you are finished, press "define." Another dialogue box will come up and you name the levels of the repeated measure (e.g., pretest, posttest, follow-up) and then name the between factor and its levels. You can also choose statistics, plots, and so forth. Your printout will show a bunch of stuff you don't need and some things you do. Under the heading of General Linear Model, you'll find a data set for within-subjects factors, listing your main effects by the names you gave them. Then there will be Multivariate Tests, which will have data you need. The first group of effects will show *F* ratio and degrees of freedom (*df*), and the second group is the real goodie, showing significance of between-subjects and within-subjects analyses. Then skip to Univariate Tests, which will show *df* and significance for your main effects.

For those interested in learning more about statistical analysis using SPSS, Bennett, Taljaard, Olaithe, Brennan-Jones, and Eikelboom (2017) published a tutorial on evaluating random error on clinician-initiated surveys, using SPSS to analyze correlation among three scorers. The appendix at the end of the article details an example of an SPSS analysis to calculate Cohen's kappa statistic for agreement between two clinician observers.

DEFINITIONS OF TERMS

Statistical inference means that we reason from characteristics of samples (statistics) in order to estimate characteristics of populations (parameters). We use statistical inference when samples have been randomly drawn from populations. Sample characteristics are incorporated in a sample distribution, but a population distribution incorporates the population characteristics that are to be estimated. A sampling distribution characterizes the likely deviations of a given statistic about a parameter.

When distributions can be approximated to the normal distribution curve, we have a basis for making probability statements about parameters and likely sampling error of statistics. In practice, there are various methods for calculating estimates of population characteristics, given sample characteristics. Distributions let us report about a body of measurements. We can present these reports as data or as graphic displays. Graphic displays make it easier to interpret how the scores cluster about a particular point or how the scores are dispersed along the measurement scale, and also how they may be skewed. Descriptive statistics are used to characterize various aspects of distributions. Indexes of how scores tend to cluster, called central tendency, include the mode, median, and mean. Indexes of how scores scatter or disperse include the range, variance, and standard deviation. The following alphabetized definitions are updated from Williams (1968):

- *Data:* (plural) the reports of observations of variables. The singular *datum* is seldom used, and data is also acceptable as a singular form.
- *Dependent variable:* a phenomenon that is affected by the researcher's manipulation of another phenomenon.
- *Descriptive method:* a research plan that defines the characteristics or relationships, or both, among variables based upon systematic observations of these variables.
- *Descriptive statistics:* calculated values that represent certain overall characteristics of a body of data.
- *Distribution:* a collection of measurements usually viewed in terms of how frequently observations are assigned to each category or point on a measurement scale.
- *Experimental method:* a research plan that tests relationships among variables based upon systematic observation of variables that are manipulated by the researcher.
- *Hypothesis:* a statement susceptible to testing by reasoning from observations.
- *Independent variable:* a phenomenon that is manipulated by the researcher and that is predicted to have an effect on another phenomenon.
- *Interval scale:* assigning numbers that identify ordered relations of some characteristic; the order has intervals that are arbitrarily assigned and equal, as well as an arbitrary zero point.
- *Mean:* the sum of the scores in a distribution divided by the number of scores (more properly called the arithmetic mean).
- *Measurement:* the assignment of numbers or symbols to specify differing characteristics of a variable.
- *Median:* the midpoint or midscore in a distribution.
- *Method:* the plan of the research, that is, how the knowledge was gained.
- *Mode:* the most frequent score in a distribution.
- *Nominal scale:* the assignment of numbers or symbols to designate subclasses that represent unique characteristics.
- *Normal distribution curve:* a particular functional relation between deviations about the mean of a distribution and the probability of these different deviations occurring.
- *Null hypothesis:* a statement that statistical differences or relationships have occurred for no reason other than laws

of chance operating in an unrestricted manner.

- *One-tailed test:* a directional hypothesis test that incorporates a rejection region in only one tail of the probability curve used for a given statistic.
- *Ordinal scale:* numbers or symbols assigned for the purpose of identifying ordered relations of some characteristic, the order having unspecified intervals.
- *Parameter:* a characteristic of a population.
- *Phenomenon:* any object or event, the characteristics of which are susceptible to observation.
- *Point-biserial correlation:* a measure of the relationship between a continuous variable (e.g., scores on a test) and a two-categorical or dichotomous variable (e.g., communication disorder or control).
- *Population distribution:* how often units or observations in a population are assigned or expected in each category or point on a measurement scale.
- *Population:* any class of phenomena arbitrarily defined on the basis of its unique and observable characteristics.
- *Power:* the probability of rejecting a null hypothesis that is false.
- *Problem:* a precise statement of what knowledge was sought and why.
- *Random sample:* phenomena selected so each phenomenon in the population has an equal chance of being selected.
- *Range:* the highest score in a distribution minus the lowest score. Total range is the highest score minus the lowest score, plus 1.
- *Ratio scale:* assigning numbers to identify ordered relations of some characteristic, the order having arbitrarily assigned and equal intervals, but an absolute zero point.
- *Rejection region (significance level):* a level of probability set by the researcher as grounds for the rejection of the null hypothesis.
- *Reliability:* the external and internal consistency of measurement.
- *Research hypothesis:* a statement expressing differences or relationships among phenomena, the acceptance or rejection of which is based upon resolving a logical alternative called a null hypothesis.
- *Results:* a precise statement of the knowledge that was gained.
- *Sample:* a collection of phenomena so selected as to represent some well-defined population.
- *Sampling distribution:* how frequently particular values of a statistic are expected when sampled randomly from a given population.
- *Sampling error:* an estimate of how statistics may be expected to deviate from parameters when sampling randomly from a given population.
- *Sampling statistics:* calculated values that represent the probable deviations of sample characteristics from population characteristics.
- *Scale:* assigning numbers or symbols to designate characteristics of a variable.

- *Significance:* the level of calculated probability low enough to reject the null hypothesis.
- *Standard deviation:* the square root of the variance, or the square root of the average value of the squares of the deviation scores from the mean of a distribution.
- *Standard error of the mean:* the standard deviation of a distribution of sample means.
- *Statistic:* a characteristic of a sample.
- *Statistical inference:* estimating parameters from statistics.
- *Statistics:* (singular) a branch of applied mathematics that specializes in ways to describe and reason from observations.
- *Two-tailed test:* a nondirectional hypothesis test that incorporates rejection regions in both tails of the probability curve used for a given statistic.
- *Type I error:* rejecting a null hypothesis when it should have been the acceptable alternative.
- *Type II error:* accepting the null hypothesis when it should have been the rejected alternative.
- *Validity:* the degree to which the researcher measures what is being claimed.
- *Variable:* a phenomenon considered in terms of how its characteristics may differ according to some well-defined classification scheme.
- *Variance:* the average value of the squares of the deviation scores from the mean of a distribution.

STATISTICS OF THE FUTURE: BAYESIAN INFERENCE

Bayesian statistics was formulated about 300 years ago by Thomas Bayes. Bayes' essential theorem refers to the likelihood of something (a belief, prediction, or trend) given some particular piece or pieces of evidence. In other words, what is the likelihood that a prior belief is supported by the facts of an actual observation? McElreath (2015) gives an example of an individual finding out if the Earth has more land or more water. A globe that is a replica of the Earth is tossed in the air and then caught. If the tip of the catcher's index finger touches water, then W is recorded; if it touches land, then L is recorded. Assume that the first toss results in W. We can now refine our hypothesis to indicate that the Earth is 100% water, but reject the hypothesis that it is 100% land. If the next toss results in L, then the hypothesis can be 50–50 land and water, and so on, with hypotheses being refined based on subsequent tosses and catches. Surprisingly, it should not take a great many tosses to reach a close approximation of the actual land and water distribution of the Earth. In the current era of big data science where there are terabytes of information, Bayesian inference has become a preferred statistical model.

Bayesian statistics calls attention to common misunderstandings and mistakes relating to *p* values and tests in general (See "Lies, Damned Lies, and Statistics: The *p* Value" at the beginning of this chapter for a critique of *p* values). Bayesian procedures make statistical inferences without *p* values. In a chapter on diagnosis of stuttering (Goldfarb, 2006), I rejected Bloodstein's (1960) continuity hypothesis that claimed the only differences between children who were normally nonfluent and those who would become individuals who stutter were persistence and severity. According to the hypothesis, diagnosis of stuttering in young children was a meaningless and futile exercise. Even without Bayesian statistical inferencing, the presence of my chapter on diagnosis of stuttering in young children, as well as many others in books and journals, represented a rejection of the continuity hypothesis, without the support of *p* values. The conclusion, and the basis for rejection of the continuity hypothesis, is that there is a likelihood of success in diagnosing stuttering in young children.

Bayesian procedures may apply to a field of education that relates to language acquisition and even treatment of child language disorders. Called statistical learning or implicit learning, it applies to learning sequential structure, where young speakers/hearers can recognize that a sound or a sequence of sounds represents a word. It is the likelihood that one element, such as a sound, syllable, or word predicts the occurrence of another. Statistical learning also applies to category structure or morphosyntax because of the predictable relation between categories and elements. For example, in English, nouns can follow an article and verbs can follow an auxiliary, but not the other way around. This predictable relation would allow the child to produce "a car" and "is kicking" but not "a kicking" or "is car" (Plante & Gómez, 2018).

Some science, including much of CSD research, can be completed using the statistical models described in this chapter, provided that they stay in well-tested contexts. McElreath (2015) asks why the traditional statistical tests are not good enough for innovative research, and answers that they tend to be both inflexible and fragile. They are inflexible in their ability to adapt to unique research contexts, and they are fragile in that they fail when applied to new contexts. To answer tomorrow's research questions using big data, CSD researchers may need to apply inferential statistical models such as the one proposed by Bayes so many years ago.

ADVANCED STUDY

The author proposes that skills in statistical methods are necessary for an individual to be granted power of professor. With new generations of scholars and researchers needed every 10 years, professors and master clinicians have an obligation to prepare individuals with adequate knowledge and skills to undertake the tasks of scholarship and research, and statistics is a key component. For evidence of the requisite statistics skills, complete the following and have your instructor, academic adviser, mentor, or CSD department chair review that you have completed the requirements and sign and date where indicated.

Student's Name: ______________________________

1. Research question: Do males and females have different preferences in judging which of three versions of a journal article is best written? The following data are observed:

	Males	Females
Version I	5	5
Version II	5	20
Version III	10	5

   Test at the .05 level of significance the hypothesis that gender is not a factor in judging quality of writing in a journal article.

2. Using the following set of data, find

   a. The mean

   b. The standard deviation to the nearest tenth

X_i measure	f_i frequency
50	4
58	4
62	3
64	6
65	2
68	1

Date of Completion: ______________________________

Faculty/Supervisor Signature ______________________________

REFERENCES

Arroyo, C., Goldfarb, R., & Sands, E. (2012). Caregiver training in an AAC intervention for severe aphasia. *Journal of Speech-Language Pathology and Applied Behavior Analysis, 5,* 59–64.

Bennett, C. M., Miller, M. B., & Wolford, G. L. (2009). Neural correlates of interspecies perspective taking in the post-mortem Atlantic salmon: An argument for multiple comparisons correction. *NeuroImage, 47,* S125.

Bennett, R. J., Taljaard, D. S., Olaithe, M., Brennan-Jones, C., & Eikelboom, R. H. (2017). Evaluating random error in clinician-administered surveys: Theoretical considerations and clinical applications of interobserver reliability and agreement. *American Journal of Audiology, 26,* 191–201.

Bloodstein, O. (1960). The development of stuttering. II. Developmental phases. *Journal of Speech and Hearing Disorders, 25,* 366–376.

Crowley, C. C. (2018). *Effects of subthalamic deep brain stimulation on communication* (Doctoral dissertation). Adelphi University, Garden City, NY.

George, D., & Mallery, P. (2007). *SPSS for windows step by step* (7th ed.). Boston, MA: Pearson Education.

Goldfarb, R. (2006). Diagnosis. In R. Goldfarb (Ed.), *Ethics: A case study from fluency* (pp. 12–29). San Diego, CA: Plural Publishing.

Goldfarb, R., & Bekker, N. (2009). Noun-verb ambiguity in chronic undifferentiated schizophrenia. *Journal of Communication Disorders, 42,* 74–88.

Goldfarb, R., DeMetropolis, S., & Friedman, D. (2013, November). *Preference of orthographic vs. semantic distinctions in aphasia.* Paper presented at the American Speech-Language-Hearing Association, Chicago, IL.

Goldfarb, R., Eisenson, J., Stocker, B., & DeSanti, S. (1994). Communicative responsibility and semantic task in aphasia and "schizophasia." *Perceptual and Motor Skills, 79,* 1027–1039.

Goldfarb, R., & Halpern, H. (2013). Time-altered word association tests (TAWAT). Appendices and Website in H. Halpern & R. Goldfarb, *Language and motor speech disorders in adults* (3rd ed.). Burlington, MA: Jones & Bartlett Learning.

Gorno-Tempini, M. L., Hillis, A. E., Weintraub, S., Kertesz, A., Mendez, M., Cappa, S. F., . . . Grossman, M. (2011). Classification of primary progressive aphasia and its variants. *Neurology, 76,* 1006–1014.

Ioannidis, J. P. A. (2005). Why most published research findings are false. *PLoS Medicine, 2,* 696–701.

Maxwell, D. L., & Satake, E. (1997). *Research and statistical methods in communication disorders.* Baltimore, MD: Williams & Wilkins.

McElreath, R. (2015). *Statistical rethinking: A Bayesian course with examples in R and Stan.* Abingdon, UK: CRC Press.

Nuzzo, R. (2014). Scientific method: Statistical errors. *Nature, 506,* 150–152.

Plante, E., & Gómez, R. L. (2018). Learning without trying: The clinical relevance of statistical learning. *Language, Speech, and Hearing Services in Schools, 49,* 710–722.

Williams, F. (1968). *Reasoning with statistics.* New York, NY: Holt, Rinehart, and Winston.

Yairi, E., & Seery, C. (2017). *Stuttering: Foundations and clinical applications* (2nd ed.). Boston, MA: Pearson.

7

Journal Article Critique

INTRODUCTION

Educated consumers of research learn to be skeptical about what they read. Just because something has been published doesn't mean that it is a good study; it may not even be correct. However, the information gained from a single research article offers new perspectives with each additional reading. This section expands on concepts that we have discussed (Goldfarb & Serpanos, 2020) concerning professional papers written in the form of a journal article. In this section, I refer to the triangle and the spiral. The triangle, with the tip pointing down and the widest part on top ▼, refers to the strategy of presenting a broad description of the problem that narrows to focus on the specific questions of the study. For example, start with general problems of language comprehension and production in specific language impairment, and then narrow your focus to the specific kind of word-finding impairment that you are investigating in your study. The spiral (think of the coils of a Slinky) never completely closes but keeps on coiling around the different sections of a study. The terms in the title are explained in the abstract; the purposes of the study stated in the abstract are explained in the introduction; methodology and results spiral back to the abstract and introduction; and the conclusion addresses the hypotheses stated at the end of the introduction. Keeping these shapes in mind may help when writing a critique of a journal article (Box 7–1). The second-person (you) voice in this discussion is deliberate, so that as you critique a journal article, you can also consider what is needed to write such an article.

Learning Objectives

After reading this chapter, the student will be able to

- identify the structure of a journal article;
- control threats to internal and external validity of experiments; and
- explain the peer-review process.

Box 7–1. Template for a Journal Article Critique

Student's Name: ______________________________

1. TITLE drew your attention and identified target population and nature of study.
2. ABSTRACT included purpose, procedures, important findings, results, and conclusions.

INTRODUCTION

3. Began with a clear statement of the general problem.
4. Broad review led to a convincing rationale. Cite evidence of ▼.
5. Literature review was current (most within the last 10 years), thorough, accurate, and critical.
6. Hypotheses were motivated by the literature review.
7. Clearly written and well organized

METHOD

8. Sample size was large enough for adequate statistical power. How do you know?
9. Inclusionary and exclusionary criteria were clear. Were other participant characteristics missing?
10. Participant selection and assignment was random. Why or why not?
11. If two or more groups, was there overall or pair matching. Why?
12. Identified threats to internal validity. Describe.
13. Identified threats to external validity. Describe.

MATERIALS

14. Instrumentation (hardware and human/behaviora1) was calibrated and appropriate.
15. Evidence of reliability and validity of hardware and tests or measurements.
16. Experimenter and human observer bias was controlled
17. Environment was controlled by S^D, S^r, and S^Δ.
18. Instructions were clear. Describe.

19. Independent variables were clear. Describe.
20. Dependent variables were clear. Describe.

PROCEDURES

21. Research design was appropriate to purpose of study.
22. Addressed threats to internal validity. Describe.
23. Addressed threats to external validity. Describe.

RESULTS

24. Results related to research problem. Cite evidence of spiral.
25. Tables and figures related to text and were clear. Organization of data was clear.
26. Statistics were appropriate for the study. Describe measures of central tendency and dispersion.

DISCUSSION

27. Discussion related to research problem. Cite evidence of spiral.
28. Note limitations of the study.
29. Conclusions related to results and literature review.
30. Results were accurately interpreted, including unexpected findings and outliers.
31. Were previous studies and theoretical explanations supported or falsified? Cite evidence of spiral.
32. Clinical implications.
33. Suggestions for future research.

STRUCTURE OF A JOURNAL ARTICLE

Empirical research follows a standard format in designing and reporting the study. The journal article critique template (see Box 7–1) indicates the general and specific areas of evaluation that are also described in detail below.

Title

Similar to the introduction in a speech, try to get the reader's attention with the title of the article. Inform the reader of both the classification variables under study and the target population. Try also to attract the reader's interest, and, where possible, to limit the title to 10 or fewer words. Here are some examples of my own articles, with comments.

Goldberg, E., & Goldfarb, R. (2005). Grammatical category ambiguity in aphasia. *Brain and Language, 95*, 293–303.

Goldfarb, R., & Bekker, N. (2009). Noun-verb ambiguity in chronic undifferentiated schizophrenia. *Journal of Communication Disorders, 42*, 74–88.

Comment: These are examples of five to seven words used effectively to fulfill the requirements of a title cited previously.

Baylow, H., Goldfarb, R., & Steinberg, R. (2014). Swallowing effect and suspected neuromuscular fatigue in adults with acute stroke: A videofluorographic analysis. *Journal of Medical Speech-Language Pathology, 21*, 333–342.

Comment: This title does go on a bit, but the authors could not select an area for deletion without sacrificing an essential element.

Goldfarb, R., & Bader, E. (1979). Espousing melodic intonation therapy in aphasia rehabilitation: A case study. *International Journal of Rehabilitation Research, 2*, 333–342.

Comment: This title is a little too cute. The focus was on training the wife of the patient in the study, and the pun indicating that the authors were both advocating use of the therapy and using the spouse as a partner in therapy was probably lost to the reader.

Abstract

The spiral begins with the abstract, where the terms used in the title are clarified, elaborated, and defined. The abstract includes purposes of the study, a brief outline of the important results, and implications of the research. Some journals include key words and learning outcomes in the abstract, which generally should be limited to 150 words.

An abstract usually presents the problem under investigation in one sentence. This is followed by pertinent characteristics of participants, such as number, type, age, and sex (add genus and species for animal studies). Next, briefly describe the experimental method, including apparatus, data-gathering procedures, and tests. Then, indicate findings, including statistical significance levels, and lastly, conclusions and clinical implications or applications.

Introduction

Think of the literature review (or introduction in a peer-reviewed journal article) as a triangle with the tip pointing down and the widest part on top ▼. The first part of the introduction will have a wide view, such as a statement about language disorders in autism. As the review progresses, the focus will be narrowed to the current field of study, and will end with the hypotheses, such as which conditions lead to more paradigmatic word associations in adolescents with autism spectrum disorders. This section should serve to review the literature relevant to your study and to motivate your hypotheses. Your literature review should not be completely uncritical; that is, you should not merely report what others have done, but provide the following:

- an original synthesis of a large body of information;

- a theoretical basis for the research you are doing;
- alternative theories on the specific or related subject;
- an indication of what is valuable in these studies; and
- an indication of what is weak or erroneous in these studies.

The information in the introduction widens the spiral by referring to previous statements and providing much more detail. Begin with a general statement of the problem, and make this the focus of the introduction. Clearly specify, at greater length than in the abstract, the purposes of the study. Present operational definitions of any terms used in the title or description which may be interpreted in more than one way. For example, you may think the word "infant" applies to a human being under the age of 12 months. In fact, an "infant of the court" is an individual younger than 21 years of age. Present your information from many points of view, using a combination of mostly recent but some classical references, where appropriate. The best references are primary sources, such as journal articles, rather than secondary sources, such as books (even this one). The problem with secondary sources is one of depending on someone else's interpretation, rather than your own. For example, if you read a summary of Smith's article as cited in Jones' book, you are depending on Jones to report Smith's work accurately. You will be following the rules of good scholarship and will more likely be accurate if you go back to the original Smith article.

Finally, all roads in the introduction lead to hypotheses. You may present your hypotheses as statements or questions, but they must be motivated by the preceding review of the literature, and they must be falsifiable (remember that hypotheses may never be proven). Although it is not required in a journal article, I recommend that a new researcher write both experimental and null hypotheses (see Chapter 4).

Levels of Evidence in Literature Reviews

Not all evidence cited in the Introduction section of a journal article should be considered equivalent in quality. Remember to be skeptical as you read this section and do not accept what you read uncritically.

As noted in Chapter 2, there are four classes of evidence, ranging from randomized controlled trials (Level I), to prospective studies with an internal control group (Level II), to other controlled trials where outcome assessment is independent of patient treatment (Level III), and to evidence from uncontrolled trials, such as case reports and expert opinion (Level IV). Communication sciences and disorders (CSD) research with a clinical focus does not often include Level I or II studies, in part because of the ethical proscription against random placement of people with language, speech, and hearing disorders into a no-treatment control group. In some medical journals, clinical research classes relating to audiology (Wasserman, Wynn, Bash, & Rosenfeld, 2006) rank retrospective studies as Level III evidence, case series without a control group as Level IV, and expert opinion as Level V. Wasserman et al. note that clinical research studies in otolaryngology would benefit from higher evidence levels.

Methods

Subjects (or More Properly, Participants)

The spiral here refers back to the individuals or groups cited in the title and abstract and described in the introduction. Clearly identify the proposed population(s), as well as the bases for participant selection. If a control group is or is not being used, explain why or why not. What variables are you controlling with regard to participants? Why have you selected these and omitted others? In other words, what are the inclusionary and exclusionary criteria for participation in the study? If the study includes participants with communication disorders, how will these disorders be assessed? Who will perform the diagnostic evaluation? How will severity and type of impairment be controlled? Remember that certain uncontrolled variables, such as age, gender, education, and socioeconomic status can confound your results because there will be alternative explanations (e.g., one group is older than the other) for the findings.

As noted above, an important aspect of participant selection relates to criteria you will require for inclusion or exclusion of the person in the study. For example, if you are assessing effects of cerumen on conductive hearing loss, then you must exclude all potential participants who have a sensorineural hearing loss. If you are studying effects of providing an initial phonemic cue on word retrieval in nonfluent aphasia, then you must exclude individuals with fluent aphasia. Common exclusionary criteria relate to uncorrected impairment of vision or hearing in studies that assume typical hearing and vision. These criteria may also be rephrased as inclusionary, as in only participants with conductive hearing loss can participate in the first study and only participants with nonfluent aphasia can participate in the second study.

Materials

Will they be standardized? If not, why not? If equipment is to be used, how will correct calibration be ensured? Who is qualified to use this equipment? As noted below in the section on threats to the internal validity of an experiment, humans can also serve as instruments that require calibration. For example, you may assume that an audiologist certified with the CCC-A is qualified to conduct a complete audiological evaluation.

Procedures

How are you conducting your research? Describe procedures in sufficient detail to permit the study to be replicated every step of the way. How will the materials be presented? Why? Who will present these materials? Why? How will your participants respond? Why? Who will score the responses? How and why? Also note how the following (described in the next section in this chapter) will be controlled:

- order of presentation;
- randomization of stimuli;
- practice effect (learning to learn);
- recording of responses; and
- reliability of and correlation between or among scorers (see Chapter 8).

Results

The Results section continues the spiral. In the Results section, key findings of the study are reported, but not interpreted. A summary of the data is presented in table or figure format, usually following American Psychological Association (APA) 2010 style. The text should explain the main outcomes in sequence to address the research questions or hypotheses and refer to information presented in tables and figures. All findings should be reported, even those that do not support the hypotheses. A description of the statistical analysis of the data and outcomes should be included; complex analyses may be presented in a visual display.

Conclusion and Discussion

For the last time, the article should spiral back to earlier sections of the article. This section should include a comparison of findings in the current study to some of the research that was reported in the introduction section. The authors should explain any similarities or differences. Are the hypotheses supported (they are never "proven") or falsified? What do the results have to do with the theories that supported the hypotheses? Did the authors consider alternative theories or explanations? Was the importance of an underlying theory woven throughout the article? In clinical research, you should also address the following question: What are the implications for clinical intervention, diagnosis and appraisal, and future research?

References

References should be presented alphabetically in APA 2010 style, unless the article is published in a medical journal. This means that references appear in alphabetical order at the end of the article and footnotes are kept to a minimum, if they are used at all. References should not include abstracts and Internet sites (although peer-reviewed, online journals are fine). Unpublished observations and personal communications should not be used as references. Manuscripts accepted but not yet published may be cited, followed by a notation of "in press" where the year of publication typically would be indicated. All references cited in the body of the paper must be included, and articles not cited in the body of the paper must not be included in the reference section.

In group studies, a major goal is for the findings to be generalizable to a larger population (see Chapter 6). For example, a successful parent-training protocol to reduce stuttering in young children that was developed in Australia (see, for example, Arnott et al., 2014; O'Brian, Smith, & Onslow, 2014) should also work in the United States. The likelihood of this happening is greater if the original study can demonstrate that is valid. The next section addresses validity in experimental research.

THREATS TO INTERNAL AND EXTERNAL VALIDITY OF EXPERIMENTS

Validity means generalizability of the data. About 40 years ago, Ira Ventry, a professor and an audiologist, was one of our consultants at the Veterans Administration (VA) Medical Center in Brooklyn, New York, and the satellite extended care center in Queens, New York. He was writing a new book on evaluating research in CSD and wanted our feedback. The book survives him and is now in a seventh edition (Orlikoff, Schiavetti, & Metz, 2015). The information that follows is based on our initial conversations that have been updated as appropriate.

Internal Validity and Factors That Affect It

We need to eliminate alternative explanations that might account for the treatment effects because the fewer the alternative explanations, the greater the internal validity of the experiment. For example, an old therapy for stuttering required the individual to pace syllable production with an arm swing. While the rhythm of the arm swing was one explanation for increased fluency, the distraction of swinging one's arm cannot be discounted.

History

History includes events occurring between the first and second measurements in addition to the experimental variable (e.g., the child also began to receive speech-language therapy in school). For example, comic strip conversations between siblings, one child with typical language development and his older brother with autism spectrum disorders, may impress caregivers as an effective dyad-specific experience (Lewandowski, Hutchins, Prelock, & Murray-Close, 2014; Vivian, Hutchins, & Prelock, 2012). The social validity of other story-based interventions done in school may be influenced by the effectiveness of the comic strip conversations at home. It is not possible to control all effects of history because we want caregivers to provide language stimulation to individuals with communication disorders. It would be unethical, for example, to tell spouses of individuals with aphasia or parents of children with specific language impairment to stop talking to their family members for the duration of the experiment.

Maturation (Similar to History)

Maturation describes changes in participants themselves that cannot be controlled by the experimenter with effects that are attributed, incorrectly, to the experimental treatment. For example, in speech sound development, most triple consonant blends are not acquired until age 6. Working on these blends for years with younger children may yield changes that are caused by typical development and not therapy. Similarly, spontaneous recovery of aphasia after a stroke, claimed here as another form of maturation, may result in improved word retrieval even without therapy for aphasia. However, in a meta-analysis of 55 reports of aphasia treatments, Robey (1998) found that outcomes for treated patients are superior to those for untreated patients in all stages of recovery.

Practice Effects

The effect of the first test on the second test is sometimes called "learning to learn." Some students take a test preparation course for the GRE to get better at timing and other strategies needed for a multiple-choice test. Scores tend to be slightly better with improvement in these strategies, even if the content of the test is not covered in the test prep courses. In a CSD example, an individual tested without a hearing aid on in a speech discrimination test later shows improvement when the test is repeated with a hearing aid. We may conclude either that the hearing aid is beneficial or that improvement is a function of practice. We try to reduce the practice effect by randomizing order of presentation. For large groups, there are tables of random numbers that may be used as guides. For smaller-sized groups, some researchers use pseudorandom ordering, where, for example, no three consecutive occurrences of the same variable can occur.

Instrumentation

Changes in the calibration of a measuring instrument or changes in the observers or scorers used may produce changes in the obtained measurements. An audiometer that has not been calibrated in five years may not present pure tones at the frequencies indicated. There are also human instruments. Individuals who give a diagnostic test without being thoroughly familiar with the manual may score responses inaccurately, in addition to behaving unethically. For example, I had to complete a 40-hr training course to be certified to use the *Porch Index of Communicative Ability* (PICA; Porch, 1981, now out of print). In addition, there may be human instrument biases, such as in identification and prediction of naturalistic speech errors in Spanish (Pérez, Santiago, Palma, & O'Seaghdha, 2007) because of the unexpected locations of phonological errors.

Statistical Regression

Atypically high or low scores tend to move, or regress, toward a more typical mean score. A way to control this threat is by cutting off the ceiling and the floor. For example, for *Time-Altered Word Association Tests* (TAWAT; Goldfarb & Halpern, 2013), we present a 10-item pretest where individuals who get more than eight items right or eight items wrong cannot participate in the study. Instead of dealing with a range of 0 to 10, the range is now 2 to 8 so that individuals with scores indicating very mild or very severe language impairments are excluded.

Differential Selection of Participants

Differences between comparison groups must be minimized with the exception of the classification variable under study. For example, researchers may need to adjust test scores or norms in diagnosis of presence or absence of aphasia (Ross & Wertz, 2001). Demographic criteria such as age, education, or gender might influence differential diagnosis. Following are two examples of ways to control potential influencing factors.

Example 1. Assuming there is equipoise between the standard and new treatments, the experimenter must assign all children with the same articulation errors randomly to a standard treatment group or a new treatment group.

Example 2. The experimenter must not intermix disorders studied, for example, no conductive hearing losses in the sensorineural group and vice versa.

Mortality

Mortality refers to differential loss of participants between experimental and control groups or between other comparison groups. This does not mean that participants have died; they may have moved or decided not to continue with the experiment. A rule of thumb is to recruit 10%

more participants than needed for adequate statistical power, so that 33 participants should be recruited if the goal is to test or treat 30 individuals.

Hawthorne Effect

A participant's behavior may change simply because of the knowledge of participation in an experiment. It is an example of observation bias. The name comes from the Hawthorne Works factory in Cicero, Illinois, where changes in lighting and work structure at the factory supposedly improved worker productivity. However, the changes in worker productivity may have resulted from the attention paid to them. Telling a child, "Let's play a game with some pictures" is less likely to generate the Hawthorne effect than a statement such as, "Let's look at some pictures to see how many words you know."

Interaction of Factors

Two or more jeopardizing factors interacting can magnify the threat that each might pose individually.

External Validity and Factors That Affect It

External validity refers to generalizability. What is the likelihood or the extent to which the results from the experiment can be generalized to other similar people or other situations? The results of a study that cannot be generalized, such as in the single-subject or case series design, are less impactful than results of a group design that has meaning beyond the population tested.

Reactive or Interactive Effects of Pretesting

Participants exposed to a pretest may react differently to the experimental treatment from those receiving the treatment without the pretest. For example, consider a pretest that measures bullying in school in adolescents who stutter. An experiment focusing on coping with bullying might not be successful without the pretest.

Participant Selection

A difference or a relationship may hold true only for certain types of participants and not for others. For example, a cue of the initial phoneme may help word retrieval for adults with Broca's aphasia but not those with Wernicke's aphasia.

Reactive Arrangements

The Hawthorne effect may operate as a threat to external validity. Language in the clinic may not generalize to school or home. I recall a child on the autism spectrum leaving the university clinic after receiving therapy to improve spontaneous production of wh- questions and saying, "Who is it? What is it? Where is it?"—to a tree.

Multiple-Treatment Interferences

When more than one experimental treatment is administered to the same participants, it is not easy to erase the effects of a prior treatment. For example, in auditory processing of spoken stimuli, increasing speed of presentation may adversely affect the ability to repeat strings of syllables. The individual is still decoding the first few syllable strings and cannot attend to the new set of syllables.

Learning Style

Learning style is a typical or preferred way to absorb, process, and retain new information or skills. While not included in most lists of threats to external validity, every learner has a style. Individuals who have communication disorders may be less likely to apply style stretching when they need approaches to learning that they resisted in the past. A style is not a strategy, and adjectives such as analytical, visual, or communicative are often used to distinguish styles from strategies that are expressed as verbs (e.g., planning or remembering). Based on preliminary research (Griffiths & Inceçay, 2016), successful university students liked to learn by hearing the target language (aural style) while interacting with others (communicative style) in a pleasant environment (environmental preference).

Threats to internal and external validity must be controlled if you hope to publish or present your research in a peer-reviewed journal or at a peer-reviewed conference or convention. In the next section there are two examples (one positive, one negative) of manuscripts I evaluated as an ad hoc peer reviewer for two different journals. The reviews follow the structure of a journal article presented at the beginning of this chapter.

PEER REVIEW

Many professors who are active in research also serve as ad hoc peer reviewers for scholarly journals (Box 7–2). We do this to help maintain standards of the journal by publishing deserving work and, where possible, to offer suggestions to strengthen the manuscript. We also get to see the newest research before anyone else.

Kreiman (2016) reviewed the purposes and benefits of peer review in a Letter to the Editor in the *Journal of Speech, Language, and Hearing Research*. She noted that while many authors consider the peer-review process to be adversarial and would hesitate to undergo peer review if it were not required, the process has the following useful functions:

- allows editors to decide what should and should not be published;
- acts indirectly to educate researchers and to improve submissions;
- filters scientific information in a negotiation between author and editor about (dis)agreement with existing knowledge of theory and practice; and
- maintains, in an imperfect way, quality control in scientific publishing

Kreiman (2016, p. 2) continues her letter by noting that everything seems to argue against reviewing. The process is always time consuming, and sometimes even takes many days. It is always hard, rarely recognized, and never paid. Authors sometimes dispute or even ignore the reviewer's recommendations, and editors sometimes overrule them. Having been an ad hoc reviewer for seven journals for many years, I can attest to all of Kreiman's plaints about perceived peer-to-peer combat. Why do we do it? The simple answer is that we review because

Box 7–2. Invitation To Be a Peer Reviewer

Peer Review: Accept with minor revisions
Ref: Journal of . . .
Title: Something to do with communication in schizophrenia
Type: Research paper

Dear Dr. Goldfarb,

We have received a copy of the revised version of the above-referenced manuscript. I would be grateful if you could give me an opinion on its suitability for publication, as you very kindly reviewed the original version.

Our goal is to provide as rapid a response as possible to our authors. Therefore, please register your response as soon as your schedule allows. If you accept this invitation, your comments will be due by . . . The original referee reports, original version of the manuscript, revised manuscript, and the author's reply, including a detailed response to the referee reports, can be found by logging into . . .

To help you review this manuscript you are granted free access to Scopus for 30 days after accepting this invitation. Scopus is the largest abstract and citation database of research literature and quality Web sources. With Scopus, it is easy to find references, similar articles, or papers by the same authors. If you will not be able to provide comments within this time frame, please contact us immediately by clicking on the following link:

Yours sincerely,
JKL, PhD
Associate Editor
Journal of . . .

we enjoy mentoring others and serving our professions.

Examples of Peer Review

Following are two examples of my ad hoc peer reviews, one positive and one negative, with identifying information deleted (see Box 7–2 for an invitation to be a peer reviewer).

Accepted with Revisions

For the article that was accepted, I served as Reviewer #1 and a few of my comments appear in italics. The review was much longer and took about a week to write.

1. Introduction

Q. The second paragraph reviews literature that is 20 to 30 years old, and begins with "more recently." It is certainly more recent than the 100-year-old references that were cited in the preceding paragraph, but not current. The authors also neglected the discussion of "schizophrenic" language by linguistics in one journal in the 1970s (Chaika, 1974; Fromkin, 1975; Lecours & Vanier-Clement, 1976). They do not mention the notion of "schizophasia," although they use tests for aphasia in identifying language disorders in their participants.

R. We have now added the literature suggested by the two referees and mentioned the notion of schizophasia, as requested. We also made clearer that our communicative assessment is focused less on language abilities than on pragmatic abilities, expressed not only by language but also through gestures, prosody, and so on. Therefore, the references to the wide literature on linguistic or aphasic deficit in schizophrenia were necessarily reduced.

Q. There are also two instances in particular which posit troubling theoretical claims. The first suggests "difficulty in patients with schizophrenia in attributing mental states toward others during every day communicative exchanges." Do the authors claim that a theory of mind disturbance may be defined as a pragmatic deficit?

R. We thank the referee for his/her comment. We modified the utterance in the paper and briefly discussed in the discussion section, as also suggested by Referee 2, the role of ToM ability in explaining the pragmatic deficit of patients with schizophrenia. We did not claim that theory of mind disturbance may be defined as a pragmatic deficit. We are in line with Sperber & Wilson (2002), who argued for the existence of a specialized mechanism for the understanding of communicative intentions. We agree with the authors that the interpretation of utterances does not simply consist of applying general mind-reading abilities to a particular domain. By contrast, we think that communication requires a dedicated component, with its own specific mechanisms and application.

Q. Second, they claim that "the current literature on communicative impairments in patients with schizophrenia mainly focuses on linguistic abilities for communicative purposes." There is a substantial literature in neurolinguistics that addresses language deficits in schizophrenia resulting from functional frontal lobe deficits and temporal lobe overactivation.

R. We have now clarified that the area of interest of our study was neither language dysfunction nor neurolinguistic dysfunctions in schizophrenia, but the pragmatic communicative domain expressed by different means. We are aware that the current literature addresses different brain areas as responsible for language deficit in schizophrenia, but we believe that this interesting domain of research was not so central for our paper.

2. Participants

Q. There were a small number of participants (17), which, although acknowledged in this section, did not stop the authors from making claims in the conclusion and discussion sections that are too broad for the data collected.

R. We have now reworked the discussion section, introducing the small number of participants as one of the principal limitations of our study and scaling back our general conclusion.

Q. Criterion for inclusion was the DSM-IV, which is also noted in section 2.2 (Procedure). Although participants were taking typical neuroleptics, atypical neuroleptics, or "other medications," as indicated in Table 1, there should be some commentary in this section about medications. Dopaminergic medications may affect the excessive dopamine activity in the mesolimbic pathway, which may be the basic neurocircuit abnormality in schizophrenia, causing delusions and hallucinations.

R. In the current version of the manuscript we added the number of patients treated with typical/atypical neuroleptics, and a brief comment on their possible role in the emotional processing of patients with schizophrenia. However, the literature does not point out a specific role of typical/atypical neuroleptics in the pragmatic task performance of patients with schizophrenia.

Q. Uncorrected vision or hearing impairments should also be cited as exclusionary criteria.

R. We now explicitly cite the presence of vision or hearing impairments as exclusionary criteria.

3. Statistical Analysis

Q. The authors used a 2 × 3 ANOVA nine times (5 for comprehension and 4 for production scales), evaluations which are based on computation of mean differences. For these types of analyses, most studies strive to obtain a sample where N = 30*, because the difference between 30 and infinity is statistically trivial. It would have been better to analyze the data according to a repeated measures design (SPSS general linear model), in order to reduce the error term. Correlations between ABaCo and PANSS yielded what was described only as "a significant negative relationship." With the finding of* $r = -.55$*, the association is real, but not strong, which would be demonstrated by squaring the r and reporting a strength of association measure.*

R. We agree with the reviewer, and actually we used a repeated measures design in the previous version of the manuscript. We now make explicit, at several locations in the Results section, that we performed repeated measures ANOVAs for each scale. We apologize for the confusion we created. Moreover, we thank the reviewer for her/his suggestion: squaring the *r* value certainly makes it easier to understand the relation between the variables. In the current version of the manuscript, we report the r^2 value and make explicit the percentage of variance shared between the variables.

4. Results and Discussion

Q. That patients with schizophrenia performed significantly worse than controls is not surprising. The claim that the findings "confirm the hypothesis of a general difficulty by patients with schizophrenia to reason," as opposed to having "a simple linguistic impairment" is not supported by the data in the present study. Similarly, the study did not target inferences, and the authors should not make a claim that errors resulted from tasks requiring more inferential ability.

R. We have now rephrased all the ambiguous sentences.

Q. Finally, the authors assert that their study "testifies to the fact" of relative difficulty of certain pragmatic phenomena. A pattern of results does not constitute a fact.

R. We have now reworded the sentence as suggested by the referee.

Rejected Article

As this was an original submission, only my comments are included. I completed the review in two days.

Reviewer Recommendation and Comments for Manuscript Number J . . .

Title: Something to do with the language of schizophrenia

Reviewer Blind Comments to Author:

J . . . Review

The author presents a method for examining the story-retelling ability of 42 adults with chronic undifferentiated schizophrenia, using text analysis. The author hopes to provide new information about the ability of individuals with schizophrenia to adhere to themes.

The article is not recommended in its present form for publication in J . . . for the following reasons: poor professional writing and lack of adherence to APA style, inadequate and outdated literature review, and lack of in-depth analysis of the linguistic content of the samples.

Specific Comments

1. Overall, professional writing is not up to the standards expected for publication in a scholarly journal. There are many grammatical and punctuation errors throughout the paper. Introduction needs reworking; much of it should be condensed or deleted. There is substantial recent literature relevant to the language of schizophrenia that was not included.
2. Paper should use the phrase, "individuals with schizophrenia," not "schizophrenics."
3. Andreasen (there are two relevant papers published in 1979) should be credited for lines 30 to 36.
4. There is inadequate justification for use of "foible" instead of "disorder" regarding the language of schizophrenia, where there is abundant evidence of disturbance (perhaps a better word than "foible"), especially in semantic and pragmatic realms.
5. Use APA style (e.g., use ampersand, not "and," as in Mitchell & Crow, 2005, in lines 41–43; references in lines 50, 57; and period after "et al." in line 47).
6. References for linguistic deficits are very dated, with only one after 2000. This section needs extensive updating.
7. Historical review (40 years ago) should include the debate in the literature about the language of schizophrenia compared to aphasia, as well as the Breslau school (German) concept of "schizophasia." This is especially necessary in light of the author's claim that the study of schizophrenic language was "data rich, theory poor."
8. What the author describes as thematic discontinuity in story retelling that differs from the sample has been explained in other studies as examples of confabulation and propagation. What makes the new framework better than previous ones?

9. Self-continuous storytelling findings in the language of schizophrenia is not novel, nor does it help differentiate the language of schizophrenia from the language of dementia or even Wernicke's aphasia.
10. The study essentially represents qualitative research, but does not employ the triangulation method typical of such studies. Efforts at quantifying the data are shown only in very cursory analysis, such as presence of self-continuity. There have been many excellent studies of schizophrenic language using linguistic analyses, but these have all been much deeper analyses than the category-driven method described in the present study.

ADVANCED STUDY

The author proposes that skills in critiquing a journal article are necessary for an individual to be granted power of professor. With new generations of scholars and researchers needed every 10 years, professors and master clinicians have an obligation to prepare individuals with adequate knowledge and skills to undertake the tasks of scholarship and research, and critiquing a journal article is a key component. For evidence of the requisite skills in critiquing a journal article, complete the following and have your instructor, academic adviser, mentor, or CSD department chair review that you have completed the requirements and sign and date where indicated.

Student's Name: ____________________

1. What is the structure of a journal article?
2. How should you organize the information in the introduction section of a journal article?
3. What do I want the triangle and the spiral to represent?
4. What is the difference between internal and external validity?
5. Choose one type of clinical intervention in language, speech, or hearing and explain how you can make the treatment more valid.
6. Cite three ways that the authors of the accepted journal article successfully responded to the peer reviewer.
7. Cite three ways that the authors of the rejected journal article could improve their manuscript.

Date of Completion: ____________________

Faculty/Supervisor Signature: ____________________

REFERENCES

American Psychological Association. (2010). *Publication manual of the American Psychological Association* (6th ed.). Washington, DC: Author.

Arnott, S., Onslow, M., O'Brian, S., Packman, A., Jones, M., & Block, S. (2014). Group Lidcombe Program treatment of early stuttering: A randomized controlled trial. *Journal of Speech, Language and Hearing Research, 57*, 1606–1618.

Goldfarb, R., & Halpern, H. (2013). Time-Altered Word Association Tests (TAWAT). In H. Halpern & R. Goldfarb (Eds.), *Language and motor speech disorders in adults* (3rd ed., appendices and website.). Burlington, MA: Jones & Bartlett Learning.

Goldfarb, R., & Serpanos, Y. (2020). *Professional writing in speech-language pathology and audiology* (3rd ed.). San Diego, CA: Plural Publishing.

Griffiths, C., & Inceçay, G. (2016). Styles and style-stretching: How are they related to successful learning? *Journal of Psycholinguist Research, 45*, 599–613.

Kreiman, J. (2016). Letter to the editor: On peer review. *Journal of Speech, Language, and Hearing Research, 59*, 1–4.

Lewandowski, J. F., Hutchins, T. L., Prelock, P. A., & Murray-Close, D. (2014). Examining the benefit of including a sibling in story-based interventions with a child with Asperger syndrome. *Contemporary Issues in Communication Science and Disorders, 41*, 179–195.

O'Brian, S., Smith, K., & Onslow, M. (2014). Webcam delivery of the Lidcombe Program for early stuttering: A Phase I clinical trial. *Journal of Speech, Language and Hearing Research, 57*, 825–830.

Orlikoff, R. F., Schiavetti, N. E., & Metz, D. E. (2015). *Evaluating research in communication disorders* (7th ed.). Boston, MA: Pearson.

Pérez, E., Santiago, J., Palma, A., & O'Seaghdha, P. G. (2007). Perceptual bias in speech error data collection: Insights from Spanish speech errors. *Journal of Psycholinguist Research, 36*, 207–235.

Porch, B. (1981). *Porch index of communicative ability*. Palo Alto, CA: Consulting Psychologists Press.

Robey, R. (1998). A meta-analysis of clinical outcomes in the treatment of aphasia. *Journal of Speech, Language, and Hearing Research, 41*, 172–187.

Ross, K. B., & Wertz, R.T. (2001). Possible demographic influences on differentiating normal from aphasic performance. *Journal of Communication Disorders, 34*, 115–130.

Vivian, L., Hutchins, T. L., & Prelock, P. A. (2012). A family-centered approach for training parents to use comic strip conversations with their child with autism. *Contemporary Issues in Communication Science and Disorders, 39*, 30–42.

Wasserman, J. M., Wynn, R., Bash, T. S., & Rosenfeld, R. M. (2006). Levels of evidence in otolaryngology journals. *Otolaryngology–Head and Neck Surgery, 134*, 717–723.

8

Diagnostic Test Critique

INTRODUCTION

An article in *The New York Times* (Carey, 2007) reported a 40-fold increase in the number of American children and adolescents who were treated for bipolar disorder in the decade from 1994 to 2003. Almost certainly, the number has grown since then. There is little concern about the likelihood of a vast spike in the incidence of bipolar disorder, as the consensus is that doctors currently use the diagnosis more aggressively than before. The startling magnitude of the increase in diagnosis intensifies the debate over the validity and reliability of the criteria used for the diagnosis. If the term *bipolar disorder* is applied as a catchall for any child exhibiting explosive or aggressive behaviors, then far too many children are being treated with powerful psychoactive drugs with few demonstrable benefits and many potentially serious side effects.

Audiology and speech-language pathology also have a history of over- and under-identifying disorders. Ours is a faddish profession. When I was a student in the 1960s and 1970s, the term *cluttering* was widely used to describe rapid-fire, indistinct speech with some word-finding difficulty and lack of awareness of difficulty by the speaker. The diagnosis was virtually absent for the next 30 years. It seems to be reviving currently, in part because of the research efforts reported at an international conference on cluttering in Bulgaria in 2007 (Bakker, Raphael, & Myers, 2010).

We have recently articulated a rule about diagnostic report writing: Say what the client does, not what the client is (Goldfarb & Serpanos, 2020). The purpose of a diagnostic test should be to identify maladaptive communicative behaviors, not to provide a label. Ideally, a test for children will indicate what aspects of communication that should be present at or below a given chronological age are present, absent, or produced inconsistently. Therapy would then first address those communicative behaviors that should have appeared at or below age level, but are being produced inconsistently.

Learning Objectives

After reading this chapter, the student will be able to

- evaluate sensitivity and specificity of diagnostic tests;
- explain what motivates his or her decision to use a particular diagnostic test; and
- identify threats to validity and reliability in tests and measurements.

LEVELS OF EVIDENCE IN DIAGNOSTIC TESTS

The staff at the Centre for Clinical Effectiveness in Australia has developed a system for evaluating studies of screenings and diagnostic tests by assigning a hierarchy of evidence (Johnston, Burrows, & Raulli, 2003). Just as there are levels of evidence for studies related to clinical intervention, there are also studies of screenings and diagnostic tests that differ in terms of scientific rigor. A study assigned Level I is considered to be the most rigorous and those rated Level IV are the least rigorous and more susceptible to bias (Box 8–1).

The next section addresses problems in diagnosis, especially when attempting to differentiate among diagnostically related groups (DRGs).

PROBLEMS IN DIAGNOSIS: DUMPING IT IN THE CHOCOLATE

I supported myself through college by working in an ice cream factory. Occasion-

Box 8–1. Levels of Evidence Regarding Studies of Diagnostic Tests

Level I—Independent, blind comparison of an appropriate spectrum* of consecutive patients, all of whom have undergone both the study test and the reference standard.

Level II—Independent, blind, or objective comparison but in a set of nonconsecutive patients, or confined to a narrow spectrum of study individuals (or both), all of whom have undergone both the study test and the reference standard.

Level III—Independent blind comparison of an appropriate spectrum, but the reference standard was not applied to all study patients.

Level IV—Either reference standard was not applied blinded or not applied independently, or no reference test was applied (case series).

*An appropriate spectrum is a cohort of patients who would normally be tested for the target disorder. An inappropriate spectrum compares patients already known to have the disease with patients diagnosed with another condition, or with a separate group of normal patients (case-control).

Source: Reprinted with permission from Harris & Turner, 2011, p. 26.

ally, at the end of the work day, there was excess ice cream mix. The next day's run would start with chocolate and the excess mix would be blended in. Chocolate was strong enough in flavor and color to absorb the leftover. Continuing the metaphor, overdiagnosis may occur when a particular classification is the "flavor of the month."

Psycholinguistic Studies

Over the past 40 years, our research groups have developed linguistic tools to assist in the differential diagnosis of language disorders of adults with Alzheimer disease, vascular (frontotemporal) dementia, the language of schizophrenia, and various classifications of aphasia, as compared to control groups of typical young adults and typical elderly. The first group of studies, using word association of time-altered stimuli, tested semantic and syntactic hypotheses (for an overview see Goldfarb & Halpern, 2013). The second group of studies of communicative responsibility and semantic tasks yielded semantic and pragmatic language data (for an overview see Stocker & Goldfarb, 1995). And the third group of investigations of noun-verb ambiguity addressed neurolinguistic and psycholinguistic theories (Goldfarb & Bekker, 2009; Goldberg & Goldfarb, 2005). Characteristic patterns of language and communicative behavior were noted for all groups; the discussion was on implications for clinical intervention.

Our research has proceeded from the premise that linguistic data can aid in the differentiation of communication disorders in diagnostically related groups. The following hypothetical case description illustrates the need for differential diagnosis (Goldfarb, 2006):

> An elderly homeless man, identified as Mr. X because he cannot say his name, has been admitted with what the emergency room physician described as "disorganized language." The patient has no identification, no documented medical history, and has not yet had brain imaging studies.
>
> You have been asked to determine if the disorganized language represents fluent aphasia, the language of schizophrenia, or the language of dementia. The patient is referred to a speech-language pathologist at University Hospital. Evaluation of Mr. X's language reveals preservation of prosody, phonology, morphology, and syntax, with disturbances in semantics and pragmatics. This still fits the pattern of the diagnostically related groups of fluent aphasia, the language of Alzheimer and vascular dementia, and the language of chronic undifferentiated schizophrenia.

Differential diagnosis of alcohol intoxication (AI) as opposed to traumatic brain injury (TBI) can lead to tragic consequences. One of my patients at the Veterans Administration (VA) Extended Care Center in St. Albans, New York, needed to travel to our acute care affiliate in Brooklyn, a distance of about 20 miles, for treatment. The patient, a man of about 50 with TBI and ataxic dysarthria, was not ambulatory and had to be driven in the hospital van. The driver of the van experienced a sudden, fatal heart attack but was able to pull over to the side of the road and turn off the engine before slumping over the steering wheel. A short while later, two policemen arrived in a cruiser and saw the slumped driver. The paralyzed patient in the back tried to explain what had happened in his severely slurred speech. The officer responded to his partner, "They're both drunk. Let them sleep it off," and drove away. It took 4 hr for the hospital to send another van to get the patient and take care of the deceased driver. Needless to say, we prepared some in-service training for the police precinct on differentiating drunkenness from a speech disorder. This is not easy to do, as Shackelford and Nale (2016) reported substantial overlap between the signs of TBI and AI.

Neuroimaging Studies

The left perisylvian region has been classically described as the zone of language (see a review by Code, 2013). Damage following occlusion or narrowing of the left middle cerebral artery (MCA) can independently cause language problems (aphasia), speech articulation disorders (apraxia of speech), and many other deficits. Medicinal, mechanical, and surgical techniques have all met with qualified success in resolving thromboembolic occlusions in the distribution of the MCA.

In 1996, the U.S. Food and Drug Administration (FDA) approved the use of tissue plasminogen activator (tPA) treatment for managing ischemic stroke within the first three hours of onset. Unfortunately, cerebrovascular accidents often occur during sleep hours, and the 3-hr window is missed. In addition, tPA treatment can be contraindicated when the stroke is hemorrhagic, where such intervention can have devastating consequences. Such an outcome received attention in the case of Israel's former Prime Minister Ariel Sharon. He was comatose for some 10 years before he died because of improper administration of "clot-busting" drugs when he was having a brain bleed.

Mechanical removal of occlusions with the Merci retriever system was approved for use in patients with stroke in 2004. The Merci retriever works as a corkscrew that inserts into the thrombosis (clot) and draws it out. In one study (Devlin, Baxter, Feintuch, & Desbiens, 2007), single-center data focused on 25 consecutive patients where most instances of acute ischemic stroke followed isolated middle cerebral artery lesions. Successful reperfusion was obtained in about half of the Merci trials, although some patients with tandem proximal carotid and intracranial lesions were treated with carotid angioplasty and stenting, and not all patients were treated within the 3-hr window.

At present, decisions regarding areas for reperfusion—whether the intervention is medical, mechanical, or surgical—are based on an examination of the brain. The following sections address some of the limitations associated with visually based information.

Threats to Accurate Diagnosis

The advent of neural imaging techniques has presented a challenge to strict localizationists who posit direct brain–behavior relationships. Evidence of reduced blood flow, narrowing, or obstruction in the left hemisphere MCA should correspond with impairments in function associated with the affected portion of the brain. That this is not always the case points to shortcomings both in localizationist theory and in neural imaging, as follows.

Hypoperfusion

Magnetic resonance perfusion weighted imaging can be useful in identifying hypoperfusion (reduced bloodflow) of specific brain regions, which may be associated with disruption of selective language functions. Pharmacological blood pressure elevation may increase regional brain perfusion and language function. Reperfusion of the ischemic and dysfunctional tissue can reveal brain/language relationships before the reorganization that follows a stroke (Hillis et al., 2001).

Localizing brain functions has been typically supported by evidence of shared areas of brain damage in individuals with a similar language deficit, and is sometimes called the "lesion overlap" approach. That is, if there is a functional deficit, then the area of the brain damaged in most of these individuals must have been responsible for that function. When the reciprocal association, the probability that the lesion caused the deficit, is evaluated, then the relationship may not be supported. Hypoperfusion does not necessarily specify area of infarct. For example, structural damage or low blood flow in the left posterior inferior frontal gyrus may result in poor drainage into the anterior insula. Reperfusion of the anterior insula will not relieve symptoms of apraxia of speech, a motor programming speech disorder associated with left frontal lobe damage (Hillis et al., 2004).

Polytypicality

Many adults with communication disorders, such as adults with poststroke aphasia, display language characteristics that cross diagnostic boundaries. The polytypic nature of aphasia highlights the limitations of classifications that require separate groupings and imply independence of individual language functions (Schwartz, 1984).

Virtually all aphasias involve reduction of available vocabulary, linguistic rules, and verbal retention span, as well as impaired comprehension and production of messages. It is not unusual for a patient with Broca's aphasia, for example, to have difficulty in auditory comprehension, an impairment listed among the principal diagnostic characteristics of Wernicke's aphasia.

The combination of severe oral expressive deficit along with severe auditory comprehension deficit would probably be indicative of a global aphasia (Damasio, 2008). Although type of language deficit is usually a reliable predictor of site of lesion, the reverse correspondence does not hold as closely. The "exceptions," where lesions corroborated by computerized tomography did not predict type of aphasia, ran about 16% or about one in six (Basso, Lecours, Moraschini, & Vanier, 1985).

Brains Versus Veins

The underlying principle of functional magnetic resonance imaging (fMRI) is that magnetic properties of oxygenated blood are different from deoxygenated blood. The scan detects alterations in brain function or physiology associated with cognitive, motor, and sensory task performance. The gold standard of blood oxygenation level dependent (BOLD) technique is better than repeated injections of gadolinium (Gd) at generating images sensitive to the oxygenation level of blood. Arterial spin tagging is an approach similar to Gd, but arterial blood water is "tagged" magnetically using an RF pulse rather than by Gd injection.

Clinical applications have been limited to attempts to guide neurosurgery or radiation therapy to spare important functional tissue. Applications in neuroscience research include brain mapping studies using BOLD fMRI to assess language lateralization, word generation, and sentence comprehension. BOLD fMRI use in disease states has focused on recovery of language ability after stroke and mapping regional changes in activity during epileptic seizures.

Publication of more than 40,000 articles reveals functional brain imaging to localize behavioral and cognitive processes to specific areas in the human brain is often not confirmed by traditional, lesion-based studies (Ross, 2010).

The "brains versus veins" issue is related to the part of the functional signal that arises not from the brain capillaries and parenchyma (presumably at the site of activation), but rather from larger draining veins; accordingly, accuracy of localizing neural activity is limited.

Dumping It in the Chocolate

There are frequent instances in our professions where we metaphorically dump the diagnosis in the chocolate. Some gratuitous examples occur in the diagnosis of "quirky" children with unspecified communication disorders. Catchall terms begin at birth, where the diagnosis of FLK (for funny-looking kid) has only recently been discontinued. In the Middle Ages, the medical diagnosis for quirky children was humors of the liver; more recently, the children were diagnosed with brain fever, minimum brain damage, and minimal cerebral dysfunction. Currently, the chocolate into which many of these children's problems are dumped is the reticulolimbic complex of the brain. Better than humors of the liver, but not by much.

Increasing Accurate Diagnosis

An accurate diagnosis depends on using a test or assessment procedure that has adequate control of several factors. The following examples are taken from a study (Baylow, Goldfarb, Taviera, & Steinberg, 2009) comparing efficacy of the chin-down posture in reducing aspiration in acute stroke via bedside evaluation or videofluoroscopy.

True and False Positives and Negatives

In any comparison of a test result with an accepted standard, the number of true and false positives and negatives is calculated from a 2 × 2 table (Rosenbek, McCullough, & Wertz, 2004). True positives in the study by Baylow et al. (2009) were operationally defined as the number of participants who were predicted to have aspirated when drinking 1 cc of thin liquid without use of the chin-down posture on the clinical/bedside examination and who subsequently aspirated on video fluoroscopy (recorded in cell "a").

True negatives were the number of participants who were not predicted to have aspirated when drinking 1 cc of thin liquid without use of the chin-down posture on the clinical/bedside examination and who subsequently did not aspirate on videofluoroscopy (recorded in cell "d").

False positives (cell "b") were those participants who were predicted by the clinician to have aspirated during the clinical/bedside examination and who subsequently did not aspirate on videofluoroscopy.

False negatives (cell "c") were those participants who were predicted by the clinician not to have aspirated during the clinical/bedside examination and who subsequently aspirated on videofluoroscopy (Box 8–2).

Sensitivity and Specificity Data Analysis

Sensitivity and specificity calculations are used to determine the value of a test. Sensitivity refers to the proportion of participants who have the sign (e.g., aspiration on videofluoroscopy) and who were also predicted to have a positive sign (e.g., aspiration with and without the chin-down posture on the clinical/bedside examination). Sensitivity is calculated by the number of true positives divided by the sum of the true positives and false negatives [SENS = a / (a + c)].

Specificity refers to the proportion of participants who did not have the sign (e.g., no aspiration on videofluoroscopy) and who were also not predicted to have a positive sign (e.g., no aspiration with and without the chin-down posture on the clinical/bedside examination). Specificity is calculated by the number of true negatives divided by the sum of the false positives and true negatives [SPEC = d / (b + d)].

Positive and Negative Predictive Values Data Analysis

The positive predictive value can be defined as the proportion of the participants who were positively predicted by the clinician to be aspirating with and without use of the chin-down posture during the clinical/bedside evaluation and who also aspirated during the videofluoroscopy. The negative predictive value can be defined as the proportion of the participants who were positively predicted by the clinician to be not aspirating with and without use of the chin-down posture during the clinical/bedside evaluation and who also did not aspirate during the videofluoroscopy.

If the diagnostic instrument or measure you select controls for the variables above, you will reduce the likelihood of dumping your findings in the chocolate.

THE DIAGNOSTIC TEST MANUAL

All diagnostic tests have manuals that must be mastered before an audiologist (A) or speech-language pathologist (SLP) can implement the test. It is important to practice on typical individuals several times before attempting to use the test on clinical, experimental, or fragile populations. Test manuals usually include the four components of theory, development, administration, and scoring. The examples that follow are taken from the two tests on which I am a coauthor (Goldfarb

Box 8–2. True and False Positives and Negatives

Cell A: True positive	Cell B: False positive
Cell C: False negative	Cell D: True negative

& Halpern, 2013; Stocker & Goldfarb, 1995), as well as other sources. The manual (e.g., Goldfarb & Halpern, 2013) may begin with uses and abuses of the test and describe diagnosis, therapy, and professional preparation.

Theory and Development

Theory

A diagnostic test usually begins with a review of the literature that includes a historic perspective of the theories that underlie the current hypothetical constructs. It is often norm-referenced for individuals with typical and disordered communication. For example, in *Time-Altered Word Association Tests* (TAWAT), Goldfarb and Halpern (2013) describe how word association tests were originally used to generate psychoanalytic data (Gordon, Silverstein, & Harrow, 1982; Merten, 1992; Shean, 1999), and then review word association tests used for linguistic purposes. In the *Stocker Probe for Fluency and Language, Third Edition*, Stocker and Goldfarb (1995, now out of print) refer to Johnson's semantogenic theory (Johnson, 1955, 1959) and Bloodstein's continuity hypothesis (Bloodstein, 1970) and then address the aspects of communicative responsibility or level of demand for creativity that form the basis for the assessment and treatment described later in the manual.

The theory underlying an articulation test may refer to typical acquisition of consonant singletons and consonant clusters, as in the *Goldman-Fristoe Test of Articulation, Third Edition* (GFTA-3; Goldman & Fristoe, 2015). Theories of language acquisition in children, as reported in the *Clinical Evaluation of Language Fundamentals, Fifth Edition* (CELF-5; Wiig, Semel, & Secord, 2013), justify the 13 subtests in the areas of language content as well as expressive and receptive language.

In essence, the theory portion of a manual describes why the test exists and why there is a need for it. Later in this chapter, I will refer to *construct validity* or the degree to which a test reflects a theory of the characteristics to be measured.

Development

In the development portion of the manual, authors typically describe how the test was constructed. For example, the *Stocker Probe* has five levels of demand (levels of communicative responsibility) to identify stuttering in response to Levels I (either-or question), II (simple wh-question), III (more complex wh-question), IV (request for attributes or sematic features), and V (request to tell a story).

Although TAWAT is primarily a research tool, we established norms based on word association responses from more than 300 undergraduate students (Goldfarb & Halpern, 1984). A form of TAWAT presented to 91 institutionalized elderly individuals with and without dementia who resided in New Jersey (Santo Pietro & Goldfarb, 1985) was replicated by an independent group in Arizona (Abeysinghe, Bayles, & Trosset, 1990) whose results with an independent population of individuals with dementia were similar to ours. Other more widely used and well-known tests have normative data from much larger samples. For example, the GFTA-3 (Goldman & Fristoe, 2015) originally reported norms for more than 39,000 children from grades 1 through 12 and expanded new norms to include ages 2 to 21 in the most recent edition of the test. Some test manuals, such as the CELF-5 (Wiig, Semel, & Secord, 2013), report results of pilot studies to evaluate new items, verify basal and ceiling scores, and review items to minimize bias. There was also tryout research to include varied races and ethnicities as well as parental education backgrounds. Funding agencies may require norm-referenced data to determine whether or not a child can be approved for intervention services.

In the research that underlies the theory and development of TAWAT (Goldfarb & Halpern, 1981, 1984; Halpern, Goldfarb, Brandon, & McCartin-Clark, 1985; Santo Pietro & Goldfarb, 1985) and the *Stocker Probe* (Goldfarb, Eisenson, Stocker, & DeSanti, 1994; Goldfarb & Goldberg, 2004), we have tried to control threats to generalizability of the data (see Chapter 7) and have addressed factors that affect both internal and external validity. Our goal was to eliminate alternative explanations that might account for the treatment effects, because the fewer the alternative explanations, the greater the internal validity of the experiments (Orlikoff, Schiavetti & Metz, 2015). By presenting the complete TAWAT in one session, three threats to internal validity are avoided.

The first threat, history, refers to events that occur between the first and second measurements in addition to the experimental variable. If one were to administer, for example, the auditory portion of TAWAT and the individual with a language disorder receives speech-language therapy focusing on word association, then this history might affect the individual's performance on the visual portion of TAWAT when given at a later date. Similarly, there is a threat of maturation, similar to history, which refers to changes in the individuals themselves that cannot be controlled by the experimenter. When working with individuals with aphasia, particularly those within six months post-onset of CVA, spontaneous recovery may be a factor of maturation. Aphasia is a disorder that may migrate, for example, from jargon to Wernicke to anomic forms. Finally, there is no effect of mortality, or differential loss of participants in comparison groups, when TAWAT is given in a single session.

We have controlled for practice effects in the construction of TAWAT by using pseudorandom ordering of the stimulus variables, so that there are no three consecutive occurrences of any of the word parameters of grammatical class, abstraction level, frequency of occurrence, and length. It is important that in administering TAWAT, the clinician vary presentation of Lists A and B, as well as auditory and visual modalities and speed of presentation.

Regarding instrumentation, the computerized version of TAWAT is available for free (http://home.adelphi.edu/~go18170/tawat/newtest/test7.html). Speed of stimulus presentation has been calibrated to present visual stimuli at 20-ms (sweep speed) and 250-ms (fixation speed) exposures. Similarly, the auditory stimuli have been prepared, using audio editing software, to play at 10 to 14 phonemes per second (normal speed) and at 5 to 7 phonemes per second (half speed). Clinicians administering TAWAT must be sure to gain facility and confidence in the ability to score the five parameters of paradigmatic, syntagmatic, repetitious, anomalous, and unclassifiable by practicing administration and scoring on typical adults before attempting to test individuals with language impairments. Changes in scorers or observers may produce changes in the obtained measurements, but this is minimized by the strict definitions of the five parameters for classification.

One use of the TAWAT pretest is to reduce the possibility of statistical regression or outlier scores. Atypically high or low scores tend to regress to a more typical mean score. By using the ceiling and floor cutoffs on the pretest as exclusionary criteria, the likelihood of atypical scores will be reduced.

The manual for the computerized version of TAWAT (Goldfarb & Halpern, 2013) indicates the efforts the authors made to minimize differential selection of participants, where the goal is to avoid differences between comparison groups with the exception of the classification variable (e.g, an individual who is typical or has aphasia, dementia, or the language of schizophrenia) under study.

The Hawthorne effect occurs when an individual is aware of participating in an experiment. This effect is minimized by carefully reciting the instructions, as indicated in the "Procedure" section.

Among the factors that affect external validity, reactive or interactive effects of pretesting is important to TAWAT. Participants exposed to a pretest may react differently to the experimental treatment from those who receive the treatment without the pretest. Do not try to save time by skipping the pretest. Everyone who is given TAWAT must also be given the pretest.

We have normed the stimuli for TAWAT and have studied its effect on various typical and atypical populations. However, the relationships we have reported relate to populations and not necessarily to individuals. There may be a threat of subject selection to the external validity of TAWAT, as we cannot make predictions about the word association behavior of an individual participant.

It is possible for the Hawthorne effect to operate as a threat to external validity, a phenomenon sometimes called *reactive arrangements*. Presenting TAWAT as a therapy task, and not as a test, may reduce the Hawthorne effect.

Administration and Scoring

Administration

Before administrating a test, the SLP or A must be familiar with the materials and setup. For example, in the GFTA-3 (Goldman & Fristoe, 2015), the materials include the picture easel, the response form, the manual, and the supplemental developmental norms booklet; the setup requires a quiet, well-lit room and the examiner and examinee sitting across from each other. For the CELF-5 (Wiig, Semel, & Secord, 2013), Record Form 1 will be used for children ages 5 to 8 and Form 2 for children ages 9 to 21. The examiner may need to make accommodations, such as allowing extra time for responses, and modifications, such as rewording or presenting the instructions in both English and the student's native language.

As noted in Box 11–3 in Chapter 11, there are rules for test administration. Expressed as S^{Δ} (pronounced "S delta"), there must be no consequence for a response by an examinee. However, some seasoned clinicians do provide input where the response is a positive affirmation for pointing or page-turning behavior, so that feedback of "Good!" refers to good pointing and not to the correctness of the response. This does not usually work, as "Good!" tends to follow a correct response and something like "Okay . . . " follows an error.

There may be special considerations for administration of computerized tests. For example, TAWAT has a functional specifications document (Appendix A; Goldfarb & Halpern, 2013) for setup instructions before, during, and after the test; a description of the page components that are loaded dynamically; and navigation requirements. There is promise and there are threats associated with computer-based language assessment (Douglas & Hegelheimer, 2007; Jamieson, 2005). These include delivery and response technologies; authoring options; and scoring, feedback, and reporting systems.

Scoring

Accurate scoring depends on mastery of the underlying theory of the test. For example, TAWAT assesses the paradigmatic shift in vocabulary development. The five scoring options depend on the type of word association produced: paradigmatic (same grammatical class, as in an association of "up–down"), syntagmatic (different grammatical class or a grammatical continuation, as in "up–stairs"), repetitious (repeating the word or adding a prefix or suffix, as in "up–upper"), anomalous (a word association that cannot be easily explained, as in "up–green"), and unclassifiable (unintelligible, a multiword response, or no response). There is a help screen in the computerized program that lists the most frequent associations for each stimulus word.

Scoring sounds in words on the GFTA-3 requires knowledge of the International Phonetic Alphabet to indicate substitutions, omissions, distortions, and additions on the response form. Adding the number of errors yields a raw score. Finally, by using the examinee's chronological age, gender, and raw score the examiner can find the standard score in the chart provided.

Recording error responses is not as easy as it seems. For example, on the *Stocker Probe*, a fluent response is indicated with a check mark and a disfluent response receives a dash. Children routinely observe the examiner closely and say, "That was bad," "That was bumpy," or "I stuttered" when they see a dash recorded. Trying to avoid an adverse reaction may take considerable ingenuity, as when I used a check mark for a fluent response and a check mark with an extra line at the top for disfluent (Child: "Why does that check have a tail?").

In the video accompanying the *Boston Diagnostic Aphasia Examination* (Goodglass, Kaplan, & Barresi, 2001), the legendary aphasiologist Harold Goodglass demonstrates test administration and scoring. There are two instances when the man with aphasia says to Dr. Goodglass, "That wasn't right," and, "I got that wrong." So don't beat yourself up when you find it difficult to master the S^{Δ} strategy.

We now turn to assessment of reliability and validity of tests and measurements. Note that a measurement or test can be reliable without being valid, but if it is considered valid, it must also be reliable.

RELIABILITY AND VALIDITY OF TESTS AND MEASUREMENTS

Reliability

The term *reliability* means precision of measurement; it also refers to consistency.

You can set your scale at home to weigh everyone at two pounds lower than they actually weigh. The scale is reliable, but not valid. It is precisely wrong in the same amount, every time. On the other hand, validity, or the degree to which a test measures what it claims to test and the truth or correctness or reality of the measurement, depends on it also being reliable.

There are three typical ways to check the reliability of a test or measurement (Orlikoff, Schiavetti & Metz, 2015): test–retest reliability, parallel or equivalent form, and split–half. There is also another measure called interrater reliability that refers to human instruments or scorers. Consumers of research must be diligent in evaluating reliability measurements in test manuals, as reliability scores are often reported as statistically significant, but are rarely reported as weak. As noted in Chapter 6, the correlation coefficient r measures straight-line association, from −1 (perfect negative association) to +1 (perfect positive association).

There is a specific way in which r measures straight-line association. The square (r^2) of the correlation coefficient is the proportion of the variance of one variable that can be explained by straight-line dependence on the other variable. This is sometimes called the strength of association measure. Because r is almost always less than 1 (or more than −1) and r^2 results from multiplying a fraction, then r^2 will be a smaller number than r. As a general rule, r^2 greater than .80 indicates a strong association and r^2 lower than .60 indicates a weaker association. That is, even though a statistical finding may be significant, it may also be weak. A test manual may report a correlation of $r = .70$ with a very low probability of sampling error ($p >$ .01). The manual should, but usually does not, indicate that r^2 is less than .50, which means that less than half of the variance of one variable can be explained by straight-line dependence on the other variable, and the association is weak.

Test–Retest Reliability

Test–retest refers to a repetition of the same test where both sets of results should be identical, or nearly so. Threats to test–retest reliability include the practice effect, history, and maturation. If the test is repeated immediately, the second score may be inflated because the test taker has just practiced taking the test. Control of the practice effect by delaying administration of the retest may increase the threat of history or maturation. There must be enough time for the stimuli in the original implementation of the test to be forgotten, but not so much time that the child will learn more about the test stimuli in therapy or in school, or that the poststroke adult will experience spontaneous recovery.

Parallel or Equivalent Forms

In this test of reliability, there are two versions of the same test. For example, Form A and Form B of the *Peabody Picture Vocabulary Test, Fourth Edition* (PPVT-4; Dunn & Dunn, 2007) measure vocabulary at the same levels of difficulty. The total of 72 words in List A and List B of TAWAT are equivalent forms, with both including the 36 words needed to represent one instance each of three parts of speech (noun, verb, adjective), three levels of abstraction (high, medium, low), two frequencies of occurrence (frequent, infrequent), and two lengths (long, short): $3 \times 3 \times 2 \times 2 = 36$. Patterns of responses to List A and List B should be identical, or nearly so, if the test is given under the same conditions.

Split–Half Reliability

In most tests for split–half reliability, a test is divided into even and odd numbered questions, but the goal is to create two equivalent parts. Even if the test progresses from easier to harder questions or tasks, as most do, patterns of responses to the odd–even split should identical, or nearly so. Most tests progress from easier to harder examples in order to make it easier to get basal and ceiling scores, as well as to motivate the individual taking the test by building in success at the beginning. However, an alternative argument is to present the hard items first, when the test taker is fresher, and the easier questions later, when fatigue may set in, but this is seldom done.

Interrater Reliability

As discussed in Chapter 7, instrumentation does not refer only to an audiometer or a speech generating device; there are also human instruments. Assuming that raters have the same credentials, such as the Certificate of Clinical Competence in SLP or A, the ratings that two or more of these individuals provide should be identical, or nearly so. Interrater reliability is a correlation measure, so it is not surprising that the value of r will often be .90 or higher.

Validity

Validity means the degree to which a test measures what it claims to measure. Validity means truth or correctness or reality of measurement. Rosenbek (2012) has observed that as group studies research dealing with clinical intervention has improved in validity by controlling multiple extraneous variables, it becomes less likely that a clinician will find a representative of the group in the typical clinical caseload. In other words, the improved quality of the intervention research may make it *less* likely to be disseminated into clinical practice. There are three ways to establish the validity of a test or measure.

Content Validity

Content validity: a subjective procedure for logically or rationally evaluating items on a test to see how well they reflect what the tester wishes to measure. This is easy to understand in an articulation test where, for example, the bilabial sounds /p/, /b/, and /m/ are presumed to measure early sound development. The author of an articulation test subjectively chooses short, concrete words with bilabial sounds in the initial position that are of a low vocabulary level and that have a high frequency of occurrence in spoken word use. My particular bone to pick in terms of the content validity of articulation tests is the widespread use of the "medial" position of sounds in words. There really are only two positions of consonants in words, prevocalic and postvocalic. The /m/ in *hammer* is postvocalic in that it follows the vowel in the first (stressed) syllable, and the /m/ in *among* is prevocalic in that it precedes the vowel in the second (stressed) syllable. However, both *hammer* and *among* would be described as words with /m/ in the medial position.

Criterion Validity

Criterion validity: an objective procedure to determine how well the test or measure correlates with some outside validating criterion. There are two types.

Concurrent Validity. Concurrent validity: administering a test or measure and an outside validating criterion at the same time. This was reported in the first edition of the *Peabody Picture Vocabulary Test* (PPVT) where IQ scores were reported in the summary sheet because the PPVT correlated well with the *Stanford-Binet Intelligence Scales,* a standard of intelligence measurement since 1916. However, the authors (Dunn & Dunn, 2007) realized that a test of receptive vocabulary was an insufficient basis for reporting IQ scores and eliminated this assessment of concurrent validity in subsequent editions.

There is a rule, often violated in diagnostic tests, that concurrent validity cannot be demonstrated by comparing yourself to yourself. The *Minnesota Test for Differential Diagnosis of Aphasia* (MTDDA) (Schuell, 1965) can take up to four hours to complete. At one time, Schuell produced a short version of the MTDDA but later disavowed it as insufficient to assess an individual with aphasia. Had she published the short version, she would not have been able to claim concurrent validity with the long version. However, authors of many current tests claim concurrent validity when they compare the most recent edition to an earlier one. Of course, subsequent editions of tests are completely permissible and should reflect improvements over earlier editions, but there must be an outside validating criterion for concurrent validity. Otherwise, the claim of concurrent validity sounds like the claim of "new and improved" breakfast cereal.

Predictive Validity. Predictive validity: when a test or measure is used to predict some future behavior. The test is administered first, time elapses, and then the criterion measure is administered. For example, predictive validity might refer to a pretherapy measure to predict how much children and adolescents might withstand bullying following therapy for stuttering. Very few communication sciences and disorders (CSD) tests demonstrate predictive validity. The High-Overall Prediction Method (HOAP slope) of the *Porch Index of Communicative Ability* (PICA; Porch, 1981) had good predictive validity, but the PICA is now out of print.

Construct Validity

Construct validity: the degree to which a test or measure reflects some theory or explanation of the characteristic to be measured. If the test is valid *and* the theory is correct, then the test will support the theory. For example, a theory might predict that children on the autism spectrum might use vocabulary differently than typical age-matched peers. If a test or measure confirmed this, then the measure would have construct validity with respect to that aspect of the theory. Problems can arise, as in the "specific abilities" theory of the *Illinois Test of Psycholinguistic Abilities* (ITPA; Kirk, McCarthy, & Kirk, 1968).

As proposed by Osgood (1957), language can be described as a set of 12 specific abilities. The ITPA assessed language in these 12 areas and then prescribed therapy in the same areas for children who did not perform at age level. The problem is that language is more than a set of specific abilities. Grammatical closure is observed in spoken language, but it contributes to language much as a ball toss contributes to a game of tennis. A tennis player must toss a ball before serving, but expertise in ball tossing does not result in a successful tennis game. The latest revised version of the ITPA (Hammill, Mather, & Roberts, 2001) still tests 12 specific abilities.

CHOOSING WHICH TEST TO GIVE

The following is a list of possible reasons to give a test. Feel free to make more than one choice. Be honest, and then complete the assignment in Box 8–3. Afterward, see if your choices on the list change.

I use the __________ (fill in your choice of test) because it

is easy to learn;

is easy to administer;

is the test I learned in clinical practicum;

is the test I learned on a clinical externship;

is written by my professor or someone I know;

is the only one I know that is geared to the age group I need to test;

is the only one I know that is geared to the disorder I need to test;

has a theory I agree with;

has a broad search of professional literature in its development;

is worth the effort to learn administration and scoring;

has clinical applications I can use;

controls threats to validity;

demonstrates good reliability; and

has good sensitivity and specificity.

Box 8–3. Instructions for Writing the Diagnostic Test Critique

p. 1: Describe theory and development of the test.

p. 2: Describe administration and scoring of the test.

p. 3: Describe target population(s) and clinical applications based on test results.

p. 4: Describe control of threats to validity and reliability. If there is no section devoted to these issues, identify what is included elsewhere and what is lacking.

p. 5: Describe how the test avoids or does not avoid "dumping it in the chocolate." For example, consider true and false positives and negatives, sensitivity and specificity, and positive and negative predictive values.

ADVANCED STUDY

The author proposes that skills in critiquing a diagnostic test are necessary for an individual to be granted power of professor. With new generations of scholars and researchers needed every 10 years, professors and master clinicians have an obligation to prepare individuals with adequate knowledge and skills to undertake the tasks of scholarship and research, and critiquing a diagnostic test is a key component. For evidence of the requisite skills in critiquing a diagnostic test, complete the following and have your instructor, academic adviser, mentor, or CSD department chair review that you have completed the requirements and sign and date where indicated.

Student's Name: ______________________________

1. Before administering your next CSD test to a child or adult with a communication disorder, remember to familiarize yourself with the test manual and do a few "dry runs" with typical children or adults.

2. Write a five-page paper including the following:

   p. 1: Describe theory and development of the test.

   p. 2: Describe administration and scoring of the test.

   p. 3: Describe target population(s) and clinical applications based on test results.

   p. 4: Describe control of threats to validity and reliability. If there is no section devoted to these issues, identify what is included elsewhere and what is lacking.

   p. 5: Describe how the test avoids or does not avoid "dumping it in the chocolate." For example, consider true and false positives and negatives, sensitivity and specificity, and positive and negative predictive values.

Date of Completion: ______________________________

Faculty/Supervisor Signature: ______________________________

REFERENCES

Abeysinghe, S., Bayles, K., & Trosset, M. (1990). Semantic memory deterioration in Alzheimer's subjects: Evidence from word association, definition, and associate ranking tasks. *Journal of Speech and Hearing Research, 33*, 574–582.

Bakker, K., Raphael, L. J., & Myers, F. M. (Eds.). (2010). *Proceedings of the first world conference on cluttering. Katerino, Bulgaria.* Retrieved from http://associations.missouristate.edu/ICA

Basso, A., Lecours, A., Moraschini, S., & Vanier, M. (1985). Anatomoclinical correlations of the aphasias as defined through computerized tomography: Exceptions. *Brain and Language, 26*, 201–229.

Baylow, H. E., Goldfarb, R., Taveira, C., & Steinberg, R. (2009). Accuracy of clinical judgment of the chin-down posture for dysphagia during the clinical/bedside assessment as corroborated by videofluoroscopy in adults with acute stroke. *Dysphagia, 24*, 423–433.

Bloodstein, O. (1970). Stuttering and normal nonfluency: A continuity hypothesis. *British Journal of Disorders of Communication, 5*, 30–39.

Carey, B. (2007, September 24). Bipolar soars as diagnosis for the young. *The New York Times*, pp. A1, A15.

Code, C. (2013). Significant landmarks in the history of aphasia and its therapy. In I. Papathanasiou, P. Coppens, & C. Potagas (Eds.), *Aphasia and related neurogenic communication disorders* (pp. 3–22). Burlington, MA: Jones & Bartlett Learning.

Damasio, H. (2008). Neural basis of language disorders. In R. Chapey (Ed.), *Language intervention strategies in aphasia and related neurogenic communication disorders* (5th ed., pp. 20–41.) Baltimore, MD: Lippincott Williams & Wilkins.

Devlin, T. G., Baxter, B. W., Feintuch, T. A., & Desbiens, N. A. (2007). The merci retrieval system for acute stroke: The southeast regional stroke center experience. *Neurocritical Care, 6*, 11–21.

Douglas, D., & Hegelheimer, V. (2007). Assessing language using computer technology. *Annual Review of Applied Linguistics, 27*, 115–132.

Dunn, L. M., & Dunn, D. M. (2007). *Peabody picture vocabulary test* (4th ed.). Hoboken, NJ: Pearson Education

Goldberg, E., & Goldfarb, R. (2005). Grammatical category ambiguity in aphasia. *Brain and Language, 95*, 293–303.

Goldfarb, R. (2006). Differential diagnosis of adults with neurogenic communication disorders. In E. M. Welsh (Ed.), *Topics in Alzheimer's disease research* (pp. 89–109). Hauppauge, NY: Nova Science.

Goldfarb, R., & Bekker, N. (2009). Noun-verb ambiguity in chronic undifferentiated schizophrenia. *Journal of Communication Disorders, 42*, 74–88.

Goldfarb, R., Eisenson, J., Stocker, B., & DeSanti, S. (1994). Communicative responsibility and semantic task in aphasia and "schizophasia." *Perceptual and Motor Skills, 79*, 1027–1039.

Goldfarb, R., & Goldberg, E. (2004). Communicative responsibility and semantic task in the language of dementia. *Perceptual and Motor Skills, 98*, 1177–1186.

Goldfarb, R., & Halpern, H. (1981). Word association of time-altered auditory and visual stimuli in aphasia. *Journal of Speech and Hearing Research, 24*, 234–247.

Goldfarb, R., & Halpern, H. (1984). Word association responses in normal adult subjects. *Journal of Psycholinguistic Research, 13*, 37–55.

Goldfarb, R., & Halpern, H. (2013). Time-altered word association tests (TAWAT). In H. Halpern & R. Goldfarb (Eds.), *Language and motor speech disorders in adults* (3rd ed., appendices and website). Burlington, MA: Jones & Bartlett Learning.

Goldfarb, R., & Serpanos, Y. (2020). *Professional writing in speech-language pathology and audiology* (3rd ed.). San Diego, CA: Plural Publishing.

Goldman, R., & Fristoe, M. (2015). *Goldman-Fristoe test of articulation* (3rd ed.). Hoboken, NJ: Pearson.

Goodglass, H., Kaplan, E., & Barresi, B. (2001). *Boston diagnostic aphasia examination* (3rd ed.). Philadelphia, PA: Lippincott Williams & Wilkins.

Gordon, R., Silverstein, M., & Harrow, M. (1982). Associative thinking in schizophrenia: A contextualist approach. *Journal of Clinical Psychology, 38*, 684–696.

Halpern, H., Goldfarb, R., Brandon, J., & McCartin-Clark, M. (1985). Word-association responses to time-altered stimuli by schizophrenic adults. *Perceptual and Motor Skills, 61*, 239-253.

Hammill, D. D., Mather, N., & Roberts, R. (2001). *The Illinois test of psycholinguistic abilities* (3rd ed.). Novarto, CA: Academic Therapy.

Harris, C., & Turner T. (2011). *Evidence-based answers to clinical questions for busy clinicians.* Melbourne, Australia: The Centre for Clinical Effectiveness, Monash Health. Retrieved from http://monashhealth.org/wp-content/uploads/2018/11/Finding-the-Evidence_BusyClinicians2018.pdf

Hillis, A. E., Kane, A., Tuffiash, E., Ulatowski, J. A., Barker, P. B., Beauchamp, N. J., & Wityk, R. J. (2001). Reperfusion of specific brain regions by raising blood pressure restores selective language functions in subacute stroke. *Brain and Language, 79*, 495–510.

Hillis, A. E., Work, M., Barker, P. B., Jacobs, M. A., Breese, E. L., & Maurer, K. (2004). Re-examining the brain regions crucial for orchestrating speech articulation. *Brain, 127*, 1479–1487.

Jamieson, J. (2005). Trends in computer-based second-language assessment. *Annual Review of Applied Linguistics, 25*, 228–242.

Johnson, W. (1955). *Stuttering in children and adults.* Minneapolis, MN: University of Minnesota Press.

Johnson, W. (1959). *The onset of stuttering.* Minneapolis, MN: University of Minnesota Press.

Johnston, R. V., Burrows, E., & Raulli, A. (2003). Assessment of diagnostic tests to inform policy decisions—Visual electrodiagnosis. *International Journal of Technology Assessment in Health Care, 9*, 373–383.

Kirk, S. A., McCarthy, J. J., & Kirk, W. D. (1968). *The Illinois test of psycholinguistic abilities.* Urbana, IL: University of Illinois Press.

Merten, T. (1992). Word association and schizophrenia: An empirical study. *Nervenarzt, 63*, 401–408.

Orlikoff, R. F., Schiavetti, N. E., & Metz, D. E. (2015). *Evaluating research in communication disorders* (7th ed.) Boston, MA: Pearson.

Osgood, C. E. (1957). Motivational dynamics of language behavior. *Nebraska symposium on motivation.* Lincoln, NE: University of Nebraska Press.

Porch, B. (1981). *Porch index of communicative ability.* Palo Alto, CA: Consulting Psychologists Press of Nebraska (1957).

Rosenbek, J. C. (2012). The science of dissemination. In R. Goldfarb (Ed.), *Translational speech-language pathology and audiology* (pp. 37–42). San Diego, CA: Plural Publishing.

Rosenbek, J. C., McCullough, G. H., & Wertz, R. T. (2004). Is the information about a test important? Applying the methods of evidence-based medicine to the clinical examination of swallowing. *Journal of Communication Disorders, 37,* 437–450.

Ross, E. D. (2010). Cerebral localization of functions and the neurology of language: Fact versus fiction or is it something else? *Stroke, 41,* 1229–1236.

Santo Pietro, M. J., & Goldfarb, R. (1985). Characteristic patterns of word association responses in institutionalized elderly with and without senile dementia. *Brain and Language, 26,* 230–243.

Schuell, H. M. (1965). *The Minnesota test for differential diagnosis of aphasia.* Minneapolis, MN: University of Minnesota Press.

Schwartz, M. (1984). What the classical aphasia categories can't do for us, and why. *Brain and Language, 21,* 3–8.

Shackelford, J., & Nale, S. (2016). Training law enforcement officers to differentiate traumatic brain injury from alcohol intoxication. *Contemporary Issues in Communication Science and Disorders, 43,* 154–163.

Shean, G. (1999). Syndromes of schizophrenia and language dysfunction. *Journal of Clinical Psychology, 55,* 233–240.

Stocker, B., & Goldfarb, R. (1995). *The Stocker probe for fluency and language* (3rd ed.). Vero Beach, FL: The Speech Bin.

Wiig, E. H., Semel, E., & Secord, W. A. (2013). *Clinical evaluation of language fundamentals* (5th ed.). Hoboken, NJ: Pearson.

PART II

Producing Research in CSD

9

Mentoring

INTRODUCTION

Communication sciences and disorders (CSD) programs need to address the lack of mentoring for undergraduate student observers, master's students engaged in clinical practicum, and their clinical supervisors who are often doctoral students. All these students could benefit from mentorship by master clinicians and academic faculty (Box 9–1).

The strategies used in graduate academic and clinical education in speech-language pathology may be termed an apprentice model. The graduate student, or apprentice, is ideally educated by speech, language, and hearing scientists as well as master clinicians who are also professors of courses in communication disorders and clinical supervisors. Mentoring is also important in undergraduate education as a means of retention and enrichment (Jacobi, 1991). Mentorship is different from apprenticeship in that the mentor may also be a benefactor. That is, the mentor may be an advocate for the student, offering solutions to problems and influence with job contacts (Siddiqui, 2014). One substantial problem is that there is no operational definition of mentoring that is agreed upon in the literature. Another is a lack of empirical data indicating the effectiveness of mentoring in helping students achieve academic success. In this chapter, these two problems will be considered as they relate to undergraduate, master's, and doctoral students. The model of mentoring developed by the American Speech-Language-Hearing Association (ASHA) will be highlighted.

Box 9–1. Academic Mentoring

Graduate
- Student may be an apprentice
- Mentor may be a benefactor

Undergraduate
- Retention and enrichment

Learning Objectives

After reading this chapter, the student will be able to

- establish mentor–student relationships;
- establish peer mentoring relationships; and
- end or advance mentoring relationships.

Box 9–2. The Mentor–Student Relationship

Traditional mentoring

From an older, more experienced person to a younger, less experienced person

An explicit or implicit transfer of knowledge, craft, and wisdom

ASHA S.T.E.P. mentoring

Other mentoring roles

Facilitating transitions in education and employment

Peer mentoring

Distance mentoring

Research mentoring

Shifting the power differential

Formal and informal mentoring

WHAT IS THE MENTOR–PROTÉGÉ OR MENTOR–MENTEE (HEREAFTER CALLED MENTOR–STUDENT) RELATIONSHIP?

Mentor was the name of an old man in Greek mythology (Homer, 1969). He took care of the boy Telemachus whose father, Odysseus (Ulysses), went on a 10-year adventure. Mentor provided emotional support and guidance to Telemachus, saving his life on occasion, and helping the boy become a young man. The concept of mentoring usually refers to a mature person who works with a younger individual (Box 9–2).

Definition of Mentoring

This discussion begins with an operational definition of mentoring. As noted above, there is a lack of universal agreement on what such a definition should be. Typically, mentoring is seen as an explicit and implicit transference of knowledge, craft, and wisdom (Siddiqui, 2014). A person with authority offers advice and opportunity to the student. The mentor has more skill and knowledge than the student, and the highest moral and professional values. Mentorship also requires time, commitment, and altruism. Eby, Allen, Evans, Ng, and DuBois (2008) summarized several concepts of mentoring appearing in the literature. They included youth, academic, and workplace areas of mentoring research, but the present text considers only the academic setting. In the academic context, research has focused on the retention, success, and academic adjustment of college students. According to the ASHA website for the S.T.E.P. (Student to Empowered Professional) mentoring program, available online at http://www.asha.org/students/gatheringplace/step/, "Mentoring is a developmental partnership through which one person shares knowledge, skills, information, and perspective to foster the personal and professional growth of someone else" (ASHA, 2004).

In the typical academic mentor–student relationship, the professor passes on knowledge of subject matter, helps the student make wise choices, and helps the student make transitions (e.g., from undergraduate to graduate student, from graduate student to clinical fellow, or from doctoral student to post-doctoral fellow or junior faculty member). Most definitions of mentoring also include facilitating personal development of the student. Ragins and Cotton (1999) reiterate the notion that a mentor is an individual who has advanced experience and knowledge, and they add that a mentor makes a commitment to provide upward support and mobility to the student's trajectory in school and in professional practice. In another broad consideration of academic mentoring, a student without a mentor will learn less well or more slowly. The mentor has also been described as an advisor, counselor, confidant, advocate, cheerleader, and listener (Inzer & Crawford, 2005).

Peer Mentoring

Another model of mentoring called peer mentoring dispenses with the requirement that the mentor is older and more experienced; rather, the peer mentor merely has more knowledge of a particular context. For example, a peer mentor may be a colleague at the university who has been in the department longer. As an example, when I accepted early retirement from the City University of New York and went to Adelphi University, I was assigned a peer mentor who was much younger and at a lower rank. However, she was helpful in my transition to a new environment and was a useful source of information about the new institution. We both recognized that there was value in and something to gain from this relationship. Indeed, we have subsequently coauthored four books. A peer mentor may also be a friend or a career guide.

Distance Mentoring

Nick et al. (2012) described a formal distance mentoring program. It incorporated the four pillars of mentoring excellence recognized as best practices in nursing, adapted here for CSD. They include the following: orientation to the faculty role; socialization to the academic community; development of teaching, research, and clinical skills; and grooming future CSD leaders (Nick et al., 2012, p. 3). Keyser et al. (2008) developed a self-assessment tool for universities to use in evaluating research mentorship. They identified the five domains of research mentorship, including the following: criteria for selecting mentors; incentives for faculty to serve as research mentors; facilitating the mentor–student relationship; strengthening the student's ability to conduct responsible research; and professional development of both mentor and student. Their self-assessment tool includes domains for research mentors (qualifications, identification, recruitment and training), for mentor incentives (promotion and tenure, recognition and awards, and evaluation), for the mentor–student relationship (matching mentors and students, guidelines and oversight, brokering and managing, conducting research, and reporting and reviewing research), and for mentor–student professional development (reporting and presenting, publishing, networking, and obtaining funding).

Mentoring of Student Clinicians by Clients

Purves, Petersen, and Puurveen (2013) proposed a unique model of mentorship, where adults with aphasia mentored student clinicians. The authors, from the University of British Columbia in Canada, partnered with 12 adults with chronic aphasia to mentor students studying speech-language pathology and other health professions. The didactic portion of the mentoring program employed panel discussions of living with aphasia, as well as smaller groups sharing stroke stories. There were other more social activities, such as field trips to places of interest on campus that were chosen by the mentors.

Perspectives of mentors at the end of the study were nuanced in that some members focused on getting better (recovering language skills), while other members focused on their roles as mentors ("helping others helps me"; Purves et al., 2013, p. S374).

Perspectives of students included an appreciation of both shifting the typical power differential between clinician and client as well as collaborative learning. They also experienced the different distribution of responsibilities in the groups. Opportunities for socialization led students to see mentors as a "persons first," rather than as aphasic adults. While students rarely described group members with aphasia as "mentors," they reported the experience as supporting student learning.

Mentor–Student Relationships

The mentor–student relationship may be formal or informal (Ragins & Cotton, 1999). Formal mentor–student relationships are usually institutionalized; for example, the student is assigned a mentor when declaring a major or when registering for clinical practicum. An informal mentoring relationship may develop spontaneously, as when a student volunteers and is chosen to be a research assistant to a faculty member. The duration of the formal relationship is usually shorter than that of the informal relationship. In informal mentoring, either person may initiate the mentoring relationship. The mentor may offer help and the student may seek to gain wisdom from a trusted person (Inzer & Campbell, 2005).

Horner and Minifie (2011) addressed the responsible conduct of research (RCR) in a series of three articles, the second of which addressed mentoring, collaboration, peer review, and data management and ownership. They began their review by stating that the responsibility to mentor new generations of researchers comes from the duty we owe to those who mentored us. They cite and review purposes and designs of mentorship as well as characteristics of mentors by referring to original sources also included in the present chapter. They also raised cautionary notes about mentoring by questioning how institutions cover the material required for RCR. In research, financial, personal, and ethics mentoring, a set of problematic behaviors were noted in the literature, including concerns about handling data, methods, policy, use of funds, outside influence, peer review, credit, and cutting corners (Horner & Minifie, 2011, p. S333).

DOES MENTORING WORK? (Box 9–3)

Eby et al. (2008) conducted a meta-analysis of more than 15,000 articles and reports of mentoring research, asking if mentoring matters, and if so, how much? A total of 112 studies and reports met all eligibility criteria.

Box 9–3. Efficacy of Mentoring

Outcomes of academic mentoring

- Behavioral
- Attitudinal
- Health related
- Relational
- Motivational
- Career

Types of mentoring for graduate students and junior faculty

- Career mentoring
- Scholarly mentoring
- Comentoring

Managing up

Academic Mentoring

Target behavioral outcomes of academic mentoring typically include an increase in academic performance and a decrease in such maladaptive behaviors as drug, alcohol, and sexual abuse. Target attitudinal outcomes might include an increase in participation in university activities as well as loyalty to the university, or school spirit. Positive health-related outcomes might occur when a mentor challenges a student's negative self-views or by engaging with the student in activities that promote better health, such as exercise. Relational outcomes reflect a mentor's impact on a student's expectations of interpersonal relationships with others. A mentor's influence on motivational outcomes might be to help a student set achievable goals and stay focused on relevant tasks, such as school assignments as opposed to video games. Lastly, career outcomes refer to the mentor's ability to enhance the student's acquisition of knowledge and skills, as reflected on the KASA (knowledge and skills assessment) forms that students maintain throughout their graduate education in ASHA-accredited master's degree programs.

In summary, Eby et al. (2008) proposed the hypothesis that mentoring is associated with positive behavioral outcomes, attitudinal outcomes, health-related outcomes, relational outcomes, motivational outcomes, and career outcomes. Effect sizes were greatest between mentoring and helping others, improving school attitudes, and in establishing positive career attitudes. The least effective associations, although they were still statistically significant, were between mentoring and reduced psychological stress and deviant behavior, and between mentoring and increases in career recognition and self-esteem.

Feldman, Arean, Marshall, Lovett, and O'Sullivan (2010; see also Johnson, Subak, Brown, Lee, & Feldman, 2010) surveyed 464 junior faculty members at the University of California, San Francisco (UCSF) to determine the characteristics of having a mentor, and 319 of the respondents reported having a mentor. Neither gender nor ethnicity had any effect on mentoring, but there were many other statistically significant findings that indicated mentoring works for faculty development in health science institutions. While the programs evaluated at UCSF were dentistry, medicine, nursing, and pharmacy, many of the findings apply to our own health profession of CSD. Feldman et al. (2010) and Johnson et al. (2010) indicated that similar programs have been developed for graduate students, medical students, and trainees at the university. UCSF established awards to recognize excellence in mentorship; there are also mentor development activities and mentoring resources.

Other Types of Mentoring

UCSF uses three different types of mentoring. The career mentor, who is not the same person as the supervisor, provides career guidance and support. The scholarly mentor, who is in the same research field, helps coordinate a feasible research plan, and helps with networking and access to potential funding resources. There is also a comentor in the junior person's area of expertise who works with the lead mentor on overall mentoring responsibilities. Feldman et al. (2010) reported that their results supported two conclusions about the positive effects of mentoring on junior faculty: they were more satisfied with the distribution of their workload; and they had higher self-efficacy than faculty who were not mentored. Feldman et al. (2010) defined self-efficacy as the belief in the ability to accomplish specific tasks and goals.

Kram (1985) proposed a mentor-role theory where the functions of mentors are in two broad categories. The first function is career development; certainly this is important, but it occurs after the mentor–student relationship is completed. In Kram's theory, the five career development functions of a mentor are sponsoring, coaching, protecting, challenging assignments, and increasing exposure and visibility. The second broad category of psychological functions charges the mentor to enhance the student's sense of competence, self-efficacy, professional development, and personal development.

Managing Up

"Managing up" is another strategy, borrowed from the business world, that has shown effectiveness in mentoring relationships with students through junior faculty (Zerzan, Hess, Schur, Phillips, & Rigotti, 2009). Adapted for graduate students in CSD, the checklist for managing up to create successful mentoring should include six categories.

Checklist for Managing Up

1. To get ready for the mentorship relationship, the student needs to have clear values; know work style and habits; recognize gaps in

knowledge and skills; understand what is needed for personal, professional, academic, skill, and research development; and list the specific opportunities sought. The student should write goals for 3 months, 1 year, and 5 years.

2. To find a mentor or mentors, the student needs to meet with peers and get recommendations, be persistent, and select multiple possible mentors. For all students, but especially those at the doctoral level, where the mentor may have many roles (adviser, dissertation chair, lead author), students should study the faculty profiles of all potential mentors to see if areas of expertise and research match their own interests.
3. The qualities of a mentor should include one who is available and accessible, has prior mentoring experience, and who will let the student establish the agenda and take risks.
4. At the first meeting, students should share their background, values, and needs; indicate how the mentor's prior research and teaching have already helped; and send an email (not a text) thank-you note after the meeting.
5. The student needs to cultivate the mentoring relationship by agreeing on the objectives and structure of the relationship, planning and setting meeting agendas, asking questions and for feedback, listening actively, and always following through on assignments. The mentor and student manage up by setting joint goals and expectations, being responsible and flexible, directing the flow of information, and following a regular meeting schedule with a specified agenda.
6. Finally, it is time for the mentor–student relationship to end. This separation should include talking about the next steps in the student's academic and professional career, as well as future mentors.

Summary

In summary, academic mentoring works, although it has been assessed only by statistical analysis of population studies and may not apply to an individual mentor–student relationship. In addition, formal versus informal mentoring and peer versus apprentice-model mentoring have not been evaluated to determine if one type is more effective than another, and to whom the mentoring model should be assigned.

DO BEING OLDER, HAVING MORE EXPERIENCE, AND HAVING GREATER PROFESSIONAL AUTHORITY QUALIFY AN INDIVIDUAL TO BE A MENTOR?

The answer to the question is, obviously, no. As noted above, a peer mentor may be less experienced and younger, but may be a successful mentor because of greater familiarity with institutional structures. There are also theories and practice guidelines regarding successful mentorship; one is not a "natural" mentor (Box 9–4). Johnson et al. (2010) discussed the need

Box 9–4. Characteristics of a Good Mentor

Theory and practice guidelines

Mentoring students in conducting research

Skills of a good mentor

for mentoring students in conducting research with the following outcomes:

- *Career commitment and satisfaction.* Mentoring at the start can avoid burnout at the end.
- *Confidence in research skills.* There can be a natural progression from being a consumer of research to designing studies as a producer of research.
- *Securing funding.* The most successful grants tend to come from laboratories that have received them in the past. Mentoring is essential to developing successive generations of grant writers.
- *Dissemination.* As Kent (2012) has noted, translational research in speech-language pathology and audiology involves bench-to-bedside and bedside-to-community research. Translational research depends on dissemination, a science in itself (Rosenbek, 2012). Kent (2012, p. 27) defined the essence of translational research as "discovery to delivery," and Rosenbek (2012, pp. 37–38) noted that clinical practice is not sufficiently altered by publication and continuing education alone. We need more ways to move new therapies from academic to nonacademic settings.

Bhagia and Tinsley (2000, p. 536) listed what they considered to be commonly recognized characteristics and skills of a good mentor. A mentor should be self-confident, inspirational, supportive, generous with time and energy, competent, friendly, honest, and respectful of the student's goals. A mentor should motivate, empathize, tolerate being a learner, be accessible, ask thought-provoking questions, build relationships, provide professional growth, and give constructive feedback.

WHAT ARE THE ETHICAL CONCERNS OF A RELATIONSHIP WITH A LARGE POWER DIFFERENTIAL? (Box 9–5)

About 20 years ago, as executive officer of the largest doctoral program in speech-language-hearing sciences in the United States (the CUNY Graduate School and University Center), I had a productive meeting with my colleagues on the issue of coercion. We were required by ASHA to end our policy of guiding our students through an en route master's degree pro-

Box 9–5. Ethical Concerns

Power differential between mentor and student

Conflicts of interest

Coercion

Autonomy of students

Informed consent

gram that would lead to the Certificate of Clinical Competence, as our program specifically led only to the doctorate. However, 14 students remained who were accepted into the program with the understanding that they would earn both the PhD and the ASHA CCC. Although we worked out an agreement with our national organization for these students, an ethical problem remained.

The 14 students would need externship placements, most likely with supervisors who did not have a PhD degree. Our concern was that some of the supervisors, who might apply for admission to our program in the future, might feel coerced to accept our student clinicians in order to curry favor for subsequent admission or to avoid possible negative feelings from our faculty if they refused to accept the student clinician. In other words, externship supervisors might feel a conflict of interest between our request for them to accept a student in a clinical placement and their own desire to pursue a doctorate at a future date. We agreed to proceed with the placements because there was no logical alternative, and the arrangements for externship placements would end once the 14 students completed their en route master's degree.

The example described previously illustrates how difficult it can be for individuals such as mentors who are in positions of power over students. We are guided in our decisions by the Belmont Report (*National Commission, 1979)* and by the ASHA Revised Code of Ethics (ASHA, 2016). Detailed discussion of both documents appear in Chapter 3, but the relevant items in the Belmont Report have to do with Respect for Persons and Informed Consent, and the relevant portions of the Code of Ethics are in Terminology ("conflict of interest" and "informed consent") and Principle of Ethics IV (Rules of Ethics E, G, H, I, J, L, and R; see Chapter 3).

Respect for persons, according to the Belmont Report has two ethical concerns, but only one applies to the mentor–student relationship. The ethical conviction that does not apply refers to individuals with diminished capacity. The conviction that is relevant to a mentoring model is that individuals should be considered as autonomous agents. This means that these individuals, students in the present case, are able to deliberate and act following this deliberation regarding their personal (and professional) goals. Mentors may not obstruct the actions of their students unless these actions are detrimental to students themselves or others. In other words, student actions should not be restricted to reflect the preferences of the mentors. In terms of clinical practicum, the Belmont Report seems to speak strongly in favor of best practices, and discourages clinical practice that is not evidence-based. Mentors must show respect for students and must not withhold information necessary for the student to make a considered judgment. However, there may be circumstances, such as when giving a student a test, when a mentor withholds necessary information temporarily.

Informed consent (see Chapter 3 for more details) requires that mentors allow students to choose what will happen to them. The elements of the informed consent process include information, comprehension, and voluntariness. In other words, the mentor is obliged to share knowledge, skills, information, and perspective with the student; make sure that the student understands what has been shared; and ensure that the subsequent actions of the student are voluntary and not coerced.

Adapted for the mentor–student relationship, the revised Code of Ethics (ASHA, 2016) considers conflict of interest to occur when private interests of the student are in opposition to those of the person (mentor) who is in a position of trust and who has greater power and authority. A mentor must provide information concerning expected outcomes and potential risks to a student. The student may consent verbally, unless written informed consent is required.

The following is adapted from Principle of Ethics IV, Rules of Ethics (ASHA, 2016) to reflect the mentor–student relationship:

E. Both mentors and students must be honest with each other. There must be no tolerance for negligence, fraud, deceit, or misrepresentation on either side.

G. Because of the power differential, mentors must strive to avoid even the appearance of harassment (physical, sexual, or emotional) or abuse their power over the student.

H. This should be obvious, but mentors and students shall not engage in sexual activities. This author recommends that individuals who are married or in a prior consensual relationship not participate in a mentor–student relationship.

I. Mentors must ensure that their students do not engage in practices that violate the Code of Ethics.

J. When a student is a mentor's research assistant, credit in subsequent convention presentations or publications will be based on the proportion of the contribution by each party. This author recommends that the mentor go further and clarify if the student will be a coauthor or will be acknowledged at the end of the paper. Typically, the mentor has the idea for the research project and designs the study; and, thus, is the first author. The mentor who is also a laboratory director is also typically the corresponding author.

L. In addition to the protected classes noted in the Belmont Report (1979), the revised Code of Ethics adds culture, language, dialect, or socioeconomic status.

R. Mentors and students must comply with all federal, state, and local laws regarding professional practice, research ethics, and the conduct of research. This author notes that ethical standards are often higher than legal standards, and that the higher standard should always prevail. For example, it may be legal to implement an outdated therapy, but it is ethically wrong.

Power Differentials

The power differential between mentor and student prompts the following list of suggestions for mentors to present to students:

Explain the rules for inviting a student to participate in the mentor–student relationship. For example, the following is an invitation that the author sent to his graduate class: Colleagues: I am in need of a research assistant for this semester. I have a contract to produce the third edition of Goldfarb and Serpanos' *Professional Writing in SLP/A* that is due in June 2018. It will require reformatting and updating from the 2014 second edition.

Responsibilities: Work for 35 hr during the semester, mostly at home.

Qualifications: Expertise in using DropBox and Microsoft Word; a strong artistic sensibility.

Compensation: One credit of tuition remission applied to the student's registration in the following semester. The student will also have access to the book that is required for SPE 670 (Year 2, Cycle III).

Decision: This week. The first matriculated student in good standing who has appropriate qualifications will be selected, based on the e-mail time stamp.

Make sure that the selection of a student is free from any discrimination identified by the participant's state. For example, Adelphi University has the following policy, based on New York State law (downloaded with permission from http://hr.adelphi.edu/title-ix/university-policy/i-statement-of-policy/):

> The University will not tolerate discrimination, harassment or retaliation based on the protected status of an individual's race, creed, color, national origin, sex, gender identity, gender expression, age, marital status, disability, ethnicity, sexual orientation, genetic predisposition or carrier status, religion, pregnancy, veteran status, or any other basis protected by applicable local, state or federal laws. With this Policy, the University prohibits not only unlawful discrimination, harassment (including sexual misconduct, dating violence, domestic violence, stalking), and retaliation, but also discourages other unprofessional and discourteous actions.

Create a contract that both mentor and student sign, with start and end dates if appropriate. Include what is expected of both mentor and student, what (if any) the compensation will be, and what the mentor or student needs to do to terminate the contract.

WHAT KINDS OF MENTORING CAN YOU EXPECT? (Box 9–6)

Throughout your college or university education, you will have different kinds of mentoring available to you. Your first exposure to the undergraduate major in CSD was probably through an academic adviser who was probably also a member of the academic or clinical faculty. Signing up as a major was very likely your first exposure to an institutional model of

Box 9–6. Academic Mentoring at Different Levels

Formal institutional mentoring at undergraduate and graduate levels

Chain of command for complaints

Clinical practicum mentoring

Teaching Assistant mentoring

mentorship in CSD, as the experience is mandated for all declaring students, is a brief exposure, and is defined as limited to registration as a CSD major.

Academic Mentorship

Your academic adviser in your undergraduate and graduate program also represents an example of formal institutional mentorship. The adviser, also probably a member of the academic or clinical faculty, makes sure that you take the correct courses in the correct sequence, and is also available for consultation about problems you may be having in these courses. The last interaction with your adviser will likely be when you file for graduation. The Council on Academic Accreditation site visitors that accredit graduate programs for ASHA and the U.S. Department of Education typically ask students if they know what to do about a complaint. Although the chain of command varies according to educational institution, the student who has a complaint about a course must first address the problem with the course instructor. Failing satisfaction on that level, the student may proceed to consult with the academic adviser, graduate program director, department chair, and divisional dean, as needed.

Clinical Mentorship

Clinical mentoring most often represents the informal model where mentorship is not codified by the institution. If you are lucky enough to have a clinical mentor, that individual will do more than supervise, modify, and grade your performance in clinical practicum. You might have discussions on best practices, evidence-based practice, setting goals based on evidence, data collection, and discharge planning. The mentorship arrangement may last throughout the practicum and even continue to help you toward the next step on your career path.

Teaching Mentorship

Lastly, your educational institution may offer opportunities for you to be a teaching or research assistant. The overall benefits (e.g., payment, tuition remission) and requirements (e.g., number of hours, amount of time spent on campus) may be specified by the institution, but the arrangement with the mentor may be formal or informal. A teaching assistant (TA) should have access to the mentor's course syllabus and the mentor should assist the student in lesson planning, preparation of assignments and tests, and grading. A TA may have specific responsibilities, such as grading exams, or broader tasks, such as preparing a lecture or supervising a class activity. A research assistant (RA; see previous section on ethics) may be guided in performing a literature review, data collection and/or analysis, and interpretation of findings. The RA, depending on the amount of the contribution to the study, may be listed as a coauthor on a subsequent presentation or publication, or listed in the acknowledgements section.

WHAT IS THE ASHA S.T.E.P. MENTOR MODEL? (Box 9–7)

The American Speech-Language-Hearing Association (ASHA) seeks to help under-

Box 9–7. ASHA S.T.E.P. Mentors

Priority for students in racial/ethnic minority groups

Goals are leadership, diversity, and retention

The ASHA community

represented minority students in communication sciences and disorders through a program of mentoring called **S.T.E.P.** (Student to Empowered Professional). ASHA (2004) developed the online program to foster collaboration, goal achievement, and problem solving. Although the program is open to all students, priority is given to students who are members of a racial/ethnic minority group, including American Indian or Alaska Native, Asian, Black or African American, Native Hawaiian or other Pacific Islander, and/or Hispanic/Latino. S.T.E.P. mentoring is open to students who are or will be enrolled in communication sciences and disorders (CSD) programs.

S.T.E.P. is a structured mentoring program where a volunteer mentor, approved by ASHA, is matched with an undergraduate or graduate student in CSD to support specific goals that include leadership, diversity, and retention. For example, the author was matched with a graduate student of color who needed advice and materials to succeed in an externship setting that dealt with adult neurogenic communication disorders. Although we never met physically, we exchanged email correspondence regularly in a one-to-one relationship. The student was self-motivated and had specific learning targets. The mentor provided guidance, professional resources, information, and cheerleading support.

The mission of S.T.E.P. is to recruit, connect, support, and retain racial/ethnic minority students in CSD programs by providing either a one-to-one setting with an experienced mentor or peer mentoring in teams. Mentors are supported by regular updates and online community networking. Typically, mentors and students exchange initial emails to get to know each other and identify their common interests. We discuss expectations, develop an action plan with goals and objectives, and set up a plan for regular communication. At the end, we evaluate our accomplishments as well as the mentoring relationship. In some cases, the relationship can continue, but is redefined as peers, colleagues, or research partners.

Mentors and students receive regular email correspondence from the membership program manager through the ASHA community. Program updates, training videos, and email correspondence to S.T.E.P. mentors and students are emailed to participants regularly.

HOW DOES GENDER AFFECT THE MENTOR–MENTEE RELATIONSHIP? (Box 9–8)

Mentoring has traditionally revolved around career advancement of males with the help of other males. Women's perspectives and experiences have not been adequately represented in the traditional mentoring model, even though we know that a woman's academic and career progress may differ from a man's. Women are often faced with family planning decisions such as child rearing and caretaking

Box 9–8. The Role of Gender in Mentoring

Inadequate representation of women's perspectives and experiences

Lack of mentors for women

Mentoring to support female academic development

Barriers for females in academia

that may lead to academic and career interruptions. Returning to school or to the workforce after a substantial interruption is a challenge that women encounter far more frequently than men do. It also may take women more time to complete their education or climb the career ladder, and the gender pay gap continues to prevail.

Academic mentoring provides psychological support and increases scholastic performance of students (Kosoko-Lasaki, Sonnino, & Voytko, 2006). Unfortunately, women are less likely to have a mentor in the educational or professional setting. Wright and Wright (1987) identified power struggles, exploitative relationships, dependency problems, sexual harassment, and professional stagnation as potential dangers for women in cross-gender mentoring relationships. There is evidence that same sex mentor–student pairs have the most comfortable interactions, but women are still at a disadvantage of finding same sex mentors due to the lower ratio of female to male faculty (Berg & Ferber, 1983).

According to the 2013 survey of the National Center for Educational Statistics, women held only 37.5% of tenured positions and nearly half (48.4%) of all tenure-track positions (U.S. Department of Education, 2013). Additionally, women made up 39.6% of all academic ranks at doctoral-level institutions. Out of those 39.6% only 8.5% of women were at the professor rank, compared to 25.6% of men (American Association of University Professors, 2015). It appears that finding a qualified female mentor, especially in traditionally male-dominated science fields, might not be an easy task. Given these difficulties, peer mentoring may become a crucial source of support for women in academia. But can this nonhierarchical support system bring women the same benefits that a traditional mentoring model would? Since women are less likely to find mentors on their own and mentors often select students based on their potential or even similarities with their younger selves, there might be a need for institutionalized mentoring programs for women in academia.

Mentoring Programs for Females

There are a few studies that explored institutionalized mentoring programs for females in academia. One of them described the mentoring efforts for women as well as minority students and faculty in their pursuit of academic success (Kosoko-Lasaki et al., 2006). The female students and junior faculty in the mentoring program agreed that mentors helped them in their professional development. Mentors provided career counseling, constructive feedback, and emotional support for personal and professional issues. The women who were mentored cited the ability to connect with other professional women and the quality of advice from their mentors as positive outcomes. The participating mentors provided positive feedback about their relationships. They reported that the mentoring relationship did not require too much of their time, and that they were most helpful in providing feedback and determining the student's career goals. The most frequent topics for discussion between mentors and women students and junior faculty during their meetings were research, promotion, and teaching.

Another study investigated the mechanisms by which mentoring might support professional development of females in academia (Dutta et al., 2011). The Institute of Psychiatry at King's College in London started a pilot mentoring program for women, where early-career employees were matched with either a male or a female mentor. Both mentors and mentees received training and completed an online survey at the beginning of the mentoring relationship, as well as at 6 months and 1 year follow-up. The study assessed job satisfaction, job-related well-being, self-esteem, self-efficacy, and work–family conflict. It was found that both mentors and mentees were able to benefit from their mutual relationships. The perceived gains for mentors included the ability to give something back, provide support and witness the mentee's development, reflect on their own career and skills, and see the Institute of Psychiatry from a different perspective. Mentees' perceptions of the benefits included confidence and assertiveness, support and encouragement, and space to reflect on careers and goals. Overall, the study found that mentoring has a positive effect on self-esteem, self-efficacy, and job-related well-being. The authors (Dutta et al., 2011) reported that theirs was a feasibility pilot study of mentoring. Missing from their analysis was any indication if gender of the mentor made a difference in the outcome of the mentoring relationships.

Both studies seem to confirm that mentoring leads to improvements in career trajectories and professional development for females in academia. Still, little is done to support women's endeavors and erase barriers to selection, promotion, and recognition. West and Curtis (2006) examined faculty gender equity indicators in a report to the AAUP and found barriers for women in higher education still in place. They concluded that these barriers raise questions of basic fairness and limit the success of educational institutions. It is clear that the efficacy of cross-gender and same gender mentor–mentee relationships needs more study. E-mentoring might be one way to address gender bias in academia.

ARE E-SUPERVISION AND E-MENTORING THE WAVE OF THE FUTURE? (Box 9–9)

E-Mentoring

E-mentoring, provided via electronic communications to establish and maintain a relationship between a mentor and a student, is an alternative to the traditional format. This form of virtual mentoring, widely used in business, professional, and academic settings tends to mirror traditional mentoring as a process that brings a senior or more experienced individual together with a less experienced one so that the latter can gain new skills, self-confidence, and knowledge from the former during the process (Colky & Young, 2006). Where the traditional academic relationship depends on the mentor's physical presence, e-mentoring can bridge the gap between the student's need and the professor's availability.

Box 9–9. Alternatives to the Traditional Mentoring Format

E-mentoring

- Virtual communication
- Decreased effects of race, gender, socioeconomic status, and disability

Challenges to establishing mentoring relationships online

- Connection may be more superficial than face-to-face
- Rules of Internet etiquette
- Technological challenges
- Perceived lack of structure

E-supervision

- Blended model
- Stages of supervision: evaluation-feedback, transitional, and self-supervision
- Guidelines for e-supervision

E-mentoring is convenient. Because the need for face-to-face meetings is eliminated, e-mentoring erases geographical and time zone barriers. It can occur either asynchronously or synchronously in a comfortable environment for both parties. Flexibility allows the participants freedom in scheduling their interactions and choosing the mode of electronic communication (e.g., e-mail, online forums, chats). E-mentoring may also offer psychological comfort to students who may feel intimidated in face-to-face interactions. Online communication may help students be more open in discussing subjects they would not feel comfortable talking about face-to-face. It also allows both participants ample time to construct responses and prepare possible questions more thoroughly and thoughtfully. Virtual communication can be saved to provide a record of progress for review. E-mentoring occurring via emails may improve the student's writing skills and research skills because it encourages sifting through resources available online and evaluating them critically. With e-mentoring, the impact of gender, race, age, socioeconomic status, and disability may be decreased.

Adding to the benefits of e-mentoring for students, it is also rewarding for the mentors in a mutually beneficial relationship (Bierema & Merriam, 2002). Mentors may receive support from their students in gaining new technological skills. Virtual mentoring offers mentors avenues for self-growth and professional development, while honing their teaching skills. Unrestricted exchange of ideas with a younger and less experienced generation may even serve as inspiration for a mentor's future research and collaboration.

There are also some unique challenges to establishing mentoring relationships online. Some people believe that it is impersonal and deprives the participants of the possibilities to connect on a deeper level that is offered in face-to-face interaction. It also entails adhering to the rules of Internet etiquette or "netiquette" (see Goldfarb & Serpanos, 2020, for examples of netiquette), social conventions that govern online communication. E-mentoring poses technological challenges, as it requires a certain level of comfort with the use of computers, applications, and the Internet. Defining roles for both mentors and students in the online space may be challenging. How much mentoring is too much? How little guidance is too little? There is a need for clear delineation of realistic goals and expectations for both participants.

There may be a perceived lack of structure that includes a defined period of time and clear learning objectives. An important consideration is that of confidentiality and privacy that can easily be breached online. Online communication raises the question of personal liability, as there may be a permanent written record of the mentor–student interactions. E-mentoring may become even more time consuming than face-to-face mentoring, if the boundaries become too blurred or the online communication is poorly executed.

E-Supervision

E-supervision: an important stage in the education and professional development of a speech-language pathology or audiology student is that of clinical supervision. During this stage, an experienced speech-language pathologist (SLP) supervises a student for the 400 hr required for national certification. In some, primarily rural areas, there is a lack of qualified professionals to guide students in their in-house and off-campus clinical practica.

A blended approach to clinical supervision can address the shortages of clinical supervisors and understaffing in high-need and/or remote areas. It combines traditional supervision with the use of technology, such as videoconferencing, video software, or other means of online communication for direct and indirect guidance. The final goal of e-supervision is the same as the traditional one—independence of the student from the supervisor. The blended model has been in practice for many years in the clinical fellowship setting. The clinical fellow is observed and evaluated by an ASHA-certified (CCC-SLP) individual 36 times during the fellowship experience, but 18 of these observations and evaluations may be virtual.

According to Anderson (1988), the process of clinical supervision includes three major stages: evaluation–feedback, transitional, and self-supervision. It also entails three supervisory styles: direct, collaborative, and consultative. The process of supervision is a continuum, across which the roles of the participants change according to the situation. Similarly, the supervisor's role moves from more direct and active to indirect or consultative as the skill set, competence, and professional self-awareness of the student develop.

The same styles and stages apply to e-supervision. ASHA's technical report on clinical supervision (2008) includes comments on the efficacy (effectiveness and efficiency) of technology in delivering supervision as one of the research directions, but only briefly mentions the topic in the main body of the report. The reader is reminded to practice caution and follow regulatory guidelines involving confidentiality (ASHA, 2008), but the report is mum on the practicality, challenges, benefits, clinical implications, or ethical considerations pertaining to e-supervision.

A qualitative study by Carlin, Milam, Carlin, and Owen (2012) described the process and outcomes of e-supervision for SLP students in Ohio. In 2003, the Ohio Department of Education (ODE) identified a need for qualified SLPs to fill school districts. This need was addressed by establishing a partnership with the local universities, who sent their graduate students to the high-need districts to work as primary practicing professionals. The practicing students required supervision, and a new challenge arose: a shortage of licensed and certified supervisors in the school districts. The ODE tackled the challenge by implementing technology. The students were connected with the supervisors via e-supervision that involved videoconferencing. The study reported positive experiences of graduate students with e-supervision. The electronic mode of supervision was found to be more convenient and less stressful. E-supervision was a practical solution that supported SLP students in four ways: timely and adequate feedback from the supervisors, supplemental materials and activities, electronic document exchange that eliminated the need to print any paperwork, and even increased likelihood of prospective employment in the school district.

A follow-up study focused on guidelines for e-supervision (Carlin, Boarman, Carlin, & Inselmann, 2013). Initially, parents, supervisors, school administration, and technology staff agree upon e-supervision. The mutual agreement is followed by a selection of a qualified SLP to supervise the graduate student. Next, the supervisor and the student receive technological training, and trials are conducted to identify any continuing needs. Lastly, the supervisors and the students schedule in-person meetings before the start of the e-supervised clinical practicum to discuss any related matters.

Conclusion

For most of its existence, face-to-face supervision has been the preferred mode of supervision in the field of communication sciences and disorders. With technological advances, e-supervision is becoming more available and acceptable. Regardless of the mode of supervision delivery, high-quality supervision is essential for the student's professional growth and success. When such guidance can be delivered electronically, there is evidence that it is a viable option. In fact, the first post-master's degree mentoring experience that most new SLP professionals have is from a clinical fellowship (CF) supervisor who holds the Certificate of Clinical Competence. As of this writing, there are 36 required CF supervisory visits, with the possibility that 18 of them are done online. Most audiology students find the CF mentoring embedded in their doctor of audiology (AuD) program.

ADVANCED STUDY

The author proposes that mentoring skills are necessary for an individual to be granted power of professor. With new generations of scholars and researchers needed every 10 years, professors and master clinicians have an obligation to prepare individuals with adequate knowledge and skills to undertake the tasks of scholarship and research, and mentoring is a key component. For evidence of the requisite mentoring skills, complete the following and have your instructor, academic adviser, mentor, or CSD department chair review that you have completed the requirements and sign and date where indicated.

Student's Name: ______________________________

Choosing a Mentor

1. Write a paragraph or two, based on an instructor's faculty profile, describing why that individual would be a suitable mentor for you.
2. Write a paragraph or two indicating what your 3-month, 1-year, and 5-year professional goals are.
3. Write a paragraph or two detailing a clinical research project that you would like to do, and how the mentor could help.
4. Write a paragraph or two detailing what you hope to accomplish in the next step of your career (master's degree program for undergraduates, clinical fellowship for master's students, post-doctoral fellowship or junior faculty position for doctoral students).

Date of Completion: ______________________________

Faculty/Supervisor Signature: ______________________________

Peer Mentorship

1. Write a paragraph or two indicating three aspects of your college or university that are excellent, and three aspects that need improvement.
2. Write a paragraph or two detailing how a student registers their major, finds an adviser, registers a complaint through the chain of command, and applies for graduation.
3. Write a paragraph or two indicating the requirements for the ASHA CCC, licensure in your state, and certification as a Teacher of Students with Speech and Language Disabilities (TSSLD or whatever your state's designation is), as well as the requirements for the bilingual extension to the TSSLD (or equivalent).
4. Write a paragraph or two indicating the rank (from lecturer to full professor) of the faculty in the CSD department, their areas of expertise, and how they wish to be addressed.

Date of Completion: ______________________________

Faculty/Supervisor Signature: ______________________________

REFERENCES

American Association of University Professors. (2015). *Table 12: Distribution of faculty, by rank, gender, category, and affiliation, 2014–15.* Retrieved from https://www.aaup.org/sites/default/files/files/2015salarysurvey/2015tab12.pdf

American Speech-Language-Hearing Association. (2004). *S.T.E.P.—Student to empowered professional mentoring program.* Retrieved from http://www.asha.org/students/gatheringplace/step/

American Speech-Language-Hearing Association. (2008). *Clinical supervision in speech-language pathology* [Technical report]. Rockville, MD: Author.

American Speech-Language-Hearing Association. (2016). *Code of ethics.* Retrieved from http://www.asha.org/Code-of-Ethics/

Anderson, J. L. (1988). *The supervisory process in speech language pathology and audiology.* Austin, TX: Pro-Ed.

Berg, H. M., & Ferber, M. A. (1983). Men and women graduate students: Who succeeds and why? *Journal of Higher Education, 54*(6), 629–648.

Bhagia, J., & Tinsley, J. A. (2000). The mentoring partnership. *Mayo Clinic Proceedings, 75,* 535–537.

Bierema, L. L., & Merriam, S. B. (2002). E-mentoring: Using computer mediated communication to enhance the mentoring process. *Innovative Higher Education, 26,* 211–227.

Carlin, C. H., Boarman, K., Carlin, E. L., & Inselmann, K. (2013). The use of e-supervision support speech-language pathologist graduate students during student teaching practica. *International Journal of Telerehabilitation, 5*(2), 21–32.

Carlin, C. H., Milam, J. L., Carlin, E. L., & Owen, A. (2012). Promising practices in E-supervision: Exploring graduate speech-language pathology interns' perceptions. *International Journal of Telerehabilitation, 4,* 25–38.

Colky, D. L., & Young, W. H. (2006). Mentoring in the virtual organization: Keys to building successful schools and businesses. *Mentoring & Tutoring, 14*(4), 433–447.

Dutta, R., Hawkes, S., Kuipers, E., Guest, D., Fear, N. T., & Iverson, A. C. (2011). One year outcomes of a mentoring scheme for female academics: A pilot study at the Institute of Psychiatry, King's College London. *BMC Medical Education, 11.* doi:10.1186/1472-6920-11-13

Eby, L. T., Allen, T. D., Evans, S. C., Ng, T., & DuBois, D. (2008). Does mentoring matter? A multidisciplinary meta-analysis comparing mentored and non-mentored individuals. *Journal of Vocational Behavior, 72,* 254–267.

Feldman, M. D., Arean, P. A., Marshall, S. J., Lovett, M., & O'Sullivan, P. (2010). Does mentoring matter: Results from a survey of faculty mentees at a large health sciences university. *Medical Education Online, 15,* 1–8. doi:10.3402/meo.v15i0.5063

Goldfarb, R., & Serpanos, Y. (2020). *Professional writing in speech-language pathology and audiology* (3rd ed.). San Diego, CA: Plural Publishing.

Homer. (1969). *The odyssey.* New York, NY: Simon and Shuster.

Horner, J., & Minifie, F. (2011). Research ethics II: Mentoring, collaboration, peer review, and data management and ownership. *Journal of Speech, Language, and Hearing Research, 54,* S330–S345.

Inzer, L. D., & Crawford, C. B. (2005). A review of formal and informal mentoring: Processes, problems, and design. *Journal of Leadership Education, 4,* 31–50.

Jacobi, M. (1991). Mentoring and undergraduate academic success: A literature review. *Review of Educational Research, 61,* 505–532.

Johnson, M. J., Subak, L. L., Brown, J. S., Lee, K. A., & Feldman, M. D. (2010). An innovative program to train health sciences researchers to be effective clinical and translational-research mentors. *Academic Medicine, 85,* 484–489.

Kent, R. D. (2012). Models and concepts of translational research. In R. Goldfarb (Ed.), *Translational speech-language pathology and audiology* (pp. 27–35). San Diego, CA: Plural Publishing.

Keyser, D. J., Lasoki, J. M., Lara-Cinisomo, S., Schultz, D. J., Williams, V. L., Zellers, D. F., & Pincus, A. (2008). Advancing institutional efforts to support research mentorship: A conceptual framework and self-assessment tool. *Academic Medicine, 83,* 217–225.

Kosoko-Lasaki, O., Sonnino, R. E., & Voytko, M. L. (2006). Mentoring for women and underrepresented minority faculty and students: Experience at two institutions of higher education. *Journal of the National Medical Association, 98,* 1449–1459.

Kram, K. E. (1985). *Mentoring at work: Developmental relationships in organizational life*. Glenview, IL: Scott Foresman.

National Commission for the Protection of Human Subjects of Biomedical and Behavioral Research. (1979). *The Belmont Report: Ethical principles and guidelines for the protection of human subjects of research.* Washington, DC: U.S. Department of Health and Human Services. Retrieved from http://www.hhs.gov/ohrp/regulations-and-policy/belmont-report/

Nick, J. M., Delahoyde, T. M., Del Prato, D., Mitchell, C., Orti, J., Ottley, C., . . . Siktberg, L. (2012). Best practices in academic mentoring: A model for excellence. *Nursing Research and Practice.* doi:10.1155/2012/937906

Purves, B. A., Petersen, J., & Puurveen, G. (2013). An aphasia mentoring program: Perspectives of speech-language pathology students and of mentors with aphasia. *American Journal of Speech-Language Pathology, 22*, S370–S379.

Ragins, B. R., & Cotton, J. L. (1999). Mentor functions and outcomes: A comparison of men and women in formal and informal mentoring relationships. *Journal of Applied Psychology, 84*, 529–550.

Rosenbek, J. C. (2012). The science of dissemination. In R. Goldfarb (Ed.), *Translational speech-language pathology and audiology* (pp. 37–42). San Diego, CA: Plural Publishing.

Siddiqui, S. (2014). Of mentors, apprenticeship, and role models: A lesson to relearn? *Medical Education Online, 19*. doi:10.3402/meo.v19.25428

U.S. Department of Education, National Center for Education Statistics, Integrated Postsecondary Education Data System (IPEDS). (2013). *Full-time instructional staff, by faculty and tenure status, academic rank, race/ethnicity, and gender (degree-granting institutions).* Retrieved from https://nces.ed.gov/programs/digest/d14/tables/dt14_315.20.asp

West, M., & Curtis, J. W. (2006). *AAUP Faculty Gender Equity Indicators 2006*. Retrieved from https://www.aaup.org/NR/rdonlyres/63396944-44BE-4ABA-9815-5792D93856F1/0/AAUPGenderEquityIndicators2006.pdf

Wright, C. A., & Wright, S. D. (1987). The role of mentors in the career development of young professionals. *Family Relations, 36*, 204–208.

Zerzan, J. T., Hess, R., Schur, E., Phillips, R. S., & Rigotti, N. (2009). Making the most of mentors: A guide for mentees. *Academic Medicine, 84*, 140–144.

10

Institutional Review Board (IRB) Research Approval

INTRODUCTION

The purpose of the Institutional Review Board (IRB) is to oversee clinical research involving human participants. It has the primary goal of ensuring participant safety. Some IRBs will have a secondary goal to ensure that research has high quality and answers important questions (Hyer, 2010). A peer-reviewed journal may not consider a manuscript for publication unless the study received IRB approval before it was conducted (Chappy & Gaberson, 2012).

This chapter will be divided into three parts: overview, history, and completing an IRB review form.

Learning Objectives

After reading this chapter, the student will be able to

- describe the history and purpose of the IRB;
- earn the certificate of completion from the National Institutes of Health (NIH) or Collaborative Institutional Training Initiative (CITI) training course on protection of human research participants; and
- prepare a research proposal that will be approved by the local IRB.

OVERVIEW

Institutional Review Boards (IRBs) began and were developed by academic institutions in the 1960s. IRB members are independent reviewers of research proposals that can be submitted for U.S. government funding. IRBs may also approve unfunded research proposals to be conducted at the academic institution. As a research ethics committee, the IRB needs to determine if the researcher can fulfill the obligations of the project and that human research participants are protected. Members of a research ethics committee usually include individuals with expertise in education, ethics, health care, and law; there is also a public member. Other members may be brought in as needed for particular expertise areas. An IRB is guided by the Belmont Report (1979) in its deliberations about the merit, accuracy, and completeness of a proposal. For example, the methodology must consider respect for persons in terms of access to participants, informed consent, and confidentiality; beneficence in terms of risk assessment; and justice in terms of access to participants and type of intervention.

The Office for Protection from Research Risks, Office of Extramural Research, National Institutes of Health (Author, 1993) defines an IRB as an administrative body established to protect the rights and welfare of human research participants recruited to engage in research activities conducted under the auspices of an affiliated institution. Research involving human participants refers to any activity intended to obtain and record information from or about individuals for research purposes.

University Policies

University policies require that all research conducted by faculty, administrators, undergraduate, and graduate students must first be reviewed by the IRB. The nature of the research includes studies that use surveys; interviews; experimental designs that involve human participants; and any research that involves children or other vulnerable populations such as the incarcerated, mentally disabled, or other protected groups (see the Belmont Report, 1979, in Chapter 3 for a list of protected groups). Study protocols that have been reviewed and approved by the IRB are usually valid for one year. If the study takes longer than one year, then the protocol must be resubmitted, using some version of a continuation form. The protocol may then get an expedited review, rather than a full review. Typically, an expedited review applies to research that involves slightly more than minimal risk, so it is not exempt from review. A protocol that has previously been approved by full board review and is resubmitted with minor revisions or for a continuation may also qualify for expedited review.

Depending on the nature of the proposed research, the IRB may require a full board review, an expedited review, or be exempt from review (Enfield & Truwit, 2008). Some student research proposals may be exempt from IRB review. After all, students write research papers for many classes and there is not enough time nor any need to wait for IRB approval. Exempted review is for research that has minimal or no risk. However, if your proposal involves human research participants, then the IRB chair or a subcommittee must review the proposal to determine if it meets federal guidelines for exemption (OHRP, 2009). Box 10–1 shows how a research project may be exempt from IRB review. All items in Part A of this section must apply AND at least one item in Part B of this section must apply. A section on food safety has been deleted as it does not apply to communication sciences and disorders (CSD) research.

Box 10–1. Exempt Research Policy

See a sample policy (used with permission) at http://research-grants.adelphi.edu/irb/

Part A (All items must apply.)

1. The research does not involve any of the following as participants: prisoners, fetuses, pregnant women, the seriously ill, or mentally or cognitively compromised adults.
2. The research does not involve any participants under the age of 18 (there is an exception in that research with participants under the age of 18 may still be considered exempt if they are participating in projects that fall under categories 1, 3, 4 and/or 5 in Part B). Studies under Part B-2 that include minors should be submitted for expedited review.
3. Study participants are not exposed to greater than minimal risks (i.e., those ordinarily encountered in daily life or during the performance of routine physical or psychological examinations or tests performed by a qualified professional).

Part B (At least one item must apply.)

1. Research is conducted in established or commonly accepted educational settings, involving normal educational practices, such as research on regular and special education instructional strategies, the effectiveness of or the comparison among instructional techniques, curricula, or classroom management methods.
2. Research involves the use of educational tests (cognitive, diagnostic, aptitude, achievement), survey procedures, interview procedures, or observation of public behavior. Participants must be de-identified and protected in the following two ways: (a) information obtained may not be recorded at any point in such a manner that human participants can be identified, directly or through identifiers linked to the subjects; and (b) disclosure of the human participants' responses outside the research may not reasonably place the participants at risk of criminal or civil liability or be damaging to the participants' financial standing, employability, or reputation.
3. Research involves the use of educational tests (cognitive, diagnostic, aptitude, achievement), survey procedures, interview procedures, or observation of public behavior under the following conditions: (a) the human participants are elected or appointed public officials or candidates for public office; and (b) federal law requires without exception that the confidentiality of the personally

identifiable information will be maintained throughout the research and thereafter.

4. Research involves the collection or study of existing data, documents, records, pathological specimens, or diagnostic specimens, if these sources are publicly available or if the information is provided to the investigator in such a manner that subjects cannot be identified directly or through identifiers linked to the subjects. We refer to this type of collection or study as retrospective research.

5. Research and demonstration projects are conducted by or subject to the approval of program directors or department heads, and are designed to study, evaluate, or otherwise examine the following: (a) public benefit or service programs; (b) procedures for obtaining benefits or services under those programs; (c) possible changes in or alternatives to those programs or procedures; or (d) possible changes in methods or levels of payment for benefits or services under those programs.

Student Research Application

A student navigating a research application for the first time needs to avoid some common errors and omissions. Poor science has ethical consequences, and poor methodology may yield unreliable results (Greaney et al., 2012). Accordingly, the researcher is required to provide an application with a description of the proposal and the data collection tools, and information about the study population and the sample size. There should be enough information to enable the research ethics committee to evaluate the scientific merit of the study.

Common errors in submissions by new applicants include the following: there is a lack of congruence among the research title, literature review, purpose of the study, hypotheses, and data collection methods and analysis; the time frame does not correspond with feasibility of completion of the study; the application lacks adequate proofreading for grammar, spelling, and content; or the application lacks certain required documentation and signatures (Greaney et al., 2012).

IRB Ethics

Moon (2009) cites Immanuel Kant's second maxim as the model for IRBs: "Act in such a way that you treat humanity, whether in your own person or in the person of any other, always at the same time as an end and never merely as a means to an end" (Kant, 1993). Human participants in research must never be merely a means to an end, or a way to find answers to research questions, but always also as ends in themselves. The IRB is necessary to ensure the welfare of human research participants, who may also be patients, colleagues, students, and community members.

Just as there is tension between the goals of research and the duty to avoid having the ends justify the means, there is an argument about the appropriate location of the IRB that can be either local or central. A local IRB functions in the academic institution that conducts the research while a central IRB is usually a for-profit entity that researchers pay for services rendered. The potential for conflicts of interest motivate arguments against both local and central forms. For example, a central IRB may be prone to grant easy approval, because investigators pay them, and the income of a central IRB depends on having a good relationship with investigators. A local IRB exists in an institution that benefits from research funding as well as the prestige garnered from a well-funded research agenda.

Location and Membership

The preferred location is probably the local IRB that exists in a physical entity—the academic institution—that has a relationship with people in a community. This relationship may include clinical care, education, and employment, in addition to research (Moon, 2009). Participants in research may also be receiving services in the university speech and hearing center, and the interests of both community and academic institution often coincide. Problems associated with research can adversely affect the community, but also the reputation of the academic institution within the community, and even the trust of the clients receiving clinical services. Local IRB members are motivated to protect the special relationship that exists between town and gown. For these reasons, many IRBs include a nonaffiliated member who represents the interests of the community. Because representing the diverse interests of a given community may be next to impossible, the main role of the nonaffiliated member often devolves into simplifying the language of consent forms.

The Federal Policy for the Protection of Human Subjects was originally promulgated as a Common Rule in 1991. The revised "final rule" became effective on January 19, 2018. Although the current document is voluminous and full of "government-speak," it is important to note that the final rule does not enable institutions to opt out of compliance with the Common Rule. Of interest to our professions is a change in the requirement that IRB approval from every site involved in multisite research can be replaced by IRB approval from a single site (Stark & Greene, 2016). Our professions have engaged in multisite research for at least forty years, beginning with cooperative studies from different Veterans Administration medical centers on efficacy of aphasia therapy (see, for example, Wertz et al., 1981), to more recent studies of a genetic basis of stuttering across different universities (see, for example, Yairi, Ambrose, & Cox, 1996). Stark and Greene (2016) note their disappointment that the final rule does not include a requirement for systematic updating of regulations in the future, so the rule remains vulnerable to obsolescence if there are changes over time in terms of standards of research, types of scientific collaboration, and political sensibilities.

HISTORY OF THE IRB

Nelson (2012) cites three historical failures to protect human research participants as motivation for the Nuremburg Code that ultimately led to our current Institutional

Review Boards (IRBs). Also included is a more recent example of ethical blindness in research.

The United States Public Health Service (USPHS) Syphilis Studies in Tuskegee, Alabama, from 1932 to 1972

During the 1920s in Macon County, Alabama, nearly 40% of adult African-American men tested positive for syphilis. The hypothesis that the USPHS developed for the study was that the black male response to syphilis would differ from the white male response. The initial plans for the study included medical treatment, but the devastating effects of the Great Depression eliminated funding for the project. The USPHS decided to proceed with a limited study, and continued the investigation (observation without treatment) well after penicillin became the treatment of choice for syphilis. As Nelson (2012, p. 101) notes, the study is a powerful reminder of what happens when researchers fail to recognize that each human participant is worthy of respect.

The Nazi Holocaust Experiments and the Resulting Doctors' Trial at Nuremberg, Germany, 1946 to 1947

After the defeat of Germany in World War II, 23 Nazi doctors and administrators were accused of war crimes and crimes against humanity. The "medical" (quotation marks mine) experiments that were exposed during the Nuremburg trials were conducted predominantly on Nazi concentration camp inmates. The experiments included, among others, sterilization to eliminate unwanted populations; high altitude exposure designed to intentionally cause death to the subject ("participant" seems to be the wrong word to use here), in order to provide information to the German air force; freezing experiments, also designed to cause death to the subject, in order to provide information about hypothermia to the German air force; forcing subjects to consume sea water, to see how much could be safe to drink, and poisons, to see their effect on food and bullets; intentionally inflicting phosphorous burns to see the potential effect of incendiary bombs; causing jaundice to test inoculations; deliberately inflicting wounds on subjects and then infecting the wounds with mustard gas; and on and on, including skeleton collection and euthanasia.

The judges of the Doctors' Trial rejected the notion that these experiments were necessary and acceptable, even in a wartime setting. The court, in condemning the experiments in the Doctors' Trial, articulated what we now know as the Nuremberg Code. The Nuremberg Code (1949; Box 10–2) is a powerful reminder of what unchecked research can become in the wrong hands.

USPHS Sexually Transmitted Diseases Inoculation Study, Guatemala, 1946 to 1948

Between 1946 and 1948, the National Institutes of Health (NIH) was a part of USPHS. NIH provided a grant in Guatemala to study if penicillin after sexual intercourse would prevent the spread of gonorrhea, syphilis, and chancroid. Researchers paid prostitutes who already had or were

Box 10–2. The Nuremberg Code

1. The voluntary consent of the human subject is absolutely essential. This means that the person involved should have legal capacity to give consent; should be so situated as to be able to exercise free power of choice, without the intervention of any element of force, fraud, deceit, duress, over-reaching, or other ulterior form of constraint or coercion; and should have sufficient knowledge and comprehension of the elements of the subject matter involved as to enable him or her to make an understanding and enlightened decision. This latter element requires that before the acceptance of an affirmative decision by the experimental subject, there should be made known to him or her the nature, duration, and purpose of the experiment; the method and means by which it is to be conducted; all inconveniences and hazards reasonable to be expected; and the effects upon his or her health or person which may possibly come from his or her participation in the experiment. The duty and responsibility for ascertaining the quality of the consent rests upon each individual who initiates, directs, or engages in the experiment. It is a personal duty and responsibility which may not be delegated to another with impunity.
2. The experiment should be such as to yield fruitful results for the good of society, unprocurable by other methods or means of study, and not random and unnecessary in nature.
3. The experiment should be so designed and based on the results of animal experimentation and a knowledge of the natural history of the disease or other problem under study that the anticipated results will justify the performance of the experiment.
4. The experiment should be so conducted as to avoid all unnecessary physical and mental suffering and injury.
5. No experiment should be conducted where there is an a priori reason to believe that death or disabling injury will occur; except, perhaps, in those experiments where the experimental physicians also serve as subjects.
6. The degree of risk to be taken should never exceed that determined by the humanitarian importance of the problem to be solved by the experiment.
7. Proper preparations should be made and adequate facilities provided to protect the experimental subject against even remote possibilities of injury, disability, or death.
8. The experiment should be conducted only by scientifically qualified persons. The highest

degree of skill and care should be required through all stages of the experiment of those who conduct or engage in the experiment.

9. During the course of the experiment, the human subject should be at liberty to bring the experiment to an end if he or she has reached the physical or mental state where continuation of the experiment seems to him or her to be impossible.

10. During the course of the experiment, the scientist in charge must be prepared to terminate the experiment at any state, if he or she has probable cause to believe, in the exercise of the good faith, superior skill, and careful judgment required of him or her, that a continuation of the experiment is likely to result in injury, disability, or death to the experimental subject.

Source: https://history.nih.gov/research/downloads/nuremberg.pdf)

deliberately infected with these diseases to have sex with three different male populations: prisoners, mental patients, and soldiers. In the end, 128 men were infected with chancroid, 234 with gonorrhea, and 427 with syphilis. Researchers attempted to develop inoculations based on the bacteria of the syphilis infection. Note that these experiments were conducted at a time that overlapped with the Doctors' Trial in Nuremberg. Note also that IRBs would consider the subjects to be vulnerable and worthy of special protections. In fact, informed consent was an established norm at the time of the Guatemala studies, and the subjects were still intentionally infected with sexually transmitted diseases. The prisoners were further coerced with offers of free cigarettes to participate in the experiments.

Pfizer Trovan Study, Nigeria, 1996

A half century after the Guatemala study, Pfizer, one of the world's largest pharmaceutical companies, sponsored a study in Kano, Nigeria, in response to an epidemic of bacterial meningitis. This disease affects the membranes of the brain and spinal cord, resulting in death in 10% of cases. Some 200 children were given doses of Trovan, an inadequately tested drug. The study did not have IRB approval, and Pfizer did not take precautions to prevent the side effects (including damage to joints, cartilage, bones, and liver) seen in the previous animal studies of the drug. An ethics committee approval letter was found to have been forged and backdated.

Dates and Events That Led to Today's Version of the IRB

- 1954: The National Institutes of Health (NIH) established an internal committee to review two kinds of research studies: those that included sick or healthy participants who might be exposed to any unusual hazard; and those that included normal (now referred to as "typical") controls in any way.

- 1974: The National Research Act that was passed in response to growing concern about the ethics violations in research created the National Commission for the Protection of Human Subjects of Biomedical and Behavioral Research. This commission produced the Belmont Report.
- 1979: The Belmont Report was published with the foundational principles of respect for persons, beneficence, and justice. Chapter 3 includes a detailed description and analysis of the Belmont Report.
- 1991: The Common Rule (Code of Federal Regulations Title 45, Part 46) was published and codified in separate regulations by 15 federal departments and agencies. It unified various policies regarding how agencies (except for the Food and Drug Administration) funded, conducted, and supported clinical research. There is a major portion, called Federal Policy or "Common Rule" (see http://www.hhs.gov/ohrp/regulations-and-policy/regulations/common-rule/index.html), and three subparts that offer additional protections for the following classes: pregnant women, fetuses, and neonates; prisoners; and children. There are basic provisions for IRBs, informed consent, and assurances of compliance. Stark and Greene (2016) noted that OHRP reported in 2011 that the Common Rule was to be overhauled to consider its burden on multisite studies that involve randomized clinical trials.

COMPLETING AN IRB REVIEW FORM

The following sections of this chapter address the parts required for completion of an IRB Review Form (Box 10–3).

Brief Description of the Project's Purposes, Methodology, and Design

What do we know about how the IRB makes its decisions? We know that, while most research proposals are not rejected outright, almost none are approved exactly as submitted. The IRB tends to conduct its work in secrecy, so there is little known about how an individual IRB deliberates, the factors that influence its decisions, or the weight given to norms and precedents. Anderson and DuBois (2012) summarized research about IRBs and found that the focus tended to be on written policies, workload, economics, and length of review time. They also considered review outcomes of multisite investigations reviewed by multiple IRBs.

The conduct of IRBs is governed by ambiguous federal research regulations. For example, there is no operational definition for minimal risk and no regulatory details regarding payment for participation in research or qualifications for nonscientist, nonaffiliated community IRB members. IRBs differ in how they apply federal guidelines; how long they take to review proposals; and how they decide to accept, reject, or require changes to research protocols. Variability does not mean that some IRBs review proposals inadequately; it signals only that there is

Box 10–3. IRB Review Form

Adelphi University Institutional Review Board Research Review Forms

IRB ID #
(to be completed by the committee)

Date submitted to IRB:

TITLE OF PROJECT:

PRINCIPAL INVESTIGATOR:

Address:

Phone:

Email:

Faculty Advisor (if not the PI):
Please note: students are required to have a faculty advisor

Address:

Phone:

Email:

You must complete a training program in the protection of human research participants before you can begin your research. Please indicate the date the training was completed (__________) and include a copy of the certification with this application. If you have not completed a training program, please contact the Office of Sponsored Programs or take the following online program: phrp.nihtraining.com

Please answer Yes or No to the following, and provide an explanation, if requested:

1. *Does this research EXCLUDE children, the elderly, prisoners, fetuses, pregnant women, the seriously ill, mentally or cognitively compromised adults, or other vulnerable groups (institutionalized populations)?*

   If your answer is NO, please explain the rationale for including the specific population(s) and the precautions you will use to protect them.

2. *Do you believe this proposal should be exempt from IRB review (see IRB Policies and Procedures Manual, section VII RESEARCH EXEMPT FROM IRB REVIEW [part A&B])?*

   If YES, please explain.

3. *Does this proposal involve the use of deception?*

   If YES, please explain.

4. *Are you requesting that written informed consent be waived (see IRB Policies and Procedures Manual, section XIII INFORMED CONSENT [B, C, and D])?*

   If YES, please explain.

I. BRIEF DESCRIPTION OF THE PROJECT'S PURPOSES:

II. PLANNED DATES FOR INITIATION AND COMPLETION OF THE PROJECT:

III. NUMBER OF SUBJECTS:

IV. CHARACTERISTICS OF SUBJECTS (e.g., age range, special populations, etc.):

V. METHOD OF SUBJECT RECRUITMENT:

VI. BRIEF DESCRIPTION OF PROJECT'S METHODS AND RESEARCH DESIGN:

VII. SEQUENCE OF ACTIVITIES REQUIRED OF THE SUBJECT (for example, advertisement, consent, debriefing, etc.):

VIII. ESTIMATED TIME COMMITMENT REQUIRED OF THE SUBJECTS:

IX. ANY POTENTIAL RISKS, DISCOMFORTS, OR STRESSES AND THE PRECAUTIONS TAKEN TO MINIMIZE THEM:

SIGNATURES AND DATE OF ALL RESEARCHERS WHO WILL BE WORKING IN DIRECT CONTACT WITH STUDY PARTICIPANTS. IN ADDITION, FACULTY ADVISORS MUST SIGN BELOW. THESE SIGNATURES INDICATE THAT ALL THE RESEARCHERS HAVE FAMILIARIZED THEMSELVES WITH UNIVERSITY POLICIES REGARDING THE LEGAL AND ETHICAL TREATMENT OF HUMAN SUBJECTS IN RESEARCH, AND ARE CERTIFIED IN HUMAN SUBJECTS PROTECTIONS TRAINING.

Principal Investigator:

Name: ______________________________ Date: ______________

Signature: ___________________________

Affiliation: __________________________
(institution/organization)

Faculty Advisor (if applicable):

Name: ______________________________ Date: ______________

Signature: ____________________________

Affiliation: ___________________________
(institution/organization)

Name: ______________________________ Date: ______________

Signature: ____________________________

Affiliation: ___________________________
(institution/organization)

ATTACHMENTS CHECKLIST:

____ 1. Informed Consent Form (Please note that the IRB has decided that all consent forms/letters should include the following statement):

This research has been reviewed and approved by the Adelphi University Institutional Review Board. If you have any questions, concerns, or comments, please contact the IRB cochairs.

____ 2. Debriefing Form (if applicable)

____ 3. Representative sample of materials/test/questionnaire items

____ 4. Sign-up sheet, solicitation script, or advertisement (whichever is applicable)

____ 5. Other attachments

Revised and reprinted with permission. *Source:* https://research-grants.adelphi.edu/irb/forms/ (Adelphi University, 2017)

a lack of transparency in the deliberation and review processes, and that is a cause for concern.

If IRBs are relying on intuition as much as careful analysis, then new researchers need some guidelines about what drives these gut feelings. Based on a systematic review (Abbott & Grady, 2011), we can draw some conclusions and make some suggestions. IRBs tend to

- overestimate the likelihood that survey questions can cause psychological or emotional distress;
- overestimate that individuals with psychiatric disorders are susceptible to coercion;
- underestimate that individuals with psychiatric disorders have decision-making capacity; and

- overly rely on nonscientist community members for information about stakeholder values, customs, and preferences.

If your research proposal is, for example, a survey to determine how peers react to stuttering in middle-school children, it would be wise to anticipate some IRB reaction to the survey questions, based on the first tendency above. If you want to investigate the prevalence of hearing loss in adults with chronic undifferentiated schizophrenia, then please address potential concerns based on the second and third tendencies above.

A cautionary tale illustrates the need to be thorough in reviewing the literature underlying the research protocol. In 2001, a 24-year-old woman died from respiratory distress and organ failure after participating in a nonphysiological study at Johns Hopkins Asthma and Allergy Center. The purpose of the study was to determine hyper-responsiveness in healthy participants in order to understand what goes wrong in asthma. Participants inhaled a ganglionic blocker that had potential side effects on the lungs that were identified in studies that appeared in the 1950s and 1960s. The research protocol included online electronic databases that went back only as far as the 1970s, and the principal investigator did not search the medical literature adequately. The investigator and the IRB were cited for a number of problems, and all research at Johns Hopkins was temporarily suspended.

IRBs were not designed with Scholarship of Teaching and Learning (SoTL) in mind (Martin, 2013). Research in the classroom may be considered academic freedom and not in the purview of the IRB. However, research in the classroom or the center for communication disorders poses potential risks, and IRBs must consider protection of participants in our classes or clinics. According to Martin (2013), data collection from students with the intention to publish or present the research is considered research with human participants and requires IRB approval. There is no mention of the IRB in the information about SoTL at the University of Wisconsin at Milwaukee, as cited by ASHA (https://www.asha.org/uploadedFiles/academic/teach-tools/SoTLOPID.pdf). Contact the chair of the local IRB with questions or concerns.

The Health Insurance Portability and Accountability Act of 1996 (HIPAA) was discussed in Chapter 3. The IRB may alter or waive HIPAA regulations, according to federal law, for the purpose of research. The waiver may or may not be attached to the informed consent form, depending on the nature of the research.

Dates for Initiation and Completion of the Project

In a study of 46 IRBs submitted by training programs for improving health care in geriatric facilities (Conforti, Ross, Hess, Lynn, & Holmboe, 2008), 48% (22) of the programs were unable to begin the program at what was prespecified as time zero. Time to IRB approval or exemption ranged from 1 to 56.5 weeks, with a mean time of 18.3 weeks and the median time of 18 weeks. This was an average of 7.5 weeks longer than the authors had anticipated. Starting a study nearly two months after researchers can reasonably expect to means that the completion date is also likely to be considerably later than planned.

Dyrbye et al. (2007) submitted the same multi-institutional research proposal to evaluate medical students' quality of life to six medical school IRBs. Four IRBs permitted an expedited review and two required full review. There was considerable variability in timeliness and consistency of the IRB reviews. For example, time to review by the committee ranged from 6 to 115 days. While most of the requests for revisions (36 of 53) involved the informed consent letter, many of the requested revisions (12 of 36) were for modifications that were unique to one institution and not requested by the others.

An efficient IRB can also serve as a recruitment tool for a university or even a nation. For example, Ireland has decided at the ministerial level to have the best human subjects review process (Neuhauser, Morrissey, & Votruba, 2012). The Faculty of Tropical Medicine (FTM) at Mahidol University, Thailand has been continuously registered with the U.S. Office for Human Research Protections (OHRP) since 2009 (Adams et al., 2014). A performance assessment tool developed by FTM showed that the time from submission to final approval for more than 100 research protocols decreased over the 45-month study period, from an average of 77 days to 70 days. The goal is for reviews to be completed in 60 days. In contrast, only one academic health center in the United States has a statement indicating that a student might attend there because of its excellent IRB review process.

Number and Characteristics of Participants

Universal neonatal hearing screening (see, for example, Mencher, Davis, DeVoe, Beresford, & Bamford, 2001) uses the auropalpebral reflex and otoacoustic emissions, as well as commercially available devices to identify hearing loss in the newborn. Questions about well-baby versus NICU screenings and how to deal with false positives remain. Regarding the IRB, the Department of Health and Human Services has provided guidelines about defining the term "viable infant," and these are available in the Institutional Review Board Guidebook (Office for Protection from Research Risks, 1993). The Belmont Report (1979) identified certain groups as needing special protections in terms of informed consent. Chapter VI of the Guidebook considered special characteristics of participants, identified as the following special classes of subjects: fetuses; women; children and minors; cognitively impaired persons; prisoners; comatose and traumatized persons; terminally ill patients; elderly/aged persons; minorities; as well as students, employees, and normal volunteers.

When designing an experiment (say, comparing adults with fluent aphasia to adults with nonfluent aphasia on a word retrieval task), the researcher determines the minimum number of participants that need to be enrolled in the study in order to have sufficient statistical power to detect a treatment effect. The number of proposed participants and the reason for choosing this number appear in the IRB proposal. If the design includes too few participants, a study may not have enough statistical power to detect a difference (and result in a Type II error; see Chapter 6). If the design includes too many participants, then there may be unnecessary costs in time or money.

The equations to determine adequate statistical power address several variables, including the following.

Variance and Standard Deviation

If the variance in the population is high, then more participants will be needed to find differences. For example, sensorineural (SN) hearing loss can range from mild to profound. A study that targets only moderate SN hearing loss will require fewer participants than one that examines the entire range of SN hearing loss.

Size of Treatment Effect

If there is only a small difference between the effects of two treatments, then more participants are needed to show a difference. For example, the chin-down and chin-tuck maneuver both influence the movement of swallowing-related structures. Leigh et al. (2015, p. 89) tested 20 healthy men and 20 healthy women to conclude that only the chin-tuck maneuver induced significant changes in the airway entrance, hyoid movement, and epiglottic base retraction.

Type I Error (Alpha)

This error occurs when researchers find a difference when one does not exist. The difference is a result of sampling error (see Chapter 6). Most published CSD literature uses the 0.05 level of confidence, or an alpha cutoff of 5%. This means that there is less than a 5% chance (1 in 20) that the results are due to sampling or other systematic error as opposed to a true difference. Overidentification of a communication disorder when none exists can result in treatment that is unnecessary, expensive, and time consuming.

Type II Error (Beta)

This error occurs when researchers do *not* find a difference when one *does* exist. Most medical literature uses the 0.2 level of confidence, or a beta cutoff of 20% (1 in 5) as an index that a significant difference is missed.

Method of Recruitment

Most studies published in journals use a boilerplate description of recruitment of participants, if they refer to recruitment at all. For example, the article might state something like the following: Participants were recruited voluntarily from three institutions in the greater New York City area. Even fewer articles include the cost of recruitment or the cost effectiveness of different recruitment strategies. Recruitment of special populations presents additional challenges (Buckwalter, 2009), including time to develop trust, know the culture, and engage the community. There must also be evidence of efforts to include an adequate number of women and minorities.

Sometimes, researchers must develop study designs to accommodate available sources of data, rather than having the research questions lead the design (Lysaght, Kranenburg, Armstrong, & Krupa, 2016). The initial direction of the planned research may change when low participant recruitment demands it. If samples are obtained out of convenience, then the external validity of the experiment is suspect. Especially in qualitative research, the problems associated with obtaining willing participants may introduce biases into the findings (Lysaght et al., 2016, p. 126).

Recruitment incentives are poorly regulated. It would probably be more likely for a researcher to recruit a participant by offering $1,000 in payment, rather than $10. At one time, hearing-aid manufacturers offered free trips to exotic locales if the audiologists attended presentations about the devices. This practice is now considered unethical. However, pharmaceutical giants continue to pay physicians handsome sums to recruit patients to participate in drug investigations. Lemmens and Miller (2006, p. 1238) concluded that patients have become de facto market products. Mandava and Millum (2013) reported that a subtle form of coercion can exist when a physician wears a lab coat and a stethoscope to a recruitment event. Potential participants "don't like to say no to doctors" (Mandava & Millum, 2013, p. 38).

What are some factors that influence recruitment in CSD? Researchers in autism spectrum disorders (ASD) have particular difficulties in recruiting a participant pool large enough to use as evidence for social policies. Conducting longitudinal studies with adults who have ASD is even harder. As noted above, individuals with intellectual disabilities require special protections, and informed consent may be more difficult to obtain. Haas et al. (2016) used a mixed methods (quantitative and qualitative) design to identify and explain differences in participants' responses. A total of 167 Australian adults across the range of ASD were recruited using social media; websites; support groups; and autism research groups, centers, and networks. Perhaps not surprisingly, there were common motivators and deterrents regarding participation. These included such inhibitors as travel and time, inaccessibility, and mental and physical health. Enablers included choice and access to researchers. Differentiators included extrinsic rewards (financial and other) and social interaction. However, about one-third of the adults with ASD did not care about extrinsic rewards, and some did not enjoy or were fearful of social interactions.

Haas et al. (2016) concluded that what motivated some adults with ASD, usually those higher on the spectrum, deterred others with more severe disabilities. They conclude that choice, sensitivity, and flexibility are key elements in recruiting adults with ASD to participate in research.

Potential Risks, Stresses, or Discomforts, and the Precautions Taken to Minimize Them

The Belmont Report (1979) links vulnerability to questions of justice in the selection of participants. Regulatory policy for the ethical conduct of research associates vulnerability with the limited ability to provide informed consent to participate (respect for persons, according to the Belmont Report). But what about when there are power differentials between experimenter and participant (or professor and student, supervisor and clinical fellow, sponsor and investigator, economically and politically advantaged and disadvantaged)? Having so many potentially vulnerable groups dilutes the ethical responsibility to protect them.

One definition of populations who are vulnerable refers to those who are "more likely than others to be misled, mistreated, or otherwise taken advantage of as participants in research" (Levine et al., 2004, p. 44). The IRB requires research submissions to indicate how the proposed study considers beneficence in terms of minimizing risks (consideration of the flip side of beneficence, maximizing benefits, is not required). The concept of vulnerability may be both too broad and too narrow. First, virtually all participants in research may be considered vulnerable, because there are so many categories of vulnerability. If everyone is vulnerable, then the regulation to protect them has no teeth and is meaningless. Second, the concept of vulnerability is also too narrow in its almost exclusive emphasis on characteristics of groups, to the exclusion of other factors that have the potential to harm participants. These include the research itself, the environment of the institution, and social or economic contexts. Finally, the concept of vulnerability stereotypes entire groups. For example, some members of racial or ethnic minorities are vulnerable and need special protections, and some do not.

A risk–benefit analysis guides the IRB in determining what should be disclosed to a potential participant on the consent form (Box 10–4). Of course, the risk–benefit analysis is also important for the IRB's judgment about whether or not to approve a research proposal. Researchers in CSD must pay particular attention to the informed consent process, because all individuals with communication disorders are, by the nature of their disorders, at a disadvantage in providing consent. Cascella and Aliotta (2014) considered the process of informed consent in CSD research. Potential participants may seem to lack self-determination to consent voluntarily because their communication disorder is seen as a cognitive deficit. However, they may have made self-determination decisions regarding housing, employment, and recreation, so why is it assumed that they cannot make decisions about participating in research? Excluding someone with a communication disorder from the informed consent process is inconsistent with the principle of respect for persons. Researchers need to estimate the degree of assistance—full, partial, or none—provided to the individual or surrogate (relative or friend) in obtaining informed consent.

IRBs at some universities may be more concerned with regulating scholarly behavior than protecting human research participants (Rubin & Sieber, 2006). However, human research protection programs (HRPPs) and IRBs are not the same thing. HRPPs are administrative programs and policies that specify the role of the IRB. HRPPs may also specify educational requirements for investigators, students, and IRB members. As the charge to implement research oversight belongs to the HRPP, the IRB may not be mandated to review minimal risk research or exempt research in some institutions. Rubin and Sieber reviewed three main recommendations from the American Association of University Professors (AAUP). These recommendations apply only to minimal risk research with autonomous adults. First, research on autonomous individuals done by surveys, interviews, or public observation should be exempt from IRB review. Second, there should be a separate set of procedures for research that is not federally funded. Finally, the AAUP should serve a coordinating role across academic disciplines.

Debriefing Form, Sign-Up Sheet, Advertisement

Debriefing is required by the IRB only when the experiment involved deception (Box 10–5). Deception involves deliberately misleading a participant about the

Box 10–4. Informed Consent Template

Informed Consent Template

IRB protocol title:

Principal investigator:

Coinvestigator/faculty adviser:

Research purposes: Explain the global research purpose in one or two sentences in lay language.

Description of research: Again, explain what will happen in the research in one or two sentences. Explain that you will be asked to complete a survey, take a test, participate in an interview, *and so forth,* and in sufficient detail so the participant will know what is expected and how much time it will take.

Potential risks: Explain any conceivable potential risk—explain if it will be minimal; if not minimal risk, what you are planning to do to ameliorate the risk.

Potential benefits: Explain potential benefits—both direct and indirect.

Costs/Compensation: Tell participants that there will be no compensation or explain the nature of any compensation (e.g., you will be entered into a lottery or receive a gift certificate or cash, etc.).

Additional Information

Contact persons: If you have any questions at any time about this research or want to discuss any possible study-related incidents, please contact (insert the principal investigator's name here) at (insert PI's number and email here). If a student investigator, include contact information for the faculty adviser.

Confidentiality: Explain the nature of the confidentiality that you wish to assure the participant. For example: Your identity as a participant in this research study will be kept confidential in any publication of the results of this study. The information obtained during this research (research records) will be kept confidential to the extent permitted by law. However, this research record may be reviewed by government agencies (such as the Department of Health and Human Services), the agency sponsoring this research, individuals who are authorized to monitor or audit the research or the Institutional Review Board (the committee that oversees all research in human subjects at Adelphi University), if required by applicable laws or regulations. State that the material will be maintained for up to seven years. Explain how the records will be kept confidential and who will have access as a part of the study (e.g., the principal investigator and other researchers). For focus groups add: While we cannot guarantee that all focus group members will maintain confidentiality, we are asking that you and all participants in this study not talk about the discussions that occur within the focus group session outside of the group.

Voluntary participation: Participation in this study is voluntary. For example: If you decide not to participate, this will not affect . . . Any new information that develops during this study, which might affect your decision to participate, will be given to you immediately. A signed copy of this consent form will also be given to you.

Institutional Review Board approval: This research has been reviewed and approved by the Adelphi University Institutional Review Board. If you have any questions, concerns or comments, please contact Dr. xxxx, chair of the IRB, at 516. 877.xxxx or xxxx@adelphi.edu

Consent for minors or people with legal guardians: When the study involves minors or legally incapacitated individuals, simplify the language so that it is appropriate to the target population. Also, make sure to get both the consent from the guardian and assent from the minor or legally incapacitated individual.

Person Obtaining Consent

Print name: ______________________________

Signature: ______________________________

Date: ______________

Study Coordinator

Print name: ______________________________

Signature: ______________________________

Date: ______________

Study Participant

Print name: ______________________________

Signature: ______________________________

Date: ______________

Revised and reprinted with permission. *Source:* https://research-grants.adelphi.edu/irb/forms/ (Adelphi University, 2017)

Box 10–5. Debriefing Template

Elements of a Debriefing Form

1. Thanks
2. What the Study Was About/the Hypothesis (or Hypotheses)
3. What the Participants Did
4. Practical Application of the Study
5. Compensation (if Applicable)
6. Contact Information

Debriefing Form (SAMPLE)

Thank you for your participation. The study in which you have served as a participant is concerned with how attention to words can improve auditory comprehension in individuals with a hearing loss. The hypothesis for this study was that adults with a mild hearing loss would identify words better when they thought they were wearing a hearing aid. You filled out some demographic questions and completed a hearing evaluation. The practical application of this research concerns how to help audiologists and speech-language pathologists do aural rehabilitation. For completing all parts of this study you will receive $25.00. If you have any questions about this research, or if you would like a copy of the results, please call Dr. XYZ at (999) 999-9999.

Revised and reprinted with permission. *Source:* https://research-grants.adelphi.edu/irb/forms/ (Adelphi University, 2017)

nature of the research or the experimental procedures. Research participants may be deceived about the purpose of the research. There may be fake or rigged equipment or procedures that are explained to participants differently. The experiment may include misleading play acting that may also include another individual acting as a confederate to play a deceptive role. Covert procedures, such as a one-way mirror or hidden camera may be employed. Finally, the entire experimental procedure may be staged in a public place to make it appear natural or real. The participant who was given, for example, a nonfunctional hearing aid to assess the placebo effect must be told of the deception at the end of the experiment. Of the five types of deception that appear in research (Benham, 2008; Miller, Gluck, & Wendler, 2008; Sharpe & Faye, 2009), none seem to be used in CSD research with any regularity.

Regarding advertising, attachments to the proposal submitted to the IRB should include letters of cooperation from any external organization or entity (including listserve) that are involved with the proposal, including participant recruitment.

Recruitment or solicitation materials generally include letters, postings, flyers, and scripts. There must be a statement included that is similar to the following: This research has been reviewed and approved by the (name of) University Institutional Review Board (IRB). If you have any comments, questions, or concerns, please contact the IRB chair, Dr. X at (phone number and email address).

Krusche et al. (2014) described an effort to determine the types of advertising that were most effective in recruiting participants for a study about staying well after depression. They listed the following as the cheapest forms of advertising: poster advertising, Web-based advertising, and mental health worker referrals. However, the yield in terms of enrolled randomized participants was inconsistent with these methods. The most cost-effective forms of advertising that yielded enrolled participants were the following: advertising online, by posters, and on a local radio station. An important strategy was saturation advertising across many sources.

AN EXAMPLE FROM CSD

The Tudor Study was described in Chapter 3. In 1939, under the supervision of Wendell Johnson (one of the founders of the science of speech-language pathology), graduate student Mary Tudor conducted a study to examine the effect of verbal labeling on the frequency of disfluency in both children who stuttered and children who were fluent. The subjects came from an orphanage in Davenport, Iowa. Johnson and Tudor's findings that they were allegedly able to induce stuttering in normally fluent children supported their hypothesis, but have also raised serious ethical concerns. A subsequent symposium and edited book (Goldfarb, 2006) investigated the Tudor Study and, more broadly, ethics in scientific research, diagnosis, and treatment in the field of communication sciences.

There was no IRB or comparable ethical committee at the time of the Tudor Study that could have reviewed the research proposal. If Johnson's diagnosogenic theory were correct, the fluent children in the negative feedback condition would have developed stuttering. Even if the theory were incorrect, as it subsequently has been determined to be, the negative feedback could have caused the children psychological distress. The study involved deception, and there was no poststudy debriefing.

Schwartz (2006) considered the type of study that a current IRB might have approved. To test the diagnosogenic theory, the children would have to be recruited from schools or clinics, but not orphanages. Parental permission would be required, along with the child's assent. A larger number of participants, more than in the Tudor Study, would be needed to assess effect of intervention. The pretest/posttest design of the original study would be changed to multiple-baseline or ABA withdrawal designs for the purpose of examining effects of intervention. The negative feedback condition would not be included, because of its potential for harm by causing fluent children to stutter, given the assumptions of the theory. Children who stuttered at the beginning of the study would have to be debriefed because they were deceived.

ADVANCED STUDY

The author proposes that Institutional Review Board (IRB) skills are necessary for an individual to be granted power of professor. With new generations of scholars and researchers needed every 10 years, professors and master clinicians have an obligation to prepare individuals with adequate knowledge and skills to undertake the tasks of scholarship and research, and the IRB is a key component. For evidence of the requisite IRB skills, complete the following and have your instructor, academic adviser, mentor, or CSD department chair review that you have completed the requirements and sign and date where indicated.

Student's Name: ______________________________

Assignment: Write a research proposal, and complete the IRB Review form in this chapter or the one used at your university. With your instructor's approval, you may submit it to your local IRB for feedback.

Date of Completion: ______________________________

Faculty/Supervisor Signature: ______________________________

REFERENCES

Abbott, L., & Grady, C. (2011). A systematic review of the empirical literature evaluating IRBs: What we know and what we still need to learn. *Journal of Empirical Research on Human Research Ethics, 6*, 3–20.

Adams, P., Kaewkungwal, J., Limphattharacharoen, C., Prakobtham, S., Pengsaa, K., & Khusmith, S. (2014). Is your ethics committee efficient? Using "IRB metrics" as a self-assessment tool for continuous improvement at the Faculty of Tropical Medicine, Mahidol University, Thailand. *PLoS One, 9*(11), e113356. doi:10.1371/journal.pone.0113356

Adelphi University. (2017). *Institutional Review Board. Policies and procedures.* Adelphi University, NY: Garden City. Retrieved from http://research-grants.adelphi.edu/irb/

Anderson, E. E., & DuBois, J. M. (2012). IRB decision-making with imperfect knowledge: A framework for evidence-based research ethics review. *Journal of Law, Medicine & Ethics, 40*(4), 951–969. doi:10.1111/j.1748-720X.2012.00724.x

Author. (1993). Protecting human research subjects: Institutional review board guidebook. *NIH Guide, 22*(29). Retrieved from https://grants.nih.gov/grants/guide/notice-files/not93-209.html

Benham, B. (2008). Moral accountability and debriefing. *Kennedy Institute of Ethics Journal, 18*(3), 253–273. Retrieved from https://search-proquest-com.libproxy.adelphi.edu:2443/docview/217112228?accountid=8204

Buckwalter, K. C. (2009). Recruitment of older adults: An ongoing challenge. *Research in Gerontological Nursing, 2*(4), 265–266.

Cascella, P. W., & Aliotta, F. (2014). Strategies to enhance the informed consent process for communication disorders researchers. *Communication Disorders Quarterly, 35*(4), 248–251.

Chappy, S., & Gaberson, K. B. (2012). To IRB or not to IRB: That is the question! *Association of*

Operating Room Nurses Journal, 95(6), 682–683. doi:10.1016/j.aorn.2012.03.012

Conforti, L., Ross, K., Hess, B., Lynn, L., & Holmboe, E. (2008, December). *Length of time needed for Institutional Review Board approval or exemption of quality improvement projects among subset of US training programs.* Presentation to the American Board of Internal Medicine, Nashville, TN.

Dyrbye, L. N., Thomas, M. R., Mechaber, A. J., Eacker, A., Harper, W., Massie, F. S., Jr., . . . Shanafelt, T. D. (2007). Medical education research and IRB review: An analysis and comparison of the IRB review process at six institutions. *Academic Medicine, 82*(7), 654–660.

Enfield, K. B., & Truwit, J. D. (2008). The purpose, composition and function of an institutional review board: Balancing priorities. *Respiratory Care, 53*, 1330–1336.

Goldfarb, R. (Ed.). (2006). *Ethics: A case study from fluency.* San Diego, CA: Plural Publishing.

Greaney, A.-M., Sheehy, A., Heffernan, C., Murphy, J., Ni Mhaolrúnaigh, S., Heffernan, E., & Brown, G. (2012). Research ethics application: A guide for the novice researcher. *British Journal of Nursing, 21*, 38–43.

Haas, K., Costley, D., Falkmer, M., Richdale, A., Sofronoff, K., & Falkmer, T. (2016). Factors influencing the research participation of adults with autism spectrum disorders. *Journal of Autism and Developmental Disorders, 46*(5), 1793–1805.

Hyer, C. F. (2010). What is an IRB, why do we need it, and what is a private IRB? *Foot & Ankle Specialist, 3*(2), 91–94.

Kant, I. (1993). *Grounding for the metaphysics of morals* (3rd ed., p. 30.). Indianapolis, IN: Hackett.

Krusche, A., Rudolf von Rohr, I., Muse, K., Duggan, D., Crane, C., & Williams, J. M. G. (2014). An evaluation of the effectiveness of recruitment methods: The staying well after depression randomized controlled trial. *Clinical Trials, 11*(2), 141–149. doi:10.1177/1740774514521905

Leigh, J-H., Oh, B-M., Seo, H. G., Lee, G. J., Min, Y., Kim, K., . . . Han, T. R. (2015). Influence of the chin-down and chin-tuck maneuver on the swallowing kinematics of healthy adults. *Dysphagia, 30*, 89–98.

Lemmens, T., & Miller, P. B. (2006). Regulating the market in human research participants. *PLoS Medicine, 3*(8), e330. doi:10.1371/journal.pmed.0030330

Levine, C., Faden, R., Grady, C., Hammerschmidt, D., Eckenwiler, L., & Sugarman, J. (2004). The limitations of "vulnerability" as a protection for human research participants. *American Journal of Bioethics, 4*(3), 44–49.

Lysaght, R., Kranenburg, R., Armstrong, C., & Krupa, T. (2016). Participant recruitment for studies on disability and work: Challenges and solutions. *Journal of Occupational Rehabilitation, 26*(2), 125–140. doi:10.1007/s10926-015-9594-1

Mandava, A., & Millum, J. (2013). Manipulation in the enrollment of research participants. *Hastings Center Report, 43*(2), 38–47.

Martin, R. C. (2013). Navigating the IRB: The ethics of SoTL. *New Directions for Teaching & Learning, 2013*(136), 59–71. doi:10.1002/tl.20076

Mencher, G. T., Davis, A. C., DeVoe, S. J., Beresford, D., & Bamford, J. M. (2001). Universal neonatal hearing screening. *American Journal of Audiology, 10*, 3–12.

Miller, F. G., Gluck, J. P., Jr., & Wendler, D. (2008). Debriefing and accountability in deceptive research. *Kennedy Institute of Ethics Journal, 18*(3), 235–251.

Moon, R. M. (2009). The history and role of institutional review boards. *Virtual Mentor, American Medical Association Journal of Ethics, 11*, 311–321.

National Commission for the Protection of Human Subjects of Biomedical and Behavioral Research. (1979). *The Belmont Report: Ethical principles and guidelines for the protections of human subjects of research* [GPO Office 887-890]. Washington, DC: Government Printing Office.

Nelson, C. R. (2012). In remembrance there is prevention: A brief review of four historical failures to protect human subjects. *Journal of Research Administration, 43*(1), 98–111.

Neuhauser, D., Morrissey, M., & Votruba, M. (2012). Your human subjects review process: A road block or a competitive advantage? *Journal of Clinical Research & Bioethics, 3*(130). doi:10.4172/2155-9627.1000130

Nuremberg Code. (1949). *Trials of war criminals before the Nuremberg military tribunals under Control Council Law, 10, 82*. Retrieved from http://www.ushmm.org/research/doctors/Nuremberg_Code.htm

Office for Human Research Protections. (2009). *Protection of human subjects. Title 45, Code of Federal Regulations, Part 46.* Retrieved from https://www.hhs.gov/ohrp/sites/default/files/ohrp/humansubjects/regbook2013.pdf

Office for Protection from Research Risks. (1993). *Protecting human research subjects: Institutional review board guidebook (Chapter VI).* Washington, DC: U. S. Government Printing Office. Retrieved from https://archive.hhs.gov/ohrp/irb/irb_chapter6.htm

Rubin, P., & Sieber, J. E. (2006). Empirical research on IRBs and methodologies usually associated with minimal risk. *Journal of Empirical Research on Human Research Ethics, 1*(4), 1–4. doi:10.1525/jer.2006.1.4.1

Schwartz, R. G. (2006). Would today's IRB approve the Tudor study? Ethical considerations in conducting research involving children with communication disorders. In R. Goldfarb (Ed.), *Ethics: A case study from fluency* (pp. 83–96). San Diego, CA: Plural Publishing.

Sharpe, D., & Faye, C. (2009). A second look at debriefing practices: Madness in our method? *Ethics & Behavior, 19*(5), 432–447. doi:10.1080/10508420903035455

Stark, L., & Greene, J. A. (2016). Clinical trials, healthy controls, and the birth of the IRB. *New England Journal of Medicine, 375*, 1013–1015.

Wertz, R., Collins, M., Weiss, D., Kurtzke, J., Friden, T., Brookshire, R., . . . Resurreccion, E. (1981). Veterans administration cooperative study in aphasia: A comparison of individual and group treatment. *Journal of Speech and Hearing Research, 24*, 580–594.

Yairi, E., Ambrose, N., & Cox, N. (1996). Genetics of stuttering. *Journal of Speech, Language, and Hearing Research, 39*, 771–784.

11

Conducting Clinical Research

INTRODUCTION

Now that you have your research proposal approved by the Institutional Review Board (IRB) and your academic, peer, or professional mentor is helping you conduct your first project as a clinical researcher, it is time to get started. Assume that your first research project with be with a single client who has a communication disorder (n = 1). Also assume that this project will have something to do with diagnosis or treatment of the communication disorder. In Chapter 5 and at the end of the present chapter, you will find information about n = 1 studies. In general, the case report design should be limited to low-incidence disorders (e.g., primary progressive aphasia) or cases of high interest due to unusual circumstances (e.g., an aphasiologist reporting the journal of his stroke). Most likely, your n = 1 study will be a variation of an A-B-A design where A indicates baseline and baseline recovery and B indicates the experimental intervention.

You will first need to develop a clinical hypothesis and then set goals. Write your clinical hypothesis as indicated in Box 11–1, and check that you have full evidence in all areas in the rubric for the clinical hypothesis as indicated in Box 11–2. If you are assessing the efficacy of an experimental clinical intervention, then ethics of practice requires that your clinical hypothesis include evidence that there is equipoise between the standard treatment and the experimental intervention (see Chapter 3). The goals that you set will be based on the nature of the disorder and type of intervention. Compare the two types of goals that Yairi and Seery (2015) show in the section on setting goals as an inadequate and an excellent example.

Learning the operant condition paradigm is a foundation for data collection, such as whether or not the research project uses applied behavior analysis for intervention in autism spectrum disorders. Our professional charge is to modify maladaptive communicative behavior, so a solid grounding in behavior modification seems appropriate.

Learning Objectives

After reading this chapter, the student will be able to

- apply the scientific method to clinical practice;
- develop a capstone project in evidence-based practice; and
- set clinical goals.

DEVELOPING A CLINICAL HYPOTHESIS

As noted in Chapter 4, the term *hypothesis* is used to refer to a statement—either descriptive or explanatory—that has not yet been adequately tested. A hypothesis suggests, with varying levels of certainty, why certain phenomena or behavior might have occurred (Nickels, 2008). An initial or working hypothesis may be little more than a provisional conjecture, while a theory uses accumulated facts to propose an explanation that is highly probable. Experienced clinicians observe the language behavior of a client to develop a hypothesis about the language impairment by comparing the behavior to an "internal database" of similar observations from previous cases (Nickels, 2008, p. 14). Validation in a clinical process depends on two activities (Tuckett, 1994): clarifying what is asserted as true, and distinguishing the actual (the facts of a clinical situation) from the theoretical (the hypothesis of what is happening in a clinical situation).

How do you develop a research question that leads to a hypothesis? At first, you must become familiar with the subject that will lead to the research question; that is, you must learn the boundary between the known and the unknown. The hardest parts will be in deciding which of the uncertainties is worthy of study and in rationalizing the need for the investigation (Farrugia, Petrisor, Farrokhyar, & Bhandari, 2010). So search the literature, paying particular attention to systematic reviews and meta-analyses, and essentially conduct your own systematic review with your research question in mind. Establish a single primary research question that specifies the population being tested and the intervention being implemented before you start any testing. Conduct a pilot study or a feasibility study to identify problems with your primary or secondary questions or errors in your protocol before applying for a grant or running a full trial.

A clinical hypothesis form, such as the type in Box 11–1 proposed by Santo Pietro and Goldfarb (1995, p. 8), is filled in to test the efficacy of descriptive or explanatory statements used in therapy. Items I through III, while not part of the hypothesis, are included as information that motivates the hypothesis. The main difference between a clinical hypothesis and a therapy plan (or the incorrectly termed "lesson plan") is the inclusion of rationales for VI and VIII. A typical therapy plan indicates the answers to *who* (the patient or client), *what* (the problem and treatment goals), *when* (schedule of intervention), *where* (location of treatment), and *how* (methodology) questions. A clinical hypothesis adds *why* questions: Why has the clinician chosen these goals, selected this treatment, chosen to implement the procedure in this particular way, and chosen these materials?

All best practices models require a literature search to determine evidence on

Box 11–1. Clinical Hypothesis

I. Identifying information: Patient's name, age, schedule of appointments, communication disorder.

II. Background information: Brief accounts of patient's background and history including pertinent information about family as well as developmental, medical, educational, psychological, occupational, and treatment histories. Note current interests, activities, and talents.

III. Recent diagnostic results: Brief statement of patient's most recent evaluation and test results.

IV. Statement of the problem: Brief statement of the particular clinical problem to be treated.

V. Treatment goals: Statement of behaviors patient is expected to achieve.

VI. Rationale for treatment goals: Reasons for choosing these goals (why the goals are appropriate for this patient).

VII. Methodology: List of procedures and materials to use to achieve the patient's treatment goals.

VIII. Rationale for methodology: Reason for choosing these procedures and materials.

IX. Bibliography: References from the literature to support the above hypothesis.

which to base clinical decisions, and references are listed in item IX. Finally, "lesson plan" is considered a misnomer, because the educational model requires the clinician to follow a curriculum even if it is not successful. Testing a clinical hypothesis follows the scientific method (see Chapter 4), where lack of success may indicate that the hypothesis has been falsified. Then the clinician can immediately try something else (test another hypothesis) that may be better suited to treating the client. There may also be less of a perceived divide between clinical intervention and clinical research when therapy involves hypothesis testing.

The only way to confirm a hypothesis is to eliminate alternative hypotheses. Simply making and verifying predictions are not the best ways to confirm a hypothesis. Make predictions with alternate hypotheses in mind, so as to eliminate as many of these hypotheses as possible. The hypothesis gains strength by defeating logical and reasonable alternatives, much as a champion athlete becomes an "all-time great" by defeating exceptionally strong challenges by rivals. Box 11–2 shows a rubric for evaluating a clinical hypothesis.

SETTING GOALS

In setting measurable therapy objectives, the clinician or clinical researcher needs to address several questions. What goals

Box 11–2. Rubric for Clinical Hypothesis

Student:	Grade:		
Topic	**Evidence**		
	Full	Partial	None
Literature Review			
References Cited			
Efficacy			
Statement of Problem			
Treatment Goals			
Rationale			
Methodology			
Rationale			
Competence in Professional Writing			
Comments:			

will impact the client's effectiveness most as a speaker? With what goals can the client expect to achieve the target behaviors? What goals are most appropriate to the client's individual background, needs, and cultural experiences? Setting specific, client-centered goals avoids a single measure of outcome that is the same in all cases. A benefit is that it allows quantification of outcomes in each case. This approach is termed *goal attainment scaling*, a method of measuring change in individual clients that was first used in learning disabilities and psychiatry, but currently also applies to rehabilitation (Wade, 2009).

It is also important that goals for clients are consistent with those of the International Classification of Functioning, Disability, and Health (ICF; WHO, 2002). Interviews with 50 persons with aphasia (PWA) poststroke were undertaken to measure the concordance between their goals and those of the ICF (Worrall et al., 2010). Of the nine goal categories articulated by PWA, the ability to return to prestroke life, as well as return of communication and physical function were expected. Regarding the word-finding deficit in aphasia, based on 100 PWA in the United Kingdom, the words considered most important to be able to say came from the category of food and drink (Palmer, Hughes, & Chater, 2017). However, there were broader life goals in the areas of social life, work, and leisure; information about aphasia and stroke; as well as altruism that are not usually addressed in rehabilitation (Worrall et al.,

2010, p. 318). The goals of PWA did link to all of those on the ICF spectrum, but particularly focused on activity and participation components.

Therapy Objectives

For clinical accountability and research purposes, it is important that goals be phrased in language that expresses what the client is doing, not thinking. For example, saying that a child with autism spectrum disorders was distracted and not compliant 40% of the time does not show what behaviors motivated the clinician to conclude that there was distraction or noncompliance. For both clinical intervention and research purposes, as indicated later in this chapter, observed behaviors following formal and informal testing are expressed as baseline data. Clinical intervention followed by baseline recovery data shows if treatment resulted in changes. A formula for writing therapy objectives that are behavioral or observable should include the following information:

> Who → will do what → to what level of accuracy → for how many trials → over how many consecutive therapy sessions → under what conditions?

Yairi and Seery (2015) compared two therapy objectives:

> John will perform his fluency targets with 95% accuracy.
>
> John will independently apply a slow, easy speech initiation on 100 utterances with 95% accuracy during spontaneous conversation with peers across two consecutive group sessions in the therapy room.

The first therapy objective includes *who* and part of *what level of accuracy*. The second goal incorporates all the behavioral or observable information required to measure progress at the end of therapy. Note that functional goals are incorporated into the second objective above. Randall and McEwen (2000) describe a 5-step process for writing functional goals in physical therapy that are easily adaptable for treatment of communication disorders. They are who → will do what → under what conditions → how well → by when. Fundamental to the ability to write functional communication goals is an understanding of functional communication in typical individuals for two reasons: the clinician needs to know whether there is a communication disorder, and communication outside the therapy room may be the ideal treatment goal. For example, individuals who have cognitive-communication disorders as a result of closed-head injury may already be able to produce social phrases and express basic personal needs, so speech-language therapy may need to focus on functional communication in daily living, community, and work environments (Hartley & Griffith, 1989).

It is important to note here that criterion levels for mastery or achievement of a goal will vary according to the client's needs. As a member of the site visit team for the Council on Academic Accreditation, I visited many communication sciences and disorders (CSD) graduate programs across the United States and found a disturbing consistency. Virtually all of the treatment goals I saw in student reports from the programs' centers for communicative disorders set a target of 80% correct responses for mastery or achievement, regardless of the task or the disorder. Another problem was that the 80% target did not indicate if it resulted from 4 out of 5 correct responses, 16 out of 20, or 80 out of 100. The "magic" 80% correct becomes ridiculous in the following case: An individual with a mild form of disfluency stutters on 15% of words spoken. The goal of 80% correct responses would be a goal to make the client worse or *more* disfluent.

A larger number of trials are necessary to show that muscle memory (striatal memory) has been developed, compared to, for example, semantic memory (hippocampal memory). Accordingly, goals for treatment of articulation disorders or treatment of dysarthria that focuses on the speech effector system—respiration, phonation, resonation, and articulation—should include many trials to criterion and a high level of accuracy. Increasing the number of trials helps statistical power in subsequent analyses, that is, the likelihood that therapy or research will detect an effect when there is one. High statistical power, the result of analyzing a large number of data points, reduces the likelihood of the Type II error of accepting a null hypothesis when it should have been the rejected alternative. Another way of saying this is that the chance of concluding there is no effect of the clinical or research treatment when there is one, goes down.

The previously described examples refer to a ratio of correct trials. The following section on operant conditioning indicates that it is sometimes more valuable to measure intervals, rather than ratios. A goal for an individual who stutters might be a percentage of words spoken with stutter-free speech, but it may also be useful to use an interval goal of three consecutive measures of 60 s of fluency at a particular task level, as is done in *The Stocker Probe for Fluency and Language, Third Edition* (Stocker & Goldfarb, 1995). Another interval goal might be three consecutive measures of 5 s of eye contact for modifying gaze aversion in a child with autism spectrum disorders.

DATA COLLECTION

We make decisions about whether or not treatment is working based on data. Good clinicians depend on data to support claims of change as a result of intervention. As the saying goes, "If you didn't document it, you didn't do it." However, accountability should not be the driving force behind data collection, because it has come to mean the involvement of a third party, often an insurance company (Olswang & Bain, 1994). Rather than only looking at data collection after the fact to demonstrate effectiveness or justify past decision making, data should be used to make ongoing clinical decisions. Data-based decision making can determine if the client is responding to treatment, if the change is significant or important, if the treatment is responsible for the change, and if the therapy target has been achieved (Olswang & Bain, 1994, p. 55).

Data can be quantitative or qualitative, and clinical research can include both. For example, an examination of how people who stutter cope with the disorder used a mixed methods approach (Swartz, Irani, & Gabel, 2015). The quantitative approach used a larger number of participants to permit generalization to a larger population of individuals who stutter, while the qualitative approach facilitated a deeper understanding of how individuals cope with stuttering. For example, a task for subsequent quantitative analysis might be completion of the question, "On a scale of 1 to 9, how well do you cope with your stuttering?," while a response to an open-ended question (e.g., "What does successfully coping with stuttering mean to you?") can be part of a qualitative analysis (Swartz et al., 2015, p. 61).

Collection of speech and language samples, whether it is in traditional orthography or by phonetic transcription, is a cumbersome and often inaccurate exercise. However, for anyone with a computer, digital data collection technology is readily available for use in research and clinical practice (Ingram, Bunta, & Ingram, 2004). Digital, as opposed to analog recording, permits access to some inexpensive and some free analysis programs. Ingram et al. note several of these options, as well as clinical options to play and edit digital audio files. Remote data collection is possible with voice and facial recognition software that is adaptable for speech-language therapy (Frost & McCrindle, 2016).

The Operant Conditioning Paradigm

Having some basic understanding of applied behavior analysis is important for accurate collection of data. The operant conditioning paradigm (Box 11–3) offers an overview of behavior modification principles. Audiologists and speech-language pathologists are in the business of modifying maladaptive behaviors in communication, cognition, and swallowing, whether the etiology of the behaviors is organic or functional.

Systematic reinforcement of operant behaviors can lead to new responses that expand a person's interactive repertoires communicatively, socially, and verbally. New reflexes cannot be learned, but operant procedures can be used to inhibit or shape released infantile oral reflexes, such as suckling and biting that may be exhibited following brain damage in adults. For example, the clinician can shape the suckling reflex for production of /w/ and /u/ sounds. Operant audiometry has been the focus of research in testing hearing of young children through localization (Primus, 1987) and visual reinforcement strategies (Thompson, Thompson, & Vethivelu, 1989).

SLPs with a limited understanding of applied behavior analysis (ABA) are at risk for modifying or evaluating maladaptive communicative behavior ineffectively. Consider the following vignette (Goldfarb, 2006): Several adults with aphasia are seated in a small group during a speech-language therapy session. One of the adult clients points to the door and says, "Go, go." When this request is ignored by the SLP, the client repeats the gesture and utterance with greater intensity. Without turning to the client, the SLP says, "Just a minute; I'm helping John now." The client then unlocks his wheelchair and rolls back and forth, ramming the chairs of the other group members. This continues until the SLP turns to the client and says, "All right, I'm coming."

This vignette illustrates important limitations in the application of the principles of reinforcement. Specifically, the client demonstrates several forms of verbal

Box 11–3. The Operant Conditioning Paradigm

$$S^D \rightarrow R \rightarrow S^{r+/-}$$

Stimuli (S^r) coming immediately *after* a performance (R) may alter that performance as follows:

	S^{r+} = Positive consequence or payoff	S^{r-} = Aversive consequence or payoff
Increase rate or probability of R	*Positive Reinforcement A. R produces or serves to turn on S^{r+} B. R prevents loss of S^{r+} (an avoidance response)	*Negative reinforcement A. R terminates S^{r-} (an escape response) B. R serves to avoid S^{r-} (an avoidance response)
Decrease rate or probability of R	A. R terminates S^{r+} (extinction)	A. R produces or serves to turn on S^{r-} (punishment) B. R terminates further escape from S^{r-} (extinction)

*Only the *upper* cells are reinforcement because to reinforce is to strengthen, that is, to increase the frequency or probability of occurrence of R.

Stimuli (S^D) coming immediately *before* a performance (R) may, by appropriate use of the relationships above, acquire control of the performance (R) as follows:

S^D serves to signal that a performance (R) *will* have a consequence (S^r) and it also signals that a consequence (S^r) will be positive or that it will be aversive. In an operant chain of performances, S^D can be a conditioned positive or aversive consequence, that is, it can serve a dual function as S^r and S^D. S^Ds exist *only* as a result of prior conditioning.

S^Δ serves to signal that a performance (R) will have NO consequence (S^r) of any kind. In an operant chain, S^Δ can be a conditioned aversive consequence, that is, it can serve a dual function as S^r and S^Δ. S^Δs exist *only* as a result of prior conditioning.

and nonverbal behavior with the potential to gain social attention (e.g., pointing, vocalizing, chair-ramming). However, the SLP responds to the one form (chair-ramming) that is the least adaptive from a social-communicative perspective. Moreover, the SLP ignores (at least twice) two conventional forms (pointing, vocalizing) with the highest level of social acceptability. If the goal is to gain the SLP's attention, then the client learns two lessons from the interaction: (1) conventional social signals are not reinforced in this context, and (2) antisocial behavior (chair-ramming) leads to reinforcement. Under these conditions, we can expect an increase in the frequence of maladaptive behaviors for communicative purposes.

The operant conditioning paradigm consists of a discriminative stimulus, an antecedent event (S^D) that sets the stage for the occurrence of a performance (R), to be followed by a consequent event that may be positive or aversive ($S^{r+/-}$). Just as the curtain goes up on a Broadway show revealing the set design before the action begins, the antecedent event includes the materials or stimulus items that the clinician brings into the therapy room. For example, an audiologist brings a spondee list and an audiometer to the test suite, or a speech-language pathologist brings a set of sequencing cards to the treatment room in order to set the occasion for the performance (R) of an activity (repeating a spondee word or sorting the cards) by the client.

The performance (R) can occur under the control of the antecedent event (S^D), the consequent event or payoff ($S^{r+/-}$), or both. The performance is specified by the clinician as the target or goal behavior and can be shaped by both antecedent and consequent events. For example, the clinician can bundle many stimulus cues into the S^D to shape a client's performance and then gradually fade them, as in the following example. The therapy session with an adult who has a severe word-finding problem due to nonfluent aphasia begins with a series of highly associative open-ended sentences. The stimulus cues include the syntax of the sentence, the initial phoneme of the target word, and an iconic or symbolic gesture. For example, the clinician raps on the top of the table while saying, "Someone is knocking at the front d___." The clinician presents 25 such sentences with the goal of having the client say 20 of them (80%) correctly over three consecutive sessions. When the goal is achieved, the clinician eliminates first the gestural and then the phonemic cue if the client maintains the target behavior of retrieving the correct word 20/25 times.

The consequent event or payoff can be positive (S^{r+}) or aversive (S^{r-}), depending on the strategy used. For example, students are told at the beginning of the semester that arriving on time to class will result in 5 points added to the final grade or that arriving late to class will result in a deduction of 5 points from the final grade. Both can be expected to increase the frequency or probability of on-time arrival to class. The consequences are, accordingly, both reinforcing, because to reinforce means to strengthen. (Remember when you used to stick reinforcers over the holes of your loose-leaf pages so they would not tear out of the binder?) The positive payoff strengthens on-time behavior because it serves to add points to your grade (see A in the upper-left cell in Box 11–3). On-time behavior can also serve to avoid the aversive consequence of points off your grade (see B in the upper-right cell in Box 11–3). A slight adjustment to the payoffs reveals the other possibilities of reinforcement. Now the class is told in the 5th week that the 5-point bonus will be added if the student comes on time for 10 consecutive weeks in the 15-week semester. Alternatively, a student who received a 5-point penalty because of lateness that occurred in the first 5 weeks could have the penalty removed with perfect punctuality for the rest of the semester. Now the payoffs are revealed in B of the top-left cell, where a student avoids the loss of the bonus by continuing to be punctual, and in A of the top-right cell, where a student can escape from the penalty by having perfect punctuality.

So the opposite of positive reinforcement is NOT negative reinforcement because they both increase the likelihood of punctuality, using the example above. However, if we look at contingencies for lateness, we can bring in the lower cells. In the lower-left cell, lateness can be extinguished when it will result in the loss of the opportunity to get 5 more points, or as in B of the lower-right cell, it triggers the 5-point penalty if lateness continues. We tend not to build A of the lower right cell into our contingency plans, as punishment is effective only to the extent that it is being delivered. Once punishment stops, it no longer has an inhibitory effect.

There are subtleties in the paradigm that the student of applied behavior analysis learns. For example, the child on the autism spectrum who exhibits tantrum behaviors (that you have defined operationally; see Chapter 4) might be expected to reduce the tantrums if they result in extinction consequences. However, extinction procedures are often accompanied by something called a compensatory rise in the maladaptive behaviors before the tantrums start to decrease. For example, extinguishing the behavior of a baby who cries to be picked up is likely to result in an increase in crying before it starts to decrease. It is crucial to keep accurate data to demonstrate that the compensatory rise in tantrums or crying is temporary.

Another subtlety about the operant conditioning paradigm is the S^{Δ} that signals that there will be no consequence following the performance (R). S^{Δ} is used when diagnostic testing is involved, an important part of pretreatment data collection in clinical research. With S^{Δ} there are consequences only for behaviors that are not being evaluated. In other words, it is incorrect to say, "Good" when a client points to the correct response on a test, unless the clinician says, "Good" for every pointing behavior. The justification is that the clinician is strengthening pointing behavior, not the consequence of the pointing. Please do not try this until you are a seasoned professional. It is hard to modulate your voice so that every utterance of "Good" sounds the same. More often, the new clinician makes the rookie mistake of saying "Good" for pointing to the correct answer, and something like "Okay" for pointing to another picture. "But I'm reinforcing pointing behavior," you say. No, you're teaching the client about correct and incorrect choices.

The design of the diagnostic test can present other problems. A frequently used design in diagnostic tests is a visual multiple-choice format, whereby the patient is shown three or four pictures, is given a stimulus word, and then has to select among the options. Heuer, Ivanova, and Hallowell (2017) noted that individuals with aphasia had a greater proportion of fixation duration for a single image than for three images in both verbal and nonverbal conditions. The more severe the aphasia, the longer was the fixation duration for nontarget singleton images following a verbal stimulus. The authors concluded that a verbal stimulus to an individual with aphasia may not override the effect of the characteristics of a visual stimulus.

Clinical intervention begins with the collection of baseline data and ends with the collection of baseline recovery data.

Simply stated, measurements before treatment starts and when treatment ends serve to support claims of change. Baseline data can include standardized testing, such as a complete audiological evaluation or a battery of tests to assess aphasia; this is called hard data. Soft data, such as that obtained by observing a child at play, is also useful as a baseline measure.

Data collection is also crucial during therapy sessions to determine achievement of target goals or evidence of mastery. The example above for meeting Yairi and Seery's (2015) goal for fluency requires baseline data (to show that the client has more than 5% disfluency) and data that documents fluency during treatment sessions.

Schedules of Reinforcement

Ideally, in an operant-based program of instruction, there should be a hierarchy that permits the client to succeed at every level, yet provides appropriate challenges along the way. We need to address antecedent events, or stimuli that set the stage for the occurrence of the target communicative behavior; what the target behavior should be at every level of therapy; and consequent events, or the types of "payoffs" that follow performance of the target behaviors. Finally, we need to decide on a schedule of reinforcement.

Reinforcement schedules can be fixed or variable ratio (number of trials) or fixed or variable interval (period of time) payoffs. In CRF, for continuous reinforcement, every correct display of the target behavior has a consequence. This is also called FR1, for fixed ratio = 1. In a fixed interval, a consequence or payoff is delivered after a prescribed period of time; for example, every 5 seconds of fluency or chair-sitting behavior. For the purpose of generalization, it is appropriate to change the schedule of reinforcement from fixed to variable. It is unlikely for a caregiver to remember to deliver a consequence exactly after, say, every 10 correct trials or every 10 seconds, but it reasonable that the consequence can be delivered after an average of 10 trials or 10 seconds. A therapy goal should be to increase the number of trials or amount of time before reinforcement is delivered. The Lidcombe Program (Onslow, Packman, & Harrison, 2003) was developed in Australia as an operant conditioning method of reinforcing fluent speech in children who stutter. While the authors view consequent events of stuttering as neutral, the fact that parents are instructed to highlight disfluencies as "bumpy speech" might lead a behaviorist to view these corrections as aversive consequences. Parents of disfluent children are trained to use variable ratio or variable interval schedules of reinforcement.

Another way to build upon an operant response is through response elaboration training (RET; Kearns, 1985), a procedure to increase verbal elaboration abilities of adults with aphasia. RET is based on shaping and chaining patient-initiated responses where the criterion level to advance to the next level is 90% correct for an individualized and predetermined number of content words per utterance. In an operant chain, the payoff (S^{r1}) becomes the antecedent event (S^{D2}) for the next link in the chain. An adaptation of RET appeared in Santo Pietro and Goldfarb (1995; Box 11–4).

Here is an example where intervention does not result in improved communication (Figure 11–1). Following is a

Box 11–4. An Application of Chaining in Response Elaboration Training

1. The patient is shown cards with line drawings giving minimal contextual cues.
2. The patient's initial responses are modeled and reinforced by the clinician, using patient's responses only.
3. The patient is asked to repeat the modeled response.
4. The clinician asks questions to prompt elaboration of patient's initial response.
5. The patient's second response is modeled and reinforced by the clinician, using patient's responses only.
6. The clinician combines initial and second responses, creating a complex sentence.
7. The patient is asked to repeat the clinician-modeled complex sentence.

Source: Based on Kearns, 1985.

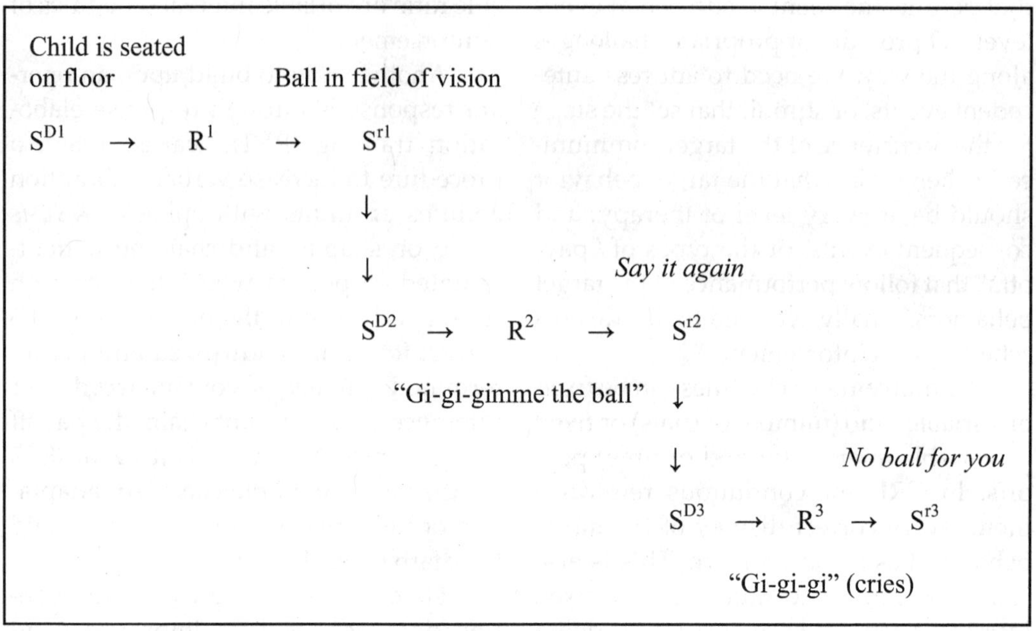

Figure 11–1. *Schematic of a behavioral chain.*

schematic of a behavioral chain for a child with disfluencies (responses in quotation marks) where the caregiver (responses in italics) may teach the child to engage in speech avoidance and escape behaviors. The child who is disfluent is seated on the floor, and turns to view a ball. The payoff of head turning is the view of the ball. Viewing the ball sets the occasion for the child to say, "Gi-gi-gimme the ball." The payoff for this utterance is the statement by the caregiver to *Say it again*. This statement sets the occasion for the child to say, "Gi-gi-gi" and to cry. The payoff for this utterance is the statement by the caregiver, *No ball for you*. The clinician–researcher who understands operant conditioning can interpret the behavioral chain as an example of a child learning to stop speaking in order to escape from an aversive consequence.

Strategies for Data Collection

The clinical practitioner and clinical researcher should have a strategy for data collection. A sample score sheet for collecting data in speech therapy for a 6-year-old child with articulation errors might be a 10 × 10 grid that includes a total of 100 boxes. Assume that the task (for example, imitation of prevocalic /r/ in a CVC context) is better suited to a ratio schedule than an interval schedule of reinforcement, and that the payoff will be one minute of play time. Scoring from left to right, write a check in pencil for every correct response and erase a check if there is a subsequent error. At the end of the row of 10 checks, stamp a smiley face and proceed to the next row. Continue until there are 100 checks (10 smiley faces) and deliver the payoff of play time. You have concentrated the child's mind and yours to expect a large number of trials in a therapy session, and have collected data that will be easy to analyze. For example, if there are 100 checks and 10 erasures, then the child has performed at a level of 100/110 correct responses, or about 91%.

An example of a scoring system using an interval schedule of reinforcement is a paired-stimulus method of increasing eye contact for a 5-year-old child with gaze aversion as part of an autism spectrum disorder. The clinician breaks a few potato chips (after determining that the child is responsive to the chips as a payoff and that the parent approves the use of chips as a reinforcer) into 25 small pieces before the therapy session starts. Assuming the goal is 5 s of eye contact over 25 trials, the clinician holds the chip between her eyes and says, "Look at me." After 5 s of eye contact, the clinician allows the child to eat the chip piece. If the child breaks eye contact before 5 s, the clinician puts the chip to the side. At the end of the task, the clinician counts how many pieces were placed to the side. For example, if there are 5 chip pieces left over, then the child accurately performed the task 20/25 times = 80% correctly.

EXPERIMENTAL DESIGN: CASE REPORT OR SINGLE-SUBJECT MULTIPLE BASELINE

Throughout this volume, the clinician–researcher has been identified as an individual who performs clinical intervention by testing hypotheses on a population of one person ($n = 1$). Using data collection strategies, such as those identified in the operant conditioning paradigm above, the clinician–researcher measures communication behaviors before, during, and after treatment.

There are several differences between case reports and single-case designs, but an important characteristic of the latter design is that the clinician collects multiple repeated measurements of the client's responses to independent variables presented by the clinician. In other words, the client's responses depend on what the clinician has presented; therefore, the client's responses are called dependent variables. By using repeated measures, the clinician can observe any changes in the dependent variables that may be caused by or be a function of clinical intervention. Ideally, the client who was first seen to have had communication problems in baseline measurements would demonstrate fewer of these problems in repeated measures of the behavior over the course of therapy, and the improvements would be maintained when baseline recovery measures were administered.

In a tutorial, Byun, Hitchcock, and Ferrin (2017) noted the high rate of Type I errors in single-case experiments and proposed ways to reduce the errors. Recall from Chapter 6 that a Type I error rejects the null hypothesis when it should have been the accepted alternative. The single-case design uses experimental controls, whereas the case study design does not. Both designs were discussed in detail in Chapter 5. Byun et al. (2017, p. 1456) referred to guidelines developed (Kratochwill et al., 2013) to improve designs in single-case methodologies. They include the following:

- The independent variable or treatment must be systematically manipulated.
- The study must not be observational or correlational.
- The study must demonstrate an effect of intervention at three different points in time.
- There must be at least five observations at each of the times noted above.
- There must be interrater reliability (see Chapter 8) of at least 80% for at least 20% of the data points in each of the times noted above.

In Chapter 1, CM was introduced as the participant in a case report to examine in-depth a specific individual in specific situations in order to illustrate important principles that might be overlooked in examining group data (Arroyo, Goldfarb, Cahill, & Schoepflin, 2010). Case study research also permits evaluation of phenomena that occur rarely and that may provide exceptions to generally accepted rules. Among weaknesses of case report research are the limitations of generalization and the increased likelihood of subjective biases on the part of the investigators. However, the factors that threaten internal validity in experimental research, especially history (events occurring between the first and second measurements in addition to the experimental variable) and maturation (changes in the subjects themselves that cannot be controlled by the experimenter and whose effects are attributed, incorrectly, to the experimental treatment), may be the substance of the case study approach (Orlikoff, Schiavetti, & Metz, 2015).

An additional problem with case report research is that, in the words of the proverb, you have put all your eggs in one basket. Here is a cautionary tale. About forty years ago, as a newly appointed head of the Audiology and Speech Pathology Service (this was before "language" became added to the title of the SLP) at the Veterans Administration Extended Care Center in St. Albans, New York, I sought to involve other professional disciplines with the veterans in our caseload. One of our outpatients was a man who had had a total laryngectomy, a radical neck dissection, and a partial glossectomy. He lost his voice, could not use a neck-placement electrolarynx effectively because of loss of neck musculature, and could not produce intelligible articulation to accompany esophageal voice. Together with a rehabilitation engineer and a dentist, we devised an artificial tongue that would fit on the patient's tongue stump and attach to the molars much like a bite plate. The four chambers of the artificial tongue would be filled with gel that would be released by biting on the molars and flow through valves to allow the tip to raise and lower. The natural tongue stump would permit protrusion and retraction of the artificial tongue.

The patient came for several fittings and then never returned. We tried our best to contact him, but he had moved from his address and gave no forwarding information. We couldn't report the results of our efforts because we didn't know if the treatment worked, and we never encountered another patient who would have been a candidate for the treatment. The good news is that a silicon tongue prosthesis has subsequently been developed and was reported to be effective for speech (Bhirangi, Somani, Dholam, & Bachher, 2012). Also, a professor of dentistry from Okayama University in Japan reportedly developed the world's first movable tongue prosthesis. It was designed to help a colleague with oral cancer speak again after a partial glossectomy. The finding was reported in the Japanese press in 2016 and is available online at https://www.rt.com/news/330913-artificial-tongue-prosthesis-cancer/, but it has not yet been published. The first human tongue transplant surgery was reported in Austria in 2003 for a patient who also had oral cancer. I'm still a little sad that we might have reported similar speech outcomes for an artificial tongue decades earlier.

Two recent case reports exemplify the benefits of studying unusual cases in detail. Full facial transplantation can result in dysphagia and reduced speech intelligibility, along with reduced ability to communicate by facial expression (Perry, Richburg, Pahomac, Bueno, & Green, 2017). A lingual strengthening program was adapted to increase lip closure pressure. Lip strength and lip mobility increased as a result of training, but speech intelligibility was not significantly changed, probably because large levels of muscle activation are not needed to produce speech, and lip weakness does not predict impairment in speech intelligibility. The second example is my own case report as an aphasiologist who had a stroke (Goldfarb, 2016) that was based on a journal I kept by keying all capital letters on a computer with my left hand during 7 days of intensive care, 21 days in a rehabilitation hospital, and subsequent outpatient treatment during the acute stage of the stroke. At the end of the journal, I was able to suggest a theory of my limited allocation of neural resources and explain my symptoms. For example, I had spasticity in the right arm and leg, but ataxic (not spastic) dysarthria because the site of lesion (a left pontine infarct) prevented cerebellar fibers from traveling through the superior cerebellar peduncle (brachium conjunctivum) and interdigitating with neural fibers in the pons.

DISSEMINATING RESULTS

In writing about dissemination of research in mental health, Fritz (2016) raised points that are equally relevant to CSD: of the hundreds of well-designed clinical studies that are reported in the literature, only a small fraction influence what happens in clinical care. There are many reasons why the translation of research into practice takes so long, and in the last three chapters of this book, the topic of dissemination is explored in detail. Among the obstacles to translating science to patient benefit, there are some common ones in every field of health care. Many of the people we care for in speech-language pathology and audiology have multiple, co-occurring problems, whereas clinical research tends to focus on a carefully selected sample of individuals with a single diagnosis. Barriers to dissemination that will be addressed in Chapters 13, 14, and 15 may be financial, institutional, social, commercial, or governmental. However, there are also special opportunities for dissemination of clinical research by students.

The student clinician–researcher has many options for dissemination unique to the status of being a student.

- Present the clinical study at a clinical internship seminar.
- Present the clinical study at a clinical externship seminar.
- Present the clinical study as a "Grand Rounds" project in a medical center placement.
- Use the research for the clinical study as part of a term paper assignment.
- Present a poster based on the study for an evidence-based therapy project in the clinic.
- Present a poster based on the study at a student research day on campus.
- Write a senior thesis, a capstone project, or a master's thesis based on the research and the results of the clinical study.

For all the projects above, except for the fourth and the seventh, students will need to prepare an oral presentation to classmates and professionals in their own as well as related disciplines. We have suggested elsewhere (Goldfarb & Serpanos, 2020) how this can be done effectively. Note that oral presentation of information is bound by the same restrictions regarding plagiarism as in a written form. Start by identifying the topic, state the purpose, indicate the main points in the body of your talk, provide supporting information and stimulate the listeners with analogies or questions, and summarize in a conclusion. Prepare by writing a topic outline or a Harvard outline, and it might be helpful to write a speaker's outline as well, with key words and phrases.

For posters or computer-generated presentations, remember that information presented orally as well as in visual form is retained longer by listeners. Use color to contrast with text to make the poster more striking; refer to the poster or slides, but never read aloud from them; limit the number of words on a slide, and separate main points on a poster; be sure that images do not become distorted when enlarged; use basic fonts and vary sizes for emphasis; and avoid too many enhancements, such as cartoons or jokes.

ADVANCED STUDY

The author proposes that clinical research skills are necessary for an individual to be granted power of professor. With new generations of scholars and researchers needed every 10 years, professors and master clinicians have an obligation to prepare individuals with adequate knowledge and skills to undertake the tasks of scholarship and research, and clinical research is a key component. For evidence of the requisite clinical research skills, complete the following and have your instructor, academic adviser, mentor, or CSD department chair review that you have completed the requirements and sign and date where indicated.

Student's Name: ______________________________

1. Write a clinical hypothesis and a null hypothesis for a client in your caseload. For the clinical hypothesis, complete sections IV through IX in Box 11–1.
2. For a simulated client with speech-language or hearing disorder, write a treatment goal using the following format: Who → will do what → to what level of accuracy → for how many trials → over how many consecutive therapy sessions → under what conditions?
3. Using the same simulated client as in #2, write how you would collect both quantitative and qualitative data.
4. Using the same simulated client, write how you would decide whether to do case report or single-subject multiple-baseline research.
5. Using the same simulated client, write three ways that you might disseminate your results.

Date of Completion: ______________________________

Faculty/Supervisor Signature: ______________________________

REFERENCES

Arroyo, C., Goldfarb, R., Cahill, D., & Schoepflin, J. (2010). AAC interventions: Case study of in-utero stroke. *Journal of Speech-Language Pathology and Applied Behavior Analysis, 5*, 32–47.

Bhirangi, P., Somani, P., Dholam, K. P., & Bachher, G. (2012). Technical considerations in rehabilitation of an edentulous total glossectomy patient. *International Journal of Dentistry, 2012*, 125–136. doi:10.1155/2012/125036

Byun, T. M., Hitchcock, E. R., & Ferrin, J. (2017). Masked visual analysis: Minimizing Type I error in visually guided single-case design for communication disorders. *Journal of Speech, Language, and Hearing Research, 60*, 1455–1466.

Farrugia, P., Petrisor, B. A., Farrokhyar, F., & Bhandari, M. (2010). Research questions, hypotheses and objectives. *Canadian Journal of Surgery, 53*, 278–281.

Fritz, G. K. (2016). Dissemination of research findings: A critical step. *Brown University Child & Adolescent Behavior Letter, 32*, 8.

Frost, S., & McCrindle, R. J. (2016). Speech development and therapy using the Kinect. *International Journal of Child Health and Human Development, 9*, 269–279.

Goldfarb, R. (2006). Operant conditioning and programmed instruction in aphasia rehabilitation. *Journal of Speech-Language Pathology and Applied Behavior Analysis, 1*, 56–65.

Goldfarb, R. (2016). An aphasiologist has a stroke. *Aphasiology, 30*, 1151–1162.

Goldfarb, R., & Serpanos, Y. (2020). *Professional writing in speech-language pathology and audiology* (3rd ed.). San Diego, CA: Plural Publishing.

Hartley, L. L., & Griffith, A. (1989). A functional approach to the cognitive-communication deficits of closed head injured clients. *Journal of Speech-Language Pathology and Audiology/Revue d'orthophonie et d'audiologie, 13*, 51–57.

Heuer, S., Ivanova, M. V., & Hallowell, B. (2017). More than the verbal stimulus matters: Visual attention in language assessment for people with aphasia using multiple-choice image displays. *Journal of Speech, Language, and Hearing Research, 60*, 1348–1361.

Ingram, K., Bunta, F., & Ingram, D. (2004). Digital data collection and analysis application for clinical practice. *Language, Speech, and Hearing Services in Schools, 35*, 112–121.

Kearns, K. P. (1985). Response elaboration training of patient initiated utterances. In R. Brookshire (Ed.), *Clinical aphasiology conference proceedings* (Vol. 15). Minneapolis, MN: BRK.

Kratochwill, T. R., Hitchcock, J. H., Horner, R. H., Levin, J. R., Odom, S. L., Rindskopf, D. M., & Shadish, W. R. (2013). Single-case intervention research design standards. *Remedial and Special Education, 34*, 26–38.

Nickels, L. (2008). The hypothesis testing approach to the assessment of language. In B. Stemmer & H. A. Whitaker (Eds.), *Handbook of the neuroscience of language* (pp. 13–22). Philadelphia, PA: Academic Press Elsevier.

Olswang, L. B., & Bain, B. (1994). Data collection: Monitoring children's treatment progress. *American Journal of Speech-Language Pathology, 3*, 55–66.

Onslow, M., Packman, A., & Harrison, E. (Eds.). (2003). *The Lidcombe Program of early stuttering intervention: A clinician's guide*. Austin, TX: Pro-Ed.

Orlikoff, R. F., Schiavetti, N. E., & Metz, D. E. (2015). *Evaluating research in communication disorders* (7th ed.). Boston, MA: Pearson.

Palmer, R., Hughes, H., & Chater, T. (2017). What do people with aphasia want to be able to say? A content analysis of words identified as personally relevant by people with aphasia. *PloS One, 12*, e0174065.

Perry, B. J., Richburg, B. D., Pahomac, B., Bueno, E. M., & Green, J. R. (2017). The effects of lip-closure exercise on lip strength and function following full facial transplantation: A case report. *American Journal of Speech-Language Pathology, 26*, 682–686.

Primus, M. A. (1987). Response and reinforcement in operant audiometry. *Journal of Speech and Hearing Disorders, 52*, 294–299.

Randall, K. E., & McEwen, I. R. (2000). Writing patient-centered functional goals. *Physical Therapy, 80*(12), 1197–1203.

Santo Pietro, M. J., & Goldfarb, R. (1995). *Techniques for aphasia rehabilitation: Generating effective treatment (TARGET)*. Vero Beach, FL: The Speech Bin.

Stocker, B., & Goldfarb, R. (1995). *The Stocker probe for fluency and language* (3rd ed.). Vero Beach, FL: The Speech Bin.

Swartz, E., Irani, F., & Gabel, R. (2015). Coping with stuttering. *Perspectives of the ASHA Special Interest Groups, SIG 4*, 58–68.

Thompson, M., Thompson, G., & Vethivelu, S. (1989). A comparison of audiometric test methods for 2-year-old children. *Journal of Speech and Hearing Disorders, 54*, 174–179.

Tuckett, D. (1994). Developing a grounded hypothesis to understand a clinical process: The role of conceptualisation in validation. *International Journal of Psychoanalytics, 75*, 1159–1180.

Wade, D. T. (2009). Goal setting in rehabilitation: an overview of what, why and how. *Clinical Rehabilitation, 23*, 291–295.

World Health Organization. (2002). *Towards a common language for functioning, disability and health: ICF*. Geneva, Switzerland: Author.

Worrall, L., Sherratt, S., Rogers, P., Howe, T., Hersh, D., Ferguson, A., & Davidson, B. (2011). What people with aphasia want: Their goals according to the ICF. *Aphasiology, 25*, 309–322.

Yairi, E., & Seery, C. H. (2015). *Stuttering: Foundations and clinical applications* (2nd ed.). Upper Saddle River, NJ: Pearson Education.

12

Conducting Academic Research

INTRODUCTION

Students conduct academic research at every stage of their education. The research may involve searches of articles and databases for the purpose of clinical treatment or completion of a course assignment. Toward the end of the undergraduate and master's degree programs, there are usually more formal assignments that require academic research. Students in the most advanced programs, including those pursuing clinical or research doctorates, can often expect to produce some form of archival document, such as a dissertation.

One purpose of the present chapter is to explore how academic research is conducted at a variety of colleges and universities throughout the United States at undergraduate, master's, and doctoral levels. The list of educational institutions that offer such programs is current, but may well have changed by the time this book is published. Navigating through http://www.asha.org will probably be useful for a student considering enrollment at institutions offering basic through advanced communication sciences and disorders (CSD) programs. Be sure that any college or university offering a master's degree in speech-language pathology (SLP) or a doctor of audiology degree (AuD) has been accredited by the Council on Academic Accreditation (CAA). The CAA is an independent body that reports to the U.S. Secretary of Education and whose recommendations for accreditation are accepted by the American Speech-Language-Hearing Association (ASHA). Program accreditation is usually granted for five to eight years, and graduation from an accredited program is required for the Certificate of Clinical Competence (CCC) in SLP/A, as well as licensure in most states as a speech-language pathologist or audiologist.

Learning Objectives

After reading this chapter, the student will be able to

- conduct research at basic and more advanced levels of education;

- decide which CSD programs in U.S. colleges and universities are the best fit; and
- explore options of funding for research.

SELECTING A RESEARCH TOPIC AND FINDING A MENTOR

Selecting a Research Topic

One of the best ways to start thinking about producing CSD research is to answer the following questions regarding the kinds of populations (e.g., age, disorder) that you want to study:

- The clinical population(s) that inspires (inspire) my most passionate feelings is (are) _____ (for example, adults with poststroke aphasia or children with cochlear implants).
- The population(s) that I related to the most in clinical observations is (are) _____.
- The clinical population(s) that I wrote about or want to write about in term papers, when given the choice is (are) _____.
- When I do clinical intervention, the population(s) that feels the least like work is (are) _____.

Now consider the area(s) of communication and its disorders that you want to study (refer to Table 12–1 or go to http://www.asha.org and fill out an ASHA Community Profile).

Once you have identified a population and a general area of inquiry, the detective work starts. Go to a database and start searching. I recommend that you begin with the database "ComDisDome" and enter the area (e.g., dysarthria) and the population (e.g., children with cerebral palsy) in the field box on the top. Make sure you click on "peer-reviewed" for articles you can trust. By entering "dysarthria in children with cerebral palsy," you are presented with 22 peer-reviewed journal articles, most of which are available in full text form. Browsing through titles or abstracts will not be enough. Read the entire articles with the goal of developing questions. For example, after reading Patel, Hustad, Connaghan, and Furr (2012), you may be inspired to ask the director of your speech science laboratory to mentor you in an investigation of fundamental frequency in middle-school children with dysarthria.

Finding a Mentor

Mentorship is crucial for new investigators (see Chapter 9). If the research topic is required by the department or the university, your first mentor may be the person who signed you up as a major in CSD. That person will likely be a member of the faculty and may also be your academic adviser; if not, then the academic adviser becomes your faculty mentor. A peer mentor, usually a CSD major who is further along in education than you are, may also be assigned to you. That person is in a good position to discuss the specific requirements for your departmental or university research project. Both your peer mentor and your faculty mentor should

Table 12–1. *Areas of Specialization in Communication Sciences and Disorders*

Speech-Language Pathology	Audiology	General
Accent modification	Audiologic rehabilitation	Accreditation
Aphasia	Auditory evoked potential	Advocacy
Apraxia	Balance assessment	Business
Augmentative and alternative communication	Central auditory processing disorders	Clinical education and supervision
Aural rehabilitation	Cerumen management	Compliance issues
Autism	Cochlear implants—programming	Continuing education
Bilingualism	Dispense over-the-counter devices	Ethics
Central auditory processing disorders	Early intervention in audiology	Evidence-based practice
Childhood language disorders	Hearing aid evaluation (pediatric)	Forensics (expert witness)
Cleft palate	Hearing aid evaluation (adults)	Global/international issues
Communication enhancement/Corporate speech-language pathology	Hearing assessment (work with adults)	Grant writing
Dementia	Hearing assessment (work with ages 3–5 year olds)	Information technology (Web/apps)
Developmental disorders	Hearing assessment (work with ages 6–18 year olds)	Interprofessional education/ interprofessional practice (IPE/IPP)
Dysarthria	Hearing assessment (work with ages 7–36 months)	Leadership in the professions (local, state, national)
Early intervention for speech	Hearing assessment (work with ages birth–6 months)	Low income populations
Fluency	Hearing assistive technology systems	Multicultural issues

continues

Table 12–1. *continued*

Speech-Language Pathology	Audiology	General
Laryngectomy	Hearing conservation	Practice issues—health care
Learning disabilities	Infant hearing aid fitting using real ear	Practice issues—private practice
Literacy	Intraoperative neurophysiological monitoring	Practice issues—schools
Oral myofunctional disorders	Real ear (verification) measures	Prevention/wellness
Resonance disorders	Tinnitus	Public health issues
Social communication disorders	Unbundle hearing aid fees	Publishing
Speech sound disorders	Validation using patient-reported outcome measures	Reimbursement and/or coding
Swallowing disorders	Vestibular rehabilitation	Research—basic
Transgender voice		Research—clinical/applied
Traumatic brain injury		Scholarship of teaching and learning (SoTL)
Voice disorders		State regulatory/licensing issues Support personnel Telepractice/telehealth

be familiar with members of the faculty who do research in your area of interest. You should also spend some time on your university's website exploring faculty profiles (mine is at http://www.adelphi.edu/faculty/profiles/profile.php?PID=0020). You will find information about the professor on the following topics: teaching, research interests, publications and presentations, grants, student work advised, and professional activities and honors. Make an appointment with the professor whose profile fits your research interests. Be prepared for the appointment by writing some of your research ideas and references you have found. Write this material professionally in a page or two, using American Psychological Association (APA) 2010 style for referencing, and offer to leave it with the professor when you arrive for your appointment. Although faculty mentors generally love to mentor students in research, we rarely get paid or earn release time for doing this. A faculty member is more likely to take responsibility for research mentorship if you show that you are prepared, committed, and organized.

Appendix 12–1 includes U.S. programs that offer undergraduate or preprofessional education at the bachelor's level. Appendix 12–2 includes U.S. programs that offer the master of arts or master of science degrees in speech-language pathology. Appendix 12–3 includes clinical and research doctoral programs in SLP or speech-language-hearing science, as well as AuD programs. Links for the PhD/AuD and BS/BA were searched through https://www.asha.org/edfind/ as well as individualized links to specific institutions, by state. Searches for the MS/MA programs were through https://caa.asha.org/

We now turn to required college and university research projects at some undergraduate, master's, and doctoral (clinical and research) levels in CSD. Not all CSD programs are represented.

CAPSTONE PROJECTS

Most CSD capstone experiences, whether they require a research-based project, a course, or some type of archival document such as an undergraduate senior thesis or a master's thesis, address evidence-based practice (EBP). Included in the framework for EBP is the ongoing assessment of evidence in the evaluation and treatment of individuals with communication disorders. EBP permits the selection of the "best possible, individualized interventions and outcomes" (Rangamani, Coppens, Greenwald, & Keintz, 2016, p. 139). A triad model for EBP training includes the following three individuals: an academic faculty member, a clinical supervisor, and a student (Rangamani et al., 2016). The goals of the model are to implement or increase use of EBP among all three stakeholders and to increase academic–clinical integration (a topic discussed in depth in Chapter 2).

Clinical Methods is a capstone course for seniors majoring in CSD at Ithaca College (see the following text). The focus is on assessment and intervention strategies in the clinical practice of speech-language pathology. Cobus-Kuo and Waller (2016) found that their students needed instruction in information literacy (IL) in order to incorporate evidence-based practice (EBP) into their clinical work. Although we have written a chapter on using library resources in a recent book on professional writing (Goldfarb & Serpanos, 2020), Cobus-Kuo and Waller identify a lack of CSD literature on teaching effective research skills as an obstacle to using evidence-based information. They note (2016, p. 36) that EBP requires IL, which they define as a synthesis of complex research skills that takes time and practice to develop. The authors reported that an effective method of teaching EBP through IL was for CSD faculty to collaborate with college librarians. The IL workshop developed at Ithaca College (Cobus-Kuo & Waller, 2016) was included in the Clinical Methods undergraduate capstone course.

In a capstone project developed for advanced CSD graduate students at

Hofstra University, Bloom (2010) had student clinicians integrate concepts of evidence-based practice (EBP) into clinical intervention for adults with motor speech disorders. Students completed the following five steps of EBP: formulating an answerable clinical question; locating the best available evidence; appraising the evidence critically; using the evidence in a client-centered way by considering biology, preferences, and values; and evaluating the EBP process and identifying ways to improve EBP skills.

In Chapter 3, I discussed the role of the U.S. Office of Research Integrity in promulgating standards for the responsible conduct of research (RCR) (U.S. Public Health Service, 2005). Chapman et al. (2013) noted that ASHA has adopted RCR standards in its guidelines (2009) and on a website (http://www.asha.org/Research/Ethics-in-Research/). Chapman et al. (2013) addressed RCR in terms of hypothetical student research. Some of the student research presented ethical concerns, such as participant recruitment, ownership and control of data, copyright, authorship, and ethics of randomized clinical trials. The purpose of the tutorial was to raise students' awareness and knowledge of RCR. The hypothetical cases were developed by graduate students at Ohio University to fulfill requirements of their capstone projects.

Following are some undergraduate capstone project requirements (from their websites, listed alphabetically):

Ithaca College

Undergraduates of speech-language pathology and audiology program at Ithaca College fulfill the capstone requirement through experiential learning. Students have the option to enroll in either the program's in-house clinical practicum, or at an approved off-campus site such as Head Start or The Center for Life Skills (https://www.ithaca.edu/hshp/clinics/lifeskills/) Concurrently, students supplement the clinical experience with a three-credit course to further discuss the principles of assessment and intervention in the field.

> http://catalog.ithaca.edu/undergrad/schools/school-health-sciences-human-performance/department-speech-language-pathology-audiology/

Saint Louis University

At Saint Louis University, students complete a capstone project as part of the general curriculum. The Senior Seminar marks the culmination of knowledge and skill from prior coursework, according to SLU's five professional dimensions. Additionally, students may enroll in a two-semester experience. Based on recommendations of faculty, selected students will enroll in Research Seminar and Research Practicum sequentially.

> http://www.slu.edu/services/registrar/catalog/pdfs/201617-CourseCatalog.pdf

SUNY Plattsburgh

SUNY Plattsburgh requires students of both the BA and BS cohorts to enroll in the designated capstone course during the spring semester of senior year. As part of the three-credit course, students will select a clinical topic of interest germane to speech-language pathology or audiology. Students are expected to research and synthesize information relative to differential diagnosis, etiology, nature, assessment, evidence-based methodologies, and prognosis. The final written product will be presented to faculty at the conclusion of the course.

https://web.plattsburgh.edu/academics/commdisorders/major.php

Previously explored topics are on display at https://digitalcommons.plattsburgh.edu/commdisorders_student_posters/index.html

University of Cincinnati
At the University of Cincinnati, the final component of the general education curriculum is a capstone experience. Students will begin planning their experience during the spring of junior year, before enrolling in the senior capstone course, which takes place over two semesters. Students may choose from the experiences of senior honors project, service learning project, portfolio, or case studies course. Further, students have the opportunity to showcase their research findings at the university's annual Presentation of Research and Innovative/Scholarly Endeavors, or "Praise," conference.

http://www.uc.edu/provost/about-us/profile/undergraduate-affairs/icl/capstone.html

http://www.cahs.uc.edu/csd/csd-news

http://www.cahs.uc.edu/csd/academic-programs/bs-in-communication-sciences-and-disorders/about-the-program

University of Maine
The senior capstone project at the University of Maine is built into the curriculum over two semesters. In the fall, students enroll in The Research Process (CSD 490), which addresses principal research methods, such as ethical decision making and professional writing. In the spring, students enroll in The Clinical Process (CSD 491), which emphasizes previously learned skills applied to the clinical context. At the conclusion of the spring semester, students will present the findings of a self-selected research topic at the Center for Undergraduate Research and University of Maine Student Research Symposium.

https://umaine.edu/comscidis/senior-capstone/

University of Minnesota
The University of Minnesota offers a three-credit course every spring in seminar format. Students will complete the capstone project within the seminar, which aims to highlight professional writing and civic engagement skills.

https://onestop2.umn.edu/pcas/viewCatalogProgram.do?programID=139&strm=1163&campus=UMNTC

Following are examples of previous capstone projects (from the university websites, listed alphabetically).

SUNY Plattsburgh: Social Communication Training for Adults with Traumatic Brain Injury and Quality of Life Improvements.

The study examines the correlation between an intervention model of social communication and improved quality of life following a closed-head injury. The location and severity of the injury produces a range of deficits in the domains of speech, language, cognition, and, most notably, pragmatics. Further, considering the age at which traumatic brain injury (TBI) is most likely, the framework of intervention must consider the social, academic, interpersonal, and occupational context of everyday life. Consequently, the student argues that social communication is the backdrop under which all other intervention should take place.

https://digitalcommons.plattsburgh.edu/commdisorders_student_posters/17/

https://digitalcommons.plattsburgh.edu/commdisorders_student_posters/

Syracuse University: Talking Hands: Does Gesture Production Help Bilingual Preschoolers Learn Words?

The study examines how gestures may or may not aid in the vocabulary acquisition of children learning two languages concurrently. Alternating treatments of a single-subject consisted of science-based vocabulary words taught through speech only, and again through speech and gesture.

https://surface.syr.edu/honors_capstone/770/

University of Maine
The following presentation titles were mentioned on the website:

The Correlation between GJB2 Gene Mutations and DFNB1

The Effect of Dysphagia Treatments on Speech Production

High Risk Infants: What Behaviors Are Displayed by the Younger Siblings of Children with Autism Spectrum Disorder?

Music Enjoyability in Post-Lingual Cochlear Implant Users

The Effects of Feelings and Awareness on Treatment in Children Who Stutter

The Social Story and Its Success with Preschool Children with Autism Spectrum Disorder

Speech Production of Children with and without Compensatory Articulation Disorder in Relation to Cleft Lip/Palate

https://umaine.edu/comscidis/features/senior-capstone-presentations/

THE MASTER'S THESIS

Research requirements are highly varied across master's programs. Many programs offer the research choice in lieu of a traditional comprehensive examination or provide an optional master's thesis. The research may be faculty directed or student directed (Blanchet, 2015). In a faculty-directed approach to research, students assist in research but take a supporting role. The student may earn an acknowledgment if the research is presented at a professional conference or published in a peer-reviewed journal, but the student usually does not contribute enough to earn authorship. The student generally gains some research experience, independent study credit, or financial compensation. In contrast, the research idea in a student-directed approach comes from the student. The research idea may or may not be well formulated, and a faculty member is recruited to supervise the project. However, the student researcher who has to maintain full course load and clinical practicum responsibilities may take longer to complete the degree than a fellow student who opts to complete a comprehensive examination instead of a master's thesis.

Graduate programs that are accredited by the Council on Academic Accreditation (CAA) may be loath to encourage the thesis option, as they can be punished for encouraging students to choose the longer route to the degree. According to the 2018 revised CAA standards, programs must report students who did not graduate on time, resulting in negative comments by the CAA on the annual report or reaccreditation report. One way to accommodate the revised standards is to offer two degree options (see Miami University in the following section), where one requires a research thesis and the other does not. The careful reader will notice that the degree of master of arts requires a thesis and the degree of master of science requires a research project, but not a thesis. This designation is consistent with other academic institutions that consider the MS to be a terminal degree and the MA a degree that is more likely to lead to doctoral study. There is still some confusion as some PhD programs offer an en route MPh (master of philosophy) degree, and some programs that award doctoral degrees may require more courses in education for PhD than for EdD (doctor of education) degrees.

Following are examples of master's-level research requirements according to university websites, listed alphabetically:

Adelphi University
Students may elect to pursue a research project as an alternative to the traditional comprehensive examination. Commensurate with a master's thesis, student research proposals are approved by a mentor, and subsequently forwarded to the department for further approval. The project is completed in the fourth semester and culminates with written documentation, proposal to a professional research conference, "friendly defense" to faculty, and presentation to students enrolled in the Research Methods course.

http://education-csd.adelphi.edu/wp-content/blogs.dir/701/files/2017/07/Graduate-SLP-Manual-2017_2018_Final.pdf

Miami University
Miami University offers both the master of arts and the master of science degree in speech-language pathology. The MA degree requires the completion of a research thesis. The MS degree requires the completion of a final research project. The thesis option is highly recommended for students planning to earn a doctoral degree or for those planning to engage in future research. Students are advised by a committee for subsequent research approval. After final documentation is submitted to the committee, the student will orally defend the research. The final research project does not require oral defense; however, it aligns with the thesis option respective to advising and approval. This type of project will be a scholarly paper prepared in the form of an article to be submitted to a peer-reviewed journal of choice.

http://www.cas.miamioh.edu/spa/GRADUATEGUIDE20062007.pdf

http://miamioh.edu/cas/academics/departments/spa/academics/graduate-studies/index.html

Penn State University
Students are required to complete a master's research paper or a master's thesis. The nonthesis option requires a paper and additional course credits in lieu of a thesis.

Both options are individually supervised and built into the curriculum.

http://bulletins.psu.edu/graduate/programs/C/GRAD%20CSD

University of Washington
University of Washington offers two specialty areas: CoreSLP and MedSP.

CoreSLP and MedSLP: A research project is not required; however, students may elect to complete a thesis. During the first year, interested students will interview with faculty to secure a research mentor. Theses will be finalized during the second year and completed by oral defense.

https://sphsc.washington.edu/master-science-coreslp

https://sphsc.washington.edu/master-science-medslp

Vanderbilt University Medical Center
The MS-SLP program does not require a research project; however, there is master's thesis option for interested students.

https://ww2.mc.vanderbilt.edu/ghss/24844

DOCTOR OF AUDIOLOGY (AUD) RESEARCH REQUIREMENTS (FROM THEIR WEBSITES, LISTED ALPHABETICALLY)

There are more than 11,000 members of the American Academy of Audiology (AAA, referred to as "Triple A"). It is the largest organization in the world whose charge is to represent audiologists, with a dedicated journal, the *Journal of the American Academy of Audiology* (JAAA). A smaller, related association is the Academy of Doctors of Audiology (ADA). The three related associations—ASHA, AAA, and ADA—all have similar but distinct Codes of Ethics. Some ethical dilemmas expressed by audiologists, in order of concern, included pay source and funding, coworkers or supervisors, compliance with federal and state regulatory guidelines, confidentiality, families and caregivers, evaluation and treatment, referrals, and caseloads (Callahan et al., 2011).

A doctoral degree (AuD) has been the entry-level degree for clinical practice since 2007, although Baylor University created the first AuD program in 1994. Baylor's program was sponsored by a $25,000 grant from the Audiology Foundation of America. It would not be enough, as a provost warned me about twenty years ago, for a proposed doctor of audiology degree to be "a master's on steroids." The AuD typically takes four years to complete, and it may also require some undergraduate prerequisite courses. The fourth year is usually dedicated to clinical externships. Based on a national survey (McNamara, 2014), students felt that the fourth year experience led to their confidence in performing complete audiological evaluations with adults and children, as well as in hearing-aid assessment and fittings. However, they felt less prepared, both academically and clinically, in the areas of vestibular rehabilitation, cochlear implants, and central auditory processing (McNamara, 2014, p. 96).

According to "AuD Facts" from the AAA's website, students who complete the degree are required to be critical consumers of research. They may also opt to participate in clinical research that focuses on efficacy of diagnosis and treatment (https://www.audiology.org/education-research/education/students/aud-facts). Students who want an academic career or who hope to do independent research in hearing science should pursue a PhD, not an AuD. Individuals with PhDs create the scientific base of the profession. Lacking a scientific base, there is no profession to practice.

Student research assignments are generally built into the AuD curriculum. Requirements are accomplished through grand rounds, clinical research, or capstone projects. Projects are completed and presented or defended prior to the fourth-year externship. Following is a sample, listed alphabetically, of AuD programs:

Auburn University
In the fall, spring, and summer semesters of the third year, students will complete a capstone experience. The student will commit to a research or clinical project for the purposes of exploring hypotheses or meeting a clinical outcome.

> http://bulletin.auburn.edu/thegraduateschool/graduatedegreesoffered/audiologyprogramaud_major/

Idaho State University
Under the supervision of the audiology faculty, students undertake a clinical project from the spring semester of their second year to the fall of their third. The clinically based scholarly project is presented in the spring of the third year.

> https://www.isu.edu/audiology/research/student/

SUNY Buffalo
During the second year of the program, the student will identify a research advisor. The research advisor will enlist two additional graduate faculty members to form a research committee. A research proposal will be approved by said committee prior to the project. At its completion, a written report will be presented to the research committee, followed by an oral presentation to the CSD department in public forum setting.

> http://arts-sciences.buffalo.edu/cds/grad/aud/degree-requirements.html

University of Iowa
Students will complete and defend a capstone project. Assignments include: A mentored research project and a mentored, non-data-based project; or a term paper that critically reviews published literature addressing a specific clinical topic assigned to the student by the AuD examination committee. Students undertaking the research and non-data-based projects will be assigned a mentor, and together will decide scope and timeline of project. At the project's completion, the student will defend the effort to an AuD examination committee, followed by a public presentation to peers. Should the student opt for the term paper option, the student will select a topic from a list of questions provided by the examination committee. On a monthly basis, the student will submit drafts and revisions to the committee, before receiving a final vote at the end of four months.

> https://clas.uiowa.edu/comsci/sites/clas.uiowa.edu.comsci/files/2017%20Grad%20Student%20Handbook%20FINAL%2011-28-17.pdf

University of Utah
Prior to the fourth-year externship, which begins over the summer, students will complete a capstone project. Mentored by

a faculty committee, projects may include a research project, literature review, or community service project over two consecutive semesters. A final paper must be written and submitted to the mentoring committee, followed by an oral presentation of the findings.

http://health.utah.edu/communication-sciences-disorders/degrees/aud/courses.php

PHD IN SPEECH-LANGUAGE-HEARING SCIENCES RESEARCH REQUIREMENTS (FROM THEIR WEBSITES, LISTED ALPHABETICALLY)

Students do or do not pursue a PhD for many reasons. I sometimes tell students that I know they have the brains for the degree, but I don't know if they have the belly for it. They will likely need to be focused on the degree for four to seven years. They won't be bored, but they may be boring during that time. Often, students pursue a PhD because they can't *not* go for it—that is, they want a career as an independent researcher and/or a position as a university professor. Based on online surveys (Davidson, Weismer, Alt, & Hogan, 2013), half the students were most deterred from pursuing a PhD because it required them to develop research projects, and half the faculty surveyed estimated that they spent half their time on research. Faculty and students agreed that being a professor was a rewarding career. The top three reasons why students said they *did not* want to pursue a PhD were length of the doctoral degree program, cost of the program, and family obligations. The top three reasons why students said they *did* want to pursue a PhD were desire for knowledge, the wish to make contributions to the profession, and their interest in higher education. Other than academia, there are rewarding careers where a PhD might be helpful, including working as a scientist in a speech research laboratory, as a service chief or rehabilitation department director in a hospital, in private practice, or in the corporate world, although 97% of respondents to an online survey of the Corporate Speech Pathology Network listed the master's degree as the highest degree (Specht & Blanchet, 2009).

Opportunities to get students interested in pursuing a PhD are more likely when they are undergraduates, rather than when they are matriculated in master's or AuD programs. Graduate students tend to be focused on their clinical careers, and while many of us in academia also hold clinical credentials, most new graduates with clinical degrees are more interested in the CCC and state license than the PhD. Witter and Brackenbury (2014) conducted a national Web-based survey about not only knowledge of the PhD in CSD but also perceptions and interest in the degree. Undergraduates seemed to know little about the PhD, and their interest in the degree was based on perceived, rather than demonstrated, knowledge.

Certainly the PhD dissertation is a considerable hurdle. The dissertation must reflect original research, make theoretical points, and be publishable in a peer-reviewed journal. The journal article based on the dissertation is generally considered the new graduate's entrée into the profession. All of us in academia have seen students who have been thwarted by the dissertation, and academic programs that invite applications for faculty membership from individuals who have completed ABD (all but dissertation) usually indicate that employment is contingent on completing the degree within a specified time. It is usually helpful when the dissertation is not the student's first attempt at independent research, and smaller research projects are often formally or informally incorporated into the requirements for the PhD.

There are abundant examples of CSD dissertations and theses online. One good source is ProQuest Dissertations &Theses (PQDT). A search of PQDT Open yields more than 40,000 open-access theses and dissertations in speech-language pathology and more than 36,000 in audiology and hearing science that are available in full-text PDF form.

The programs listed below require a dissertation at minimum, but many incorporate further research assignments into comprehensive exams or elsewhere in the curriculum:

Boston University
The doctoral program requires completion of three different research projects: directed research, qualifying project, and dissertation research. Directed research is extensively mentored and acts as a preliminary project. The qualifying project involves a substantial paper that meets the standards of peer-reviewed work in the field. Options include a systematic review, meta-analysis, and so forth. Dissertation research is the third and final assignment. Under the guidance of a dissertation committee, students will carefully construct an experimental design, collect and analyze valid data, prepare written documentation, and deliver a seminar and acceptable oral defense.

> https://www.bu.edu/academics/sar/programs/speech-language-hearing-sciences/phd/

University of Arizona
Students will complete two research rotations prior to beginning dissertation research. One rotation must be completed with a faculty member. Rotations will result in a written report or manuscript to be submitted to the appropriate publication. Students who completed a master's thesis or research equivalent may only need to complete one rotation. Initiation of dissertation research is mediated by the prospectus/dissertation committee.

> http://slhs.arizona.edu/sites/slhs/files/2017-18_phd_cactus_book.pdf

University of Florida
Students are provided several research options as part of their written qualifying examination. Further, students are expected to make at least one research presentation a year at local, state, national, or international venues in their second year and above. Upon passing the qualifying examination, a dissertation supervisory committee will guide the student through the respective processes.

> https://phhp-slhs.sites.medinfo.ufl.edu/files/2011/05/PhDHandbook-Fall2017.pdf

University of Maryland
Doctoral students will complete two primary research assignments: a candidacy research project and a dissertation. Students who completed a master's thesis or AuD capstone project may petition the faculty to accept the previous project for the candidacy paper requirement. During the first year, students will initiate their own research project under close supervision of a faculty advisor. A research plan will be implemented during the second year and culminate as the candidacy paper. This assignment must be based

on original, independent, and empirical research, guided by a faculty member. The final draft must be suitable for publication. This preliminary project determines, in part, a student's admission to candidacy and subsequent approval of dissertation research.

https://hesp.umd.edu/phd-program-hearing-and-speech-sciences#id_currec

Wayne State University
Doctoral students will complete a small research project and paper as the first of three comprehensive exams throughout the program, in addition to a dissertation. The former requires the student to collect data within the span of the semester and document findings. Results must be presented: as a submission for discussion at an appropriate national conference, as a written paper for the advisory committee, or as an oral presentation to the department. Following the completion of all three qualifying exams, students may initiate dissertation work under the guidance of a designated committee.

http://www.clas.wayne.edu/Multimedia/CSD/Files/Doctoral%20Handbook%20_August%202016.pdf

CLINICAL DOCTORATE IN SPEECH-LANGUAGE PATHOLOGY (SLP-D) RESEARCH REQUIREMENTS (FROM THEIR WEBSITES, LISTED ALPHABETICALLY)

Research includes capstone projects, clinical research studies, or applied dissertations that generally do not require an oral defense.

Kansas University
A dissertation is not required; however, students will complete a capstone project under the guidance of a mentor. Most capstone projects are completed as long-term investigative projects relative to the student's interests and clinical application. Students will prepare a written product and present the project to an advisory committee. Projects must include methodologies for communication and implementation of findings to relevant audiences.

http://www.kumc.edu/school-of-health-professions/ipcd/speech-language-pathology-(slpd)/curriculum.htm

Loma Linda University
Doctoral students will complete an applied dissertation or research capstone project. The clinical research study is based on the student's area of interest and designed under faculty mentorship. Students will complete the manuscript and perform an oral presentation of findings.

http://llucatalog.llu.edu/allied-health-professions/communication-sciences-slpd/#courseinventory

Northwestern University
During the fall and winter semesters of year two, students will complete a culminating project. This project is expected to provide an in-depth exploration of issues relevant to clinical practice. Students will explore a specialty area that may include a business proposal, process improvement plan, clinical investigation, or scholarship of teaching and learning investigation. The project will be completed under the supervision of at least one mentor; however, the final project will be submitted to and approved by the SLP-D committee.

https://slpd.northwestern.edu/courses

Nova Southeastern University
Students fulfill research requirements through an applied dissertation. Students are assigned a faculty committee to supervise and guide the project. Completion requires a detailed, accurate, and cohesive account of a scholarly investigation relative to clinical applicability and improvements in the field. Research is designed under a theory-to-practice model. There are three benchmarks in the completion of the applied dissertation: (1) the concept paper, (2) the dissertation proposal and Institutional Review Board (IRB) approval, and (3) the dissertation.

https://healthsciences.nova.edu/slp/doctoral/index.html

DOCTOR OF CLINICAL SCIENCE (CLINSCD/CSCD) RESEARCH REQUIREMENTS (FROM THE WEBSITE)

Research can include capstone projects, clinical research studies, or applied dissertations that generally do not require an oral defense.

Rocky Mountain University of Health Professions
Over three consecutive semesters, students will enroll in capstones 1, 2, and 3. Capstone 1 provides foundational knowledge for successful completion of an evidence-based practice (EBP) research project. Capstone 2 emphasizes current expectations for clinicians engaging in EBP in clinical practice and familiarizes students with project requirements. Capstone 3, the culmination, requires students to complete and present individual evidence-based projects. Students are expected to demonstrate knowledge of clinical practice through information synthesis and interpretation and application of clinical research on an expert level.

https://s3.amazonaws.com/rmu-pdfs/curriculum/SLP_Curriculum.pdf

FUNDING SOURCES

Everyone knows that undergraduate and graduate education is very expensive, sometimes prohibitively so. One advantage of being a CSD major is the likelihood of finding employment after graduation. Another is the shortage of speech-language pathologists and audiologists that is reflected in both disciplines being recognized as growth professions by the U.S. Bureau of Labor Statistics (https://www.bls.gov/). This shortage leads some school districts to support graduate education in SLP, according to the formula that the student who accepts support for graduate education must work for the school district for 2 years for each year of support.

The New York City Department of Education (DOE) offers full tuition reimbursement for master's degree students at participating colleges and universities who are matriculated in bilingual or monolingual speech-language pathology programs. Currently, most awards are going to reimburse bilingual SLP students because of the greater need for these professionals. If accepted, students must agree to work for the DOE for 2 years for each year of support. Students who do not complete the degree or who do not take a job at the DOE for 2 to 4 years, depending on the length of the award, must pay back the DOE for tuition plus interest. Check programs in school systems in your area regarding tuition reimbursement or loan forgiveness. The U.S. Department of Education offers grants and loans for personnel preparation for students with disabilities (https://ed.gov/programs/osepprep/applicant.html), with 65% of funding going to student scholarships.

Once you have found a way to pay for a CSD degree, there are other, smaller options for research and professional support. Many colleges and universities have a policy of offering start-up funding for new faculty. Student laboratory or research assistants are often included in this initial funding, sometimes referred to as "seed money." Some institutions budget for each faculty member to have a student research assistant, with the student earning a minimal amount of tuition remission for the work. It has also been my experience that faculty budgets for student research assistants are included in local grants such as the PSC-CUNY Research Foundation or the Adelphi University Faculty Development Awards, and these grants are much easier to obtain than federal funding. Student research assistants are paid an hourly rate, a flat rate, or earn tuition remission for the following semester. The Council on Undergraduate Research (CUR) supports and promotes collaborative, undergraduate, student–faculty research and scholarship. If a poster is accepted at the national conference, all travel/poster costs are covered. More than 3,000 student presenters have been supported in recent years. For more information, go to https://www.cur.org/

There also are programs to help underrepresented minority students to pursue advanced education in CSD.

Bridges-to-the-Doctorate is a federally funded (R25) grant through the National Institutes of Health to help students make a transition from master's degree to PhD programs in biomedical sciences, of which CSD is included. There must be a partnership or consortium of at least two universities and/or colleges, including the institution that makes the application. For example, as a Co-Principal Investigator of this program at the CUNY Graduate Center (doctoral granting institution), where four senior colleges of CUNY (master's degree granting institutions) participated in the consortium, the present author wrote the funded proposal for a summer research practicum for students interested in the PhD program in speech, language, and hearing sciences. Information about the Bridges program is available at https://www.nigms.nih.gov/Research/Mechanisms/Pages/Bridges-Doctoral.aspx

The Minority Biomedical Research Support (MBRS) program is administered through the National Institutes of Health with the goal of attracting underrepresented minority (UR) students to engage in biomedical research by pursuing PhD rather than MD degrees. MBRS also uses the R25 grant mechanism through its Research Initiative for Scientific Enhancement (RISE) program. The present author served as a consultant on the MBRS application at Lehman College, CUNY that met the criterion of having an enrollment of at least 50% UR students.

The National Institute on Deafness and other Communication Disorders (NIDCD) is a division of the U.S. Department of Health and Human Services, National Institutes of Health. It is the leading funder in the United States for biomedical and behavioral research and research training in the following seven areas of communication and related disorders: hearing, balance, taste, smell, voice, speech, and language. The Institute is charged to support research as well as research training related to disease prevention and health promotion. Funded projects and programs address biomedical and behavioral issues associated with communication disorders. The Institute also supports work on devices that substitutes for or improves sensory and communication function. For additional information, go to https://www.nidcd.nih.gov/funding.

Some grants through NIH are targeted to students pursuing a research doctorate as well as individuals in postdoctoral fellowships. Some of the available predoctoral awards include the following:

> Ruth L. Kirschstein Individual Predoctoral NRSA for MD/PhD and other Dual Degree Fellowships (F30)
> https://researchtraining.nih.gov/programs/fellowships/F30
>
> Ruth L. Kirschstein Predoctoral Individual National Research Service Award (F31)
> https://researchtraining.nih.gov/programs/fellowships/F31 (while conducting dissertation research)

Another NRSA award includes the following:

> Agency for Healthcare Research and Quality (AHRQ)-Sponsored National Research Service Award (NRSA) Individual Postdoctoral Fellowship (F32)
> https://grants.nih.gov/grants/guide/pa-files/PA-17-481.html

There is an award from NIDCD geared to AuD audiologists who are interested in a research dissertation:

> NIDCD Research Dissertation Fellowship for AuD Audiologists (F32)
> https://grants.nih.gov/grants/guide/pa-files/PA-18-700.html

There is also a Dissertation Award (R36) to support dissertation research costs of students in accredited research doctoral programs in the United States (including Puerto Rico and other U.S. territories or possessions).

> https://researchtraining.nih.gov/programs/other-training-related/R36

Some postdoctoral awards fall under the category of the Ruth L. Kirschstein National Research Service Award (NRSA). Among relevant NRSA Awards are the following for postdoctoral research:

> BRAIN Initiative Fellows: Ruth L. Kirschstein National Research Service Award (NRSA) Individual Postdoctoral Fellowship (F32)
> https://grants.nih.gov/grants/guide/rfa-files/RFA-MH-18-510.html
>
> Ruth L. Kirschstein National Research Service Award (NRSA) Individual Postdoctoral Fellowship (Parent F32)
> https://grants.nih.gov/grants/guide/pa-files/PA-18-670.html

The National Science Foundation offers the following fellowships:

SBE Postdoctoral Research Fellowships (SPRF)
https://www.nsf.gov/funding/pgm_summ.jsp?pims_id=504810

Robert Wenthold Postdoctoral Research Fellowship
https://www.nidcd.nih.gov/training/wenthold-fellowship

The American Association of University Women (https://www.aauw.org/) offers fellowships to women engaged in doctoral dissertation research and provides career development grants to women engaged in science, technology, engineering, and mathematics (STEM) fields, including speech-language pathology and audiology. The National Science Foundation (NSF) provides support for undergraduate students majoring in STEM fields through its S-STEM program (https://www.nsf.gov/funding/pgm_summ.jsp?pims_id=5257), while the NSF-Noyce program (https://www.nsf.gov/funding/pgm_summ.jsp?pims_id=5733) supports undergraduate students who plan to teach STEM subjects in schools.

Peer Review for Grant Applications

Applying for a research grant is not a process recommended for the thin skinned. The competition is fierce, and even some approved proposals are not funded because of budget limitations. Scholars in the bench sciences are dependent on grant support to fund their laboratories and staff, and colleges and universities depend on funding of what is called indirect costs associated with successful grant applications to support personnel, administrative, and building costs. There is an apparent paradox in that most NIH support goes to established laboratories; that is, the grants go to institutions that have a good track record of securing grants.

The following illustrates how the peer-review process works in two kinds of grant applications. The first example applies to junior faculty who often include a budget item for student research assistants, and the second example refers to senior faculty who may supervise student research abroad.

Example #1: For several years, I have served as both a primary and secondary reviewer for the Adelphi University Faculty Development Awards. These awards, generally not exceeding $5,000, support new and untenured faculty to develop a research agenda that can lead to external funding. Check with your Office of Grants and Contracts to see if your college or university offers seed money to faculty. The budget request generally includes funding for undergraduate or graduate students to work as research assistants. The grant applications that I review can earn up to 30 points as shown in Box 12–1.

Example #2: As a peer reviewer for the Fulbright Specialist Program for several years, I am asked to read and score applications and provide recommendations on which Fulbright Specialist applicants should be added to the Specialist Roster and be eligible to be matched with future grant projects. The applications provided for review had already been screened and confirmed that the applicants had met the basic eligibility requirements.

A program of the U.S. Department of State, Bureau of Educational and Cultural Affairs, the Fulbright Specialist Program allows U.S. academics and established professionals to engage in 2- to 6-week

Box 12–1. Example of a University Faculty Development Grant Review Form

On the scale indicated, please rate the proposal on the following criteria, with the highest number (1–10) indicating excellence:

The scholarly merit of the proposed activities:

(1–10) ________

The potential for the proposed scholarship to lead to future external funding, or to bring external recognition to the faculty member and/or to Adelphi University:

(1–10) ________

The importance of the project for the PI's (principal investigator) career development, commensurate with years of experience of the faculty member:

(1–10) ________

TOTAL POINTS:

(30 maximum) ________

COMMENTS: Please make any comments regarding the strengths of the proposal, or suggestions for improving weak areas. In addition, include suggestions to help mentor the principal investigator in his/her research career.

consultancies in a range of disciplines at host institutions in over 150 countries worldwide. As indicated on the Specialist Program's website (https://exchanges.state.gov/us/program/fulbright-specialist-program), through collaborative projects, Fulbright Specialists share their expertise, strengthen institutional linkages, hone their skills, gain international experience, and learn about other cultures while building capacity at their overseas host institutions. For example, during my stint as a Fulbright Specialist in applied linguistics/TEFL (a category of specialization that is no longer used) at the National Pedagogical University, Bogotá, Colombia, I mentored graduate students on their master's theses and gave presentations on research design and professional writing.

The five evaluation criteria for the Fulbright Specialist Program are professional qualifications, suitability for specialist grant activity, cross-cultural communication skills and adaptability, overall benefit to stakeholders, and personal qualities. The program encourages individuals in both academia as well as other professional spheres to apply. Peer reviewers use a scoring rubric with a 5-point scale:

5–Strongly agree with the statement

4–Agree with the statement

3–Neutral; neither agree nor disagree with the statement

2–Disagree with the statement

1–Strongly disagree with the statement

For example: The first evaluation criterion is, "The applicant displays significant experience in the selected professional field." A score of 5 indicates strong agreement with that statement.

If the peer reviewer affirms that the applicant is a strong candidate, then that person moves forward for placement on the specialist roster. At least two of the three peer reviewers must indicate scores that are high enough for the candidate to pass the peer-review process. If the decision is not to recommend the applicant, then there are guidelines (e.g., letters of recommendation are weak, professional record is weak) for the peer reviewer to use. A successful outcome of peer review does not mean that the candidate will be sent to a foreign country as a Fulbright Specialist; there has to be a match between a need at an institution in a foreign country and the skills of the applicant.

ADVANCED STUDY

The author proposes that academic research skills are necessary for an individual to be granted power of professor. With new generations of scholars and researchers needed every 10 years, professors and master clinicians have an obligation to prepare individuals with adequate knowledge and skills to undertake the tasks of scholarship and research, and academic research is a key component. For evidence of the requisite academic research skills, complete the following and have your instructor, academic adviser, mentor, or CSD department chair review that you have completed the requirements and sign and date where indicated.

Student's Name: ____________________

1. List the degrees in CSD available to students attending your college or university. For the most current information, navigate through http://www.asha.org.
2. Explain the capstone project requirement for the undergraduate degree at your college or university.
3. Explain the research requirement for the MA/MS-SLP degree at your college or university or at another university you might like to attend.
4. Explain the research requirement for the AuD degree at your college or university or at another university you might like to attend.
5. Explain the research requirement for the clinical doctorate in SLP at your college or university or at another university you might like to attend.
6. Explain the research requirement for the PhD in speech, language, and hearing science degree at your college or university or at another university you might like to attend.
7. What kind of funding or tuition remission for student research is available at your college or university?
8. Look up and describe three funding sources for doctoral students or post-doctoral fellows.

Date of Completion: ____________________

Faculty/Supervisor Signature: ____________________

REFERENCES

American Speech-Language-Hearing Association. (2009). *Guidelines for the responsible conduct of research: Ethics and the publication process* [Guidelines]. Retrieved from http://www.asha.org/docs/html/GL2009-00308.html

Blanchet, P. G. (2015). The apprentice: A model for mentoring students in research in communication sciences and disorders. *Contemporary Issues in Communication Science and Disorders, 42*, 26–32.

Bloom, R. L. (2010). A case-based approach to teaching evidence-based practice and motor speech disorders. *Contemporary Issues in Communication Science and Disorders, 37*, 123–130.

Callahan, A. J., Lass, N. J., Richards, K. L., Yost, A. B., Porter, K. S., Schrock, J. J., & Vetica, M. D. (2011). Ethical dilemmas in audiology. *Contemporary issues in Communication Science and Disorders, 38*, 76–86.

Chapman, L. R., Hassan, F. H., Modayil, M., Oommen, E., Park, T., & Horner, J. (2013). Responsible conduct of research: For students, by students. *Contemporary Issues in Communication Science and Disorders, 40*, 15–30.

Cobus-Kuo, L., & Waller, J. (2016). Teaching information literacy and evidence-based practice in an undergraduate speech-language pathology program: A student reflection. *Contemporary Issues in Communication Science and Disorders, 43*, 35–49.

Davidson, M. M., Weismer, S. E., Alt, M., & Hogan, T. P. (2013). Survey on perspectives of pursuing a PhD in communication sciences and disorders. *Contemporary Issues in Communication Science and Disorders, 40*, 98–115.

Goldfarb, R., & Serpanos, Y. (2020). *Professional writing in speech-language pathology and audiology* (3rd ed.). San Diego, CA: Plural.

McNamara, T. L. (2014). Procedures and perspectives of the 4th-year experience for the Doctor of Audiology degree. *Contemporary Issues in Communication Science and Disorders, 41*, 96–109.

Patel, R., Hustad, K. C., Connaghan, K. P. & Furr, W. (2012). Relationship between prosody and intelligibility in children with dysarthria. *Journal of Medical Speech-Language Pathology, 20*, 95–99.

Rangamani, G., Coppens, P., Greenwald, M., & Keintz, C. (2016). Collaborative methods for training evidence-based practice: The triad model. *Contemporary Issues in Communication Science and Disorders, 43*, 139–153.

Specht, N. M., & Blanchet, P. G. (2009). A survey of corporate speech pathologists' demographic characteristics, professional activities, and career satisfaction. *Contemporary Issues in Communication Science and Disorders, 36*, 118–132.

U.S. Public Health Service. (2005, May 17). Public Health Service policies on research misconduct [Final rule]. *Federal Register, 70*(94), 28370–28400, codified at Code of Federal Regulations, Title 42, Part 93.

Witter, E. A., & Brackenbury, T. (2014). Undergraduates' knowledge and interest in the doctorate of philosophy degree for communication sciences and disorders. *Contemporary Issues in Communication Science and Disorders, 41*, 252–274.

APPENDIX 12–1

BA or BS CSD Programs

Communication Disorders Undergraduate Programs	Link
Alabama	
Alabama A&M University	http://www.aamu.edu/csd
Auburn University	http://www.cla.auburn.edu/communicationdisorders/
Auburn University, Montgomery	http://conhs.aum.edu/academic-programs/undergraduate-programs/comdisorders
Samford University	http://www.samford.edu/commdisorders
University of Alabama, Tuscaloosa	http://www.cd.ua.edu/
University of Montevallo	http://www.montevallo.edu/academics/colleges/college-of-arts-sciences/communication-science-disorders/b-s-in-speech-language-pathology/
University of South Alabama	http://www.southalabama.edu/alliedhealth/speech andhearing
Arizona	
Arizona State University	http://chs.asu.edu/programs/schools/department-speechand-hearing-science
University of Arizona	http://slhs.arizona.edu
Arkansas	
Arkansas State University	http://www.astate.edu/college/conhp/departments/communicationdisorders
Harding University	http://www.harding.edu/csd/
Ouachita Baptist University	http://www.obu.edu/commdisorders/
University of Arkansas, Fayetteville	http://cdis.uark.edu/degree-programs/bse-communication-disorders/index.php
University of Arkansas for Medical Sciences/ University of Arkansas at Little Rock	http://healthprofessions.uams.edu/programs/audand speechpathology/
University of Central Arkansas	http://www.uca.edu/chbs

continues

APPENDIX 12–1. *continued*

Communication Disorders Undergraduate Programs	*Link*
California	
Biola University	http://academics1.biola.edu/communication-disorders
California Baptist University	http://www.calbaptist.edu/programs/master-of-science-speech-language-pathology/
California State University, Chico	http://www.csuchico.edu/cmsd
California State University, East Bay	http://www20.csueastbay.edu/class/departments/commsci/index.html
California State University, Fresno	http://www.csufresno.edu/cdds/
California State University, Fullerton	http://communications.fullerton.edu/hcom/hcom-cd-ma.php
California State University, Long Beach	http://www.csulb.edu/colleges/chhs/departments/communicativedisorders/
California State University, Los Angeles	http://www.calstatela.edu/dept/com_dis/
California State University, Northridge	http://hhd.csun.edu/comdis/
California State University, Sacramento	http://www.csus.edu/hhs/csad
California State University, San Marcos	http://www.csusm.edu/slp
Loma Linda University	http://www.llu.edu
San Diego State University	http://slhs.sdsu.edu/
San Francisco State University	http://www.sfsu.edu/~comdis/index.html
San Jose State University	http://www.sjsu.edu/cds/
University of Redlands	http://www.redlands.edu/study/schools-and-centers/college-of-arts-and-sciences/truesdail-center/communicative-disorders/
University of the Pacific–SLP Program	http://www.pacific.edu/Academics/Schools-and-Colleges/Thomas-J-Long-School-of-Pharmacy-and-Health-Sciences/Academics/Speech-Language-Pathology

Communication Disorders Undergraduate Programs	*Link*
Colorado	
Metropolitan State University of Denver	http://www.msudenver.edu/programs/speech-language-hearing-sciences-major-ba.shtml
University of Colorado, Boulder	http://admissions.colorado.edu/graduate/programs/slhs
University of Northern Colorado	http://www.unco.edu/nhs/asls
Connecticut	
Southern Connecticut State University	http://www.southernct.edu/cmd
University of Connecticut	http://slhs.uconn.edu/
District of Columbia	
George Washington University	http://speechhearing.columbian.gwu.edu/
Florida	
Florida State University	http://www.commdisorders.cci.fsu.edu
Jacksonville University	http://www.ju.edu/chs/
Nova Southeastern University–SLP Program	http://healthsciences.nova.edu/slp
University of Central Florida	http://www.cohpa.ucf.edu/comdis
University of Florida, Gainesville	http://www.slhs.phhp.ufl.edu
University of South Florida	http://www.usf.edu/cbcs/csd
Georgia	
Georgia Southern University (formerly Armstrong State U)	http://www.armstrong.edu/Health_professions/rehabilitation_sciences/rehab_sci_welcome
University of Georgia	http://www.coe.uga.edu/csse/
University of West Georgia	http://www.westga.edu/academics/education/program_page.php?program_id=74
Valdosta State University	http://www.valdosta.edu/colleges/education/communication-sciences-and-disorders/programs/

continues

APPENDIX 12–1. *continued*

Communication Disorders Undergraduate Programs	*Link*
Idaho	
Idaho State University, Pocatello	http://www.isu.edu/departments/csed/
Illinois	
Augustana College (IL)	http://www.augustana.edu/academics/majors--areas-of-study/communication-sciences-and-disorders
Aurora University	http://www.aurora.edu/academics/undergraduate/communication-sciences-and-disorders/index.html#axzz3mZwRtG1a
Eastern Illinois University	http://www.eiu.edu/commdis/
Elmhurst College	http://www.elmhurst.edu/academics/departments/csd
Governors State University	http://www.govst.edu/chhs/dcd
Illinois State University	http://csd.illinoisstate.edu/
Northern Illinois University	http://chhs.niu.edu/ahcd/programs/communicative-disorders/index.shtml
Northwestern University	http://www.northwestern.edu/csd
Southern Illinois University, Carbondale	http://cola.siu.edu/communicationstudies/undergraduate/
Southern Illinois University, Edwardsville	http://www.siue.edu/education/khe/undergrad/speech-pathology-audiology/index.shtml
St. Xavier University	http://www.sxu.edu
University of Illinois, Urbana-Champaign	http://www.shs.uiuc.edu
Western Illinois University	http://www.wiu.edu/csd
Indiana	
Ball State University	http://cms.bsu.edu/academics/collegesanddepartments/spaa/
Butler University	http://www.butler.edu/communication-disorders/
Indiana State University	http://www.indstate.edu/coe/cd/
Indiana University, Bloomington	http://www.indiana.edu/~sphs/

Communication Disorders Undergraduate Programs	*Link*
Purdue University	http://www.purdue.edu/hhs/slhs/
Purdue University, Fort Wayne	http://www.ipfw.edu/csd
Saint Mary's College	http://www.saintmarys.edu/majors/communicative-disorders
Iowa	
University of Iowa	http://clas.uiowa.edu/comsci/
University of Northern Iowa	http://comdis.uni.edu/
Kansas	
Fort Hays State University	http://www.fhsu.edu/commdis/
Kansas State University	http://www.he.k-state.edu/fshs/academics/csd/ugrad/
University of Kansas	http://www.ipcd.ku.edu
Wichita State University	http://www.wichita.edu/csd/
Kentucky	
Brescia University	http://www.brescia.edu
Eastern Kentucky University	http://www.cd.eku.edu
Murray State University	http://www.murraystate.edu/cdi
University of Kentucky	http://www.mc.uky.edu/CommDisorders/
Western Kentucky University	http://www.wku.edu/communicationdisorders/
Louisiana	
Louisiana State University and A&M College	http://sites01.lsu.edu/wp/comd/
Louisiana Technical University	http://liberalarts.latech.edu/communication/language/ba.php
Southeastern Louisiana University	http://www.southeastern.edu/acad_research/degrees/csd_ms.html
Southern University and A&M College	http://www.subr.edu/speechpathology

continues

APPENDIX 12–1. *continued*

Communication Disorders Undergraduate Programs	*Link*
University of Louisiana, Lafayette	http://speechandlanguage.louisiana.edu/
University of Louisiana, Monroe	http://www.ulm.edu/slp
Xavier University of Louisiana	http://www.xula.edu/speechpathology
Maine	
University of Maine, Orono	http://www.umaine.edu/comscidis
Maryland	
Loyola University Maryland	http://www.loyola.edu/academics/speech/undergraduate
Towson University	http://www.towson.edu/chp/departments/asld/undergrad/
University of Maryland, College Park	http://hesp.umd.edu/landing/Undergraduate
Massachusetts	
Boston University	http://www.bu.edu/academics/sar/programs/speech-language-hearing-sciences/bs/
Bridgewater State University	http://my.bridgew.edu/departments/CommunicationSciencesandDisorders/SitePages/Home.aspx
Elms College	http://www.elms.edu/academics/academic-divisions/communication-sciences-and-disorders.xml
Emerson College	http://www.emerson.edu/communication_disorders/
Northeastern University	http://www.northeastern.edu/bouve/csd/
Springfield College	http://www.spfldcol.edu/homepage/dept.nsf/academics/hsrs
University of Massachusetts, Amherst	http://www.umass.edu/sphhs/communication-disorders
Worcester State University	http://www.worcester.edu/Communication-Sciences-and-Disorders/
Michigan	
Andrews University	http://www.andrews.edu/undergrad/academics/programs/speechpath/

Communication Disorders Undergraduate Programs	*Link*
Calvin College	http://www.calvin.edu/academics/departments-programs/speech-pathology-audiology/
Central Michigan University	http://www.cmich.edu/colleges/CHP/hp_academics/communications_disorders/Pages/default.aspx
Eastern Michigan University	http://www.emich.edu/coe/departments/special-education/speech-language-pathology/
Grand Valley State University	http://www.gvsu.edu/csd/
Northern Michigan University	http://www.nmu.edu/cls
Wayne State University	http://www.clas.wayne.edu/csd/
Western Michigan University	http://www.wmich.edu/speech-audiology
Minnesota	
Minnesota State University, Mankato	http://ahn.mnsu.edu/cd/undergraduate/
Minnesota State University, Moorhead	http://www.mnstate.edu/slhs/
University of Minnesota, Duluth	http://www.d.umn.edu/csd
University of Minnesota, Minneapolis	http://cla.umn.edu/slhs
Mississippi	
Delta State University	http://www.deltastate.edu/artsandsciences/speech-and-hearing-sciences/
Jackson State University	http://www.jsums.edu/commdisorders
Mississippi University for Women	http://www.muw.edu/speech
University of Mississippi	http://csd.olemiss.edu/
University of Southern Mississippi	http://www.usm.edu/shs/
Missouri	
Fontbonne University	http://www.fontbonne.edu

continues

APPENDIX 12–1. *continued*

Communication Disorders Undergraduate Programs	*Link*
Maryville University	http://www.maryville.edu/hp/speech-language-pathology/
Missouri State University	http://www.missouristate.edu/csd
Rockhurst University	http://www.rockhurst.edu
Saint Louis University	http://www.slu.edu/doisy/degrees/undergraduate/communication-sciences-and-disorders.php
Southeast Missouri State University	http://www.semo.edu/commdisorders/
Truman State University	http://comdis.truman.edu/
University of Central Missouri	http://www.ucmo.edu
University of Missouri	http://healthprofessions.missouri.edu/communication-science-and-disorders
Montana	
University of Montana	http://coehs.umt.edu
Nebraska	
University of Nebraska, Kearney	http://www.unk.edu/academics/cdis/
University of Nebraska, Lincoln	http://cehs.unl.edu/secd
University of Nebraska, Omaha	http://www.unomaha.edu/college-of-education/special-education-communication-disorders/graduate/speech-language-pathology.php
Nevada	
Nevada State College	http://nsc.nevada.edu/
University of Nevada, Reno	http://www.unr.edu/degrees/speech-pathology
New Hampshire	
University of New Hampshire	http://chhs.unh.edu/csd/communication-sciences-and-disorders-bs
New Jersey	
Kean University of New Jersey	http://www.kean.edu/academics/college-education/school-communication-disorders-deafness/b.a.-speech-language-hearing-sciences

Communication Disorders Undergraduate Programs	*Link*
William Paterson University of New Jersey	http://www.wpunj.edu/cosh/departments/communication-disorders/
New Mexico	
Eastern New Mexico University	http://www.enmu.edu/cdis
New Mexico State University	http://spedcd.nmsu.edu/
University of New Mexico	http://shs.unm.edu
New York	
Adelphi University	http://education-csd.adelphi.edu/
Buffalo State College	http://www.buffalostate.edu/speech/
College of Saint Rose	http://www.strose.edu/communication-sciences-disorders/
CUNY, Brooklyn College	http://www.brooklyn.cuny.edu
CUNY, Lehman College	http://www.lehman.edu/deanhum/splanghearing/
CUNY, Queens College	http://www.qc.cuny.edu/academics/degrees/dah/lcd/pages/ma-slp.aspx
Elmira College	http://www.elmira.edu/
Hofstra University	http://www.hofstra.edu
Iona College	http://www.iona.edu/Academics/School-of-Arts-Science/Departments/Speech-Communication.aspx
Ithaca College	http://departments.ithaca.edu/slpa/
LIU Brooklyn	http://www.brooklyn.liu.edu/new_csd
LIU Post	http://www.cwpost.liunet.edu
Marymount Manhattan College	http://marymount.mmm.edu/
Mercy College	http://www.mercy.edu
Molloy College	http://www.molloy.edu
Nazareth College	http://www.naz.edu
New York University	http://steinhardt.nyu.edu/csd/
Pace University	http://www.pace.edu/

continues

APPENDIX 12–1. *continued*

Communication Disorders Undergraduate Programs	*Link*
St. John's University	http://www.stjohns.edu/
St. Joseph's College, Long Island	http://www.sjcny.edu/long-island/academics/programs-departments/communication-studies
SUNY at Buffalo	http://cdswebserver.med.buffalo.edu/drupal/
SUNY at Cortland	http://www.cortland.edu
SUNY at Fredonia	http://www.fredonia.edu
SUNY at New Paltz	http://www.newpaltz.edu/commdis
SUNY at Plattsburgh	http://web.plattsburgh.edu/academics/commdisorders/
Syracuse University	http://csd.syr.edu/about-us/speech-pathology.html
Touro College	http://shs.touro.edu/programs/speech-language-pathology/
Yeshiva University Katz School of SLP	http://www.yu.edu/stern/ug/speech-pathology-audiology
North Carolina	
Appalachian State University	http://comdis.appstate.edu/
East Carolina University	http://www.ecu.edu/csd/
North Carolina A&T State University	http://www.ncat.edu/academics/schools-colleges1/cas/index.html
Shaw University	http://www.shawuniversity.edu/
University of North Carolina, Greensboro	http://www.uncg.edu/csd/
Western Carolina University	http://csd.wcu.edu
North Dakota	
Minot State University	http://www.minotstateu.edu/enroll/programs/communications-disorders.shtml
University of Mary	http://www.umary.edu/academics/programs/communication-sciences-disorders.php
University of North Dakota	http://arts-sciences.und.edu/communication-sciences-disorders/

Communication Disorders Undergraduate Programs	*Link*
Ohio	
Baldwin Wallace University	http://www.bw.edu/academics/undergraduate/communication-sciences-disorders/
Bluffton University	http://www.bluffton.edu/edu/speech.html
Bowling Green State University	http://www.bgsu.edu/cdis
Case Western Reserve University	http://psychsciences.case.edu/undergraduate/communication-sciences/
Cleveland State University	http://www.csuohio.edu/sciences/health-sciences/graduate-programs
College of Wooster	http://academics.wooster.edu/programs/communication/default.php
Kent State University	http://www.kent.edu/ehhs/hs/spa
Miami University	http://www.muohio.edu/spa
Ohio State University	http://sphs.osu.edu/
Ohio University	http://www.ohio.edu/chsp/csd
University of Akron	http://www.uakron.edu/sslpa
University of Cincinnati	http://www.cahs.uc.edu/csd
University of Toledo	http://www.utoledo.edu/hhs/speech/
Oklahoma	
Northeastern State University	http://www.nsuok.edu
Oklahoma State University	http://cdis.okstate.edu
University of Central Oklahoma	http://www.uco.edu
University of Oklahoma–Health Sciences Center	http://alliedhealth.ouhsc.edu/Departments/CommunicationSciencesandDisorders.aspx
University of Science & Arts of Oklahoma	http://usao.edu/academics/speech-language-pathology
University of Tulsa	http://healthsciences.utulsa.edu/departments-schools/communication-disorders/

continues

APPENDIX 12–1. *continued*

Communication Disorders Undergraduate Programs	*Link*
Oregon	
Portland State University	http://www.pdx.edu/sphr/home
University of Oregon	http://education.uoregon.edu/cds
Pennsylvania	
Bloomsburg University of Pennsylvania	http://www.bloomu.edu
California University of Pennsylvania	http://www.calu.edu
Clarion University of Pennsylvania	http://www.clarion.edu/academics/colleges-andschools/college-of-health-and-human-services/department-of-communication-sciences-and-disorders/
Duquesne University	http://www.duq.edu/academics/schools/health-sciences/academic-programs/speech-language-pathology
East Stroudsburg University	http://www.esu.edu
Edinboro University of Pennsylvania	http://www.edinboro.edu/academics/schools-and-departments/cshp/departments/speech/
Geneva College	http://www.geneva.edu/object/communication_disorders
Indiana University of Pennsylvania	http://www.iup.edu/special-ed/
La Salle University	http://www.lasalle.edu/
Lebanon Valley College	http://www.lvc.edu/academics/programs-of-study/communication-sciences-disorders/
Marywood University	http://www.marywood.edu
Misericordia University	http://www.misericordia.edu/slp
Pennsylvania State University	http://csd.hhdev.psu.edu/
Temple University	http://cph.temple.edu/commsci/home
Thiel College	http://www.thiel.edu/academics/csd/index.htm
University of Pittsburgh	http://www.shrs.pitt.edu/csd
West Chester University	http://www.wcupa.edu

Communication Disorders Undergraduate Programs	Link
	Puerto Rico
Carlos Albizu University	http://www.albizu.edu/Academics/Degrees-in-Speech-and-Language
Universidad del Turabo	http://ut.suagm.edu/es/ut/programas
	Rhode Island
Rhode Island College	http://www.ric.edu/communication/index.php
University of Rhode Island	http://web.uri.edu/cmd/
	South Carolina
Bob Jones University	http://www.bju.edu
Columbia College	http://www.columbiasc.edu/academics/education/speech-language-pathology
South Carolina State University	http://www.scsu.edu/academicprograms/speechpathologyaudiology.aspx
	South Dakota
Augustana College (SD)	http://www.augie.edu/
University of South Dakota	http://www.usd.edu/csd
	Tennessee
Middle Tennessee State University	http://www.mtsu.edu/commdis/index.php
University of Tennessee Health Science Center	http://uthsc.edu/health-professions/asp/aud/index.php
	Texas
Abilene Christian University	http://www.acu.edu/graduate/academics/speech-language-pathology.html
Baylor University	http://www.baylor.edu/csd
Hardin-Simmons University	http://www.hsutx.edu/academics/holland/speechpathology
Lamar University	http://www.lamar.edu/fine-arts-communication/speech-and-hearing-sciences/index.html
Our Lady of the Lake University	http://www.ollusa.edu

continues

APPENDIX 12–1. *continued*

Communication Disorders Undergraduate Programs	*Link*
Stephen F. Austin State University	http://www.sfasu.edu/humanservices/720.asp
Texas A&M University, Kingsville	http://www.tamuk.edu/artsci/csdo
Texas Christian University	http://www.csd.tcu.edu
Texas State University	http://www.health.txstate.edu/cdis/cdis.html
Texas Tech University–Health Sciences Center	http://www.ttuhsc.edu
Texas Woman's University	http://twu.edu/communication-sciences/
University of Houston	http://www.uh.edu/class/comd/
University of North Texas	http://aslp.hps.unt.edu/
University of Texas at Dallas	http://www.utdallas.edu
University of Texas, Austin	http://csd.utexas.edu/
University of Texas Rio Grande Valley	http://www.utrgv.edu/communication-disorders/index.htm
West Texas A & M University	http://www.wtamu.edu/academics/communication-disorders.aspx
Utah	
Brigham Young University	http://education.byu.edu/comd
University of Utah	http://health.utah.edu/communication-sciences-disorders/
Utah State University	http://www.comd.usu.edu
Vermont	
University of Vermont	http://www.uvm.edu/
Virginia	
Hampton University	http://science.hamptonu.edu/csad/
James Madison University	http://www.csd.jmu.edu
Longwood University	http://www.longwood.edu/socialworkcsds/index.html

Communication Disorders Undergraduate Programs	*Link*
Old Dominion University	http://www.odu.edu/cdse
Radford University	http://www.radford.edu/content/wchs/home/cosd.html
University of Virginia	http://curry.virginia.edu/academics/speech-communication-disorders
West Virginia	
Marshall University	http://www.marshall.edu/communication-disorders/
West Liberty University	http://westliberty.edu/health-sciences/
West Virginia University	http://admissions.wvu.edu/academics/majors/speech-pathology-and-audiology
Wisconsin	
Concordia University, Wisconsin	http://www.cuw.edu
Marquette University	http://www.marquette.edu/speech-pathology-audiology/undergraduate.shtml
University of Wisconsin, Eau Claire	http://www.uwec.edu/academics/college-education-human-sciences/departments-programs/communication-sciences-disorders/
University of Wisconsin, Madison	http://csd.wisc.edu/
University of Wisconsin, Milwaukee	http://uwm.edu/healthsciences/academics/communication-sciences-disorders/
University of Wisconsin, River Falls	http://www.uwrf.edu/csd/index.cfm
University of Wisconsin, Stevens Point	http://www.uwsp.edu/csd/
University of Wisconsin, Whitewater	http://www.uww.edu/coeps/departments/comdis
Wyoming	
University of Wyoming	http://www.uwyo.edu/comdis/

APPENDIX 12–2

MA or MS SLP Programs

Institution Offering MA/MS in SLP	*Link*
Alabama	
Alabama A&M University	http://www.aamu.edu/csd
Auburn University	http://cla.auburn.edu/communicationdisorders/speech-language-pathology/
University of Alabama, Tuscaloosa	http://www.cd.ua.edu/
University of Montevallo	http://www.montevallo.edu
University of South Alabama	http://www.southalabama.edu/alliedhealth/speechand hearing
Arizona	
Arizona State University	http://chs.asu.edu/programs/schools/department-speechand-hearing-science
Northern Arizona University	http://www.nau.edu/chhs/csd
University of Arizona	http://slhs.arizona.edu
Arkansas	
Arkansas State University	http://www.astate.edu/college/conhp/departments/communicationdisorders
Harding University	http://www.harding.edu/csd/
University of Arkansas, Fayetteville	http://www.uark.edu
University of Arkansas for Medical Sciences/ University of Arkansas at Little Rock	http://healthprofessions.uams.edu/programs/audandspeechpathology/
University of Central Arkansas	http://www.uca.edu/chbs
California	
California State University, Chico	http://www.csuchico.edu/cmsd

Institution Offering MA/MS in SLP	*Link*
California State University, East Bay	http://www20.csueastbay.edu/class/departments/commsci/index.html
California State University, Fresno	http://www.csufresno.edu/cdds/
California State University, Fullerton	http://communications.fullerton.edu/hcom/hcom-cd-ma.php
California State University, Long Beach	http://www.csulb.edu/colleges/chhs/departments/communicativedisorders/
California State University, Los Angeles	http://www.calstatela.edu/dept/com_dis/
California State University, Northridge	http://hhd.csun.edu/comdis/
California State University, Sacramento	http://www.csus.edu/hhs/csad
California State University, San Marcos	http://www.csusm.edu/slp
Chapman University	http://www.chapman.edu/crean/academic-programs/graduate-programs/ms-communication-sciences-and-disorders/index.aspx
Loma Linda University	http://www.llu.edu
San Diego State University	http://slhs.sdsu.edu/
San Francisco State University	http://www.sfsu.edu/~comdis/index.html
San Jose State University	http://www.sjsu.edu/cds/
University of Redlands	http://www.redlands.edu/study/schools-and-centers/college-of-arts-and-sciences/truesdail-center/communicative-disorders/
University of the Pacific–SLP Program	http://www.pacific.edu/Academics/Schools-and-Colleges/Thomas-J-Long-School-of-Pharmacy-and-Health-Sciences/Academics/Speech-Language-Pathology
Colorado	
University of Colorado, Boulder	http://admissions.colorado.edu/graduate/programs/slhs

continues

APPENDIX 12–2. *continued*

Institution Offering MA/MS in SLP	*Link*
University of Northern Colorado	http://www.unco.edu/nhs/asls
Connecticut	
Southern Connecticut State University	http://www.southernct.edu/cmd
University of Connecticut	http://slhs.uconn.edu/
District of Columbia	
Gallaudet University	http://www.gallaudet.edu/department-of-hearing-speech-and-language-sciences/
George Washington University	http://www.gwu.edu/~sphr
Howard University	http://www.howard.edu
University of the District of Columbia	http://www.udc.edu
Florida	
Florida International University	http://www.csd.fiu.edu
Florida State University	http://www.commdisorders.cci.fsu.edu
Nova Southeastern University–SLP Program	http://healthsciences.nova.edu/slp
University of Central Florida	http://www.cohpa.ucf.edu/comdis
University of Florida, Gainesville	http://www.slhs.phhp.ufl.edu
University of South Florida	http://www.usf.edu/cbcs/csd
Georgia	
Georgia Southern University (formerly Armstrong State University)	http://www.armstrong.edu/academic-departments/rs-communication-sciences-ms
Georgia State University	http://education.gsu.edu/epse/
University of Georgia	http://www.coe.uga.edu/csse/

Institution Offering MA/MS in SLP	*Link*
University of West Georgia	https://www.westga.edu/academics/education/program_page.php?program_id=74
Valdosta State University	http://www.valdosta.edu/colleges/education/communication-sciences-and-disorders/programs/
Hawaii	
University of Hawaii at Manoa	http://csd.jabsom.hawaii.edu
Idaho	
Idaho State University, Pocatello	http://www.isu.edu/departments/csed/
Illinois	
Eastern Illinois University	http://www.eiu.edu/commdis/
Elmhurst College	http://www.elmhurst.edu/academics/departments/csd
Governors State University	http://www.govst.edu/chhs/dcd
Illinois State University	http://csd.illinoisstate.edu/
Northern Illinois University	http://www.chhs.niu.edu/ahcd/programs/slp/graduate/
Northwestern University	http://www.northwestern.edu/csd
Rush University	http://www.rush.edu/slp
Southern Illinois University, Carbondale	http://www.coe.siu.edu/cds/
Southern Illinois University, Edwardsville	http://www.siue.edu/education/khe/graduate/speech-pathology-audiology/index.shtml
St. Xavier University	http://www.sxu.edu
University of Illinois, Urbana-Champaign	http://www.shs.uiuc.edu
Western Illinois University	http://www.wiu.edu/csd
Indiana	
Ball State University	http://cms.bsu.edu/academics/collegesanddepartments/spaa/
Indiana State University	http://www.indstate.edu/coe/cd/

continues

APPENDIX 12–2. *continued*

Institution Offering MA/MS in SLP	*Link*
Indiana University, Bloomington	http://www.indiana.edu/~sphs/
Purdue University	http://www.purdue.edu/hhs/slhs/
Iowa	
St. Ambrose University	http://www.sau.edu/mslp
University of Iowa	http://clas.uiowa.edu/comsci/
University of Northern Iowa	http://comdis.uni.edu/
Kansas	
Fort Hays State University	http://www.fhsu.edu/commdis/
Kansas State University	http://www.he.k-state.edu/fshs/programs/grad/csd-grad.php
University of Kansas	http://www.ipcd.ku.edu
Wichita State University	http://www.wichita.edu/csd/
Kentucky	
Eastern Kentucky University	http://www.cd.eku.edu
Murray State University	http://www.murraystate.edu/cdi
University of Kentucky	http://www.mc.uky.edu/CommDisorders/
University of Louisville	http://louisville.edu/medicine/degrees
Western Kentucky University	http://www.wku.edu/communicationdisorders/
Louisana	
Louisiana State University and A&M College	http://sites01.lsu.edu/wp/comd/
Louisiana State University–Health Science Center, New Orleans	http://www.lsuhsc.edu
Louisiana State University–Health Sciences Center, Shreveport	http://www.medcom.lsuhscshreveport.edu/ah/page.php?id=35

Institution Offering MA/MS in SLP	***Link***
Louisiana Technical University	http://liberalarts.latech.edu/communication/language/index.php
Southeastern Louisiana University	http://www.selu.edu
Southern University and A&M College	http://www.subr.edu/speechpathology
University of Louisiana, Lafayette	http://speechandlanguage.louisiana.edu/
University of Louisiana, Monroe	http://www.ulm.edu/slp
Maine	
University of Maine	http://www.umaine.edu/comscidis
Maryland	
Loyola University Maryland	http://www.loyola.edu/speech
Towson University	http://www.towson.edu/chp/departments/asld/
University of Maryland, College Park	http://hesp.umd.edu
Massachusetts	
Boston University	http://www.bu.edu/academics/sar/programs/speech-language-hearing-sciences/ms-phd/
Emerson College	http://www.emerson.edu/communication_disorders/
MGH Institute of Health Professions	http://www.mghihp.edu/academics/communication-sciences-and-disorders/
Northeastern University	http://www.northeastern.edu/bouve/csd/
University of Massachusetts, Amherst	http://www.umass.edu/sphhs/communication-disorders
Worcester State University	http://www.worcester.edu/MS-Speech-Language-Pathology
Michigan	
Calvin College	http://www.calvin.edu/academics/departments programs/speech-pathology-audiology/

continues

APPENDIX 12–2. *continued*

Institution Offering MA/MS in SLP	*Link*
Central Michigan University	http://www.cmich.edu/colleges/CHP/hp_academics/communications_disorders/Pages/default.aspx
Eastern Michigan University	http://www.emich.edu/coe/departments/special-education/speech-language-pathology/
Michigan State University	http://cas.msu.edu/departments/csd
Wayne State University	http://www.clas.wayne.edu/csd/
Western Michigan University	http://www.wmich.edu/speech-audiology
Minnesota	
Minnesota State University, Mankato	http://ahn.mnsu.edu/cd/
Minnesota State University, Moorhead	http://www.mnstate.edu/slhs/
St. Cloud State University	http://www.stcloudstate.edu/csd/
University of Minnesota, Duluth	http://www.d.umn.edu/csd
University of Minnesota, Minneapolis	http://cla.umn.edu/slhs
Mississippi	
Jackson State University	http://www.jsums.edu/commdisorders
Mississippi University for Women	http://www.muw.edu/speech
University of Mississippi	http://csd.olemiss.edu/
University of Southern Mississippi	http://www.usm.edu/shs/
Missouri	
Fontbonne University	http://www.fontbonne.edu/academics/departments/communication-disorders-and-deaf-education-department/master-of-science-in-speech-language-pathology/
Missouri State University	http://www.missouristate.edu/csd
Rockhurst University	http://ww2.rockhurst.edu/communication-sciences-disorders/program-options

Institution Offering MA/MS in SLP	*Link*
Saint Louis University	http://www.slu.edu/doisy/degrees/undergraduate/communication-sciences-and-disorders.php
Southeast Missouri State University	http://www.semo.edu/commdisorders/
Truman State University	http://comdis.truman.edu/
University of Central Missouri	http://www.ucmo.edu
University of Missouri	http://healthprofessions.missouri.edu/communication-science-and-disorders
Montana	
University of Montana	http://coehs.umt.edu
Nebraska	
University of Nebraska, Kearney	http://www.unk.edu/academics/cdis/
University of Nebraska, Lincoln	http://cehs.unl.edu/secd
University of Nebraska, Omaha	http://www.unomaha.edu/college-of-education/special-education-communication-disorders/graduate/speech-language-pathology.php
Nevada	
University of Nevada, Reno	http://www.unr.edu/degrees/speech-pathology
New Hampshire	
University of New Hampshire	http://chhs.unh.edu/csd/communication-sciences-and-disorders-ms
New Jersey	
Kean University of New Jersey	http://grad.kean.edu/slp
Montclair State University	http://www.montclair.edu/chss/communication-sciences-disorders
Seton Hall University	http://www.shu.edu/go/slp
Stockton University	http://www2.stockton.edu/
William Paterson University of New Jersey	http://www.wpunj.edu/cosh/departments/communication-disorders/

continues

Institution Offering MA/MS in SLP	*Link*
New Mexico	
Eastern New Mexico University	http://www.enmu.edu/cdis
New Mexico State University	http://www.nmsu.edu
University of New Mexico	http://shs.unm.edu
New York	
Adelphi University	http://education-csd.adelphi.edu/
Buffalo State College	http://www.buffalostate.edu/speech/
College of Saint Rose	https://www.strose.edu/communication-sciences-disorders-ms/
CUNY, Brooklyn College	http://www.brooklyn.cuny.edu
CUNY, Hunter College	http://www.hunter.cuny.edu/comsc
CUNY, Lehman College	http://www.lehman.edu/deanhum/splanghearing/
CUNY, Queens College	http://www.qc.cuny.edu/academics/degrees/dah/lcd/pages/ma-slp.aspx
Hofstra University	http://www.hofstra.edu
Ithaca College	http://departments.ithaca.edu/slpa/
LIU Brooklyn	http://www.brooklyn.liu.edu/new_csd
LIU Post	http://www.cwpost.liunet.edu
Mercy College	http://www.mercy.edu
Molloy College	http://www.molloy.edu
Nazareth College	http://www.naz.edu
New York Medical College	http://www.nymc.edu/departments/academic-departments/school-of-health-sciences-and-practice/speech-language-pathology/
New York University	http://steinhardt.nyu.edu/csd/
St. John's University	http://www.stjohns.edu/
SUNY at Buffalo	http://cdswebserver.med.buffalo.edu/drupal/
SUNY at Fredonia	http://www.fredonia.edu

Institution Offering MA/MS in SLP	*Link*
SUNY at New Paltz	http://www.newpaltz.edu/commdis
SUNY at Plattsburgh	http://web.plattsburgh.edu/academics/commdisorders/
Syracuse University	http://csd.syr.edu/about-us/speech-pathology.html
Teachers College, Columbia University	http://www.tc.edu/bbs/speech/
Touro College	http://shs.touro.edu/programs/speech-language-pathology/
North Carolina	
Appalachian State University	http://comdis.appstate.edu/
East Carolina University	http://www.ecu.edu/csd/
North Carolina Central University	http://www.nccu.edu
University of North Carolina, Chapel Hill	http://www.med.unc.edu/ahs/sphs/
University of North Carolina, Greensboro	http://www.uncg.edu/csd/
Western Carolina University	http://csd.wcu.edu
North Dakota	
Minot State University	http://www.minotstateu.edu/graduate/future_students/pages/communication-disorders.shtml
University of North Dakota	http://arts-sciences.und.edu/communication-sciences-disorders/
Ohio	
Bowling Green State University	http://www.bgsu.edu/cdis
Case Western Reserve University	http://psychsciences.case.edu/graduate/graduate-comm-sciences-programs/
Cleveland State University	http://www.csuohio.edu/sciences/health-sciences/graduate-programs
Kent State University	http://www.kent.edu/ehhs/hs/spa
Miami University	http://www.muohio.edu/spa

continues

Institution Offering MA/MS in SLP	*Link*
Ohio State University	http://sphs.osu.edu/
Ohio University	http://www.ohio.edu/chsp/csd
University of Akron	http://www.uakron.edu/sslpa
University of Cincinnati	http://www.cahs.uc.edu/csd
University of Toledo	http://www.utoledo.edu/hhs/speech/
Oklahoma	
Northeastern State University	http://www.nsuok.edu
Oklahoma State University	http://cdis.okstate.edu
University of Central Oklahoma	http://www.uco.edu
University of Oklahoma–Health Sciences Center	http://alliedhealth.ouhsc.edu/Departments/CommunicationSciencesandDisorders.aspx
University of Tulsa	http://healthsciences.utulsa.edu/departmentsschools/communication-disorders/
Oregon	
Pacific University	http://www.pacificu.edu/coe/csd/
Portland State University	http://www.pdx.edu/sphr/home
University of Oregon	http://education.uoregon.edu/cds
Pennsylvania	
Bloomsburg University of Pennsylvania	http://www.bloomu.edu
California University of Pennsylvania	http://www.calu.edu
Clarion University of Pennsylvania	http://www.clarion.edu/academics/colleges-and schools/college-of-health-and-human-services/department-of-communication-sciences-and-disorders/
Duquesne University	http://www.duq.edu/academics/schools/health-sciences/academic-programs/speech-language-pathology
East Stroudsburg University	http://www.esu.edu

Institution Offering MA/MS in SLP	*Link*
Edinboro University of Pennsylvania	http://www.edinboro.edu/academics/schools-and-departments/cshp/departments/speech/
Indiana University of Pennsylvania	http://www.iup.edu/special-ed/
La Salle University	http://www.lasalle.edu/
Marywood University	http://www.marywood.edu
Misericordia University	http://www.misericordia.edu/slp
Pennsylvania State University	http://csd.hhdev.psu.edu/
Temple University	http://cph.temple.edu/commsci/home
University of Pittsburgh	http://www.shrs.pitt.edu/csd
West Chester University	http://www.wcupa.edu
Puerto Rico	
Carlos Albizu University	http://www.albizu.edu/Academics/Degrees-in-Speech-and-Language
Universidad del Turabo	http://ut.suagm.edu/
University of Puerto Rico, San Juan	http://www.upr.edu/
Rhode Island	
University of Rhode Island	http://web.uri.edu/cmd/
South Carolina	
South Carolina State University	http://www.scsu.edu/academicprograms/speechpathologyaudiology.aspx
University of South Carolina	http://www.sc.edu/study/colleges_schools/public_health/study/areas_of_study/communication_sciences_and_disorders/index.php
South Dakota	
University of South Dakota	http://www.usd.edu/csd
Tennessee	
East Tennessee State University	http://www.etsu.edu/cpah/commdis

continues

APPENDIX 12–2. *continued*

Institution Offering MA/MS in SLP	*Link*
Tennessee State University	http://www.tnstate.edu
University of Memphis	http://www.memphis.edu/csd
University of Tennessee–Health Science Center	http://uthsc.edu/health-professions/asp/aud/index.php
Vanderbilt University	http://ww2.mc.vanderbilt.edu/GHSS/
Texas	
Abilene Christian University	http://www.acu.edu/graduate/academics/speech-language-pathology.html
Baylor University	http://www.baylor.edu/csd
Lamar University	http://www.lamar.edu/fine-arts-communication/speech-and-hearing-sciences/index.html
Our Lady of the Lake University	http://www.ollusa.edu
Stephen F. Austin State University	http://www.sfasu.edu/humanservices/69.asp
Texas A&M University, Kingsville	http://www.tamuk.edu/artsci/csdo
Texas Christian University	http://www.csd.tcu.edu
Texas State University	http://www.health.txstate.edu/cdis/cdis.html
Texas Tech University–Health Sciences Center	http://www.ttuhsc.edu
Texas Woman's University	https://twu.edu/communication-sciences/
University of Houston	http://www.uh.edu/class/comd/
University of North Texas	http://aslp.hps.unt.edu/
University of Texas at Dallas	http://www.utdallas.edu
University of Texas, Austin	http://csd.utexas.edu/
University of Texas, Rio Grande Valley	http://www.utrgv.edu/communication-disorders/index.htm
University of Texas, El Paso	https://www.utep.edu/chs/slp/

Institution Offering MA/MS in SLP	*Link*
West Texas A & M University	http://www.wtamu.edu/academics/communication-disorders.aspx
Utah	
Brigham Young University	http://education.byu.edu/comd
University of Utah	http://health.utah.edu/communication-sciences-disorders/
Utah State University	http://www.comd.usu.edu
Vermont	
University of Vermont	http://www.uvm.edu/
Virginia	
Hampton University	http://science.hamptonu.edu/csad/
James Madison University	http://www.csd.jmu.edu
Longwood University	http://www.longwood.edu/socialworkcsds/index.html
Old Dominion University	http://www.odu.edu/cdse
Radford University	http://www.radford.edu/content/wchs/home/cosd.html
University of Virginia	http://curry.virginia.edu/academics/speech-communication-disorders
Washington	
Eastern Washington University	http://www.ewu.edu/csd
University of Washington	https://sphsc.washington.edu/ms-med-slp
Washington State University	https://medicine.wsu.edu/research/dcp/speech-and-hearing-sciences/
Western Washington University	http://www.wwu.edu/
West Virginia	
Marshall University	http://www.marshall.edu/communication-disorders/
West Virginia University	https://graduateadmissions.wvu.edu/academics/graduate-programs/speech-pathology-m

continues

APPENDIX 12–2. *continued*

Institution Offering MA/MS in SLP	*Link*
Wisconsin	
Marquette University	http://www.marquette.edu/speech-pathology-audiology/
University of Wisconsin, Eau Claire	http://www.uwec.edu/academics/college-education-human-sciences/departments-programs/communication-sciences-disorders/
University of Wisconsin, Madison	http://csd.wisc.edu
University of Wisconsin, Milwaukee	http://uwm.edu/healthsciences/academics/communication-sciences-disorders/
University of Wisconsin, River Falls	http://www.uwrf.edu/csd/index.cfm
University of Wisconsin, Stevens Point	http://www.uwsp.edu/csd/
University of Wisconsin, Whitewater	http://www.uww.edu/coeps/departments/comdis
Wyoming	
University of Wyoming	http://www.uwyo.edu/comdis/

APPENDIX 12–3

PhD and AuD Programs

SLP/SHS PhD	AuD
Alabama	
University of South Alabama (SHS)	Auburn University University of South Alabama
Arizona	
Arizona State University (SHS) University of Arizona (SHS)	Arizona State University A.T. Still University–Arizona School of Health Sciences University of Arizona
Arkansas	
University of Arkansas for Medical Sciences/University of Arkansas at Little Rock (SHS) University of Central Arkansas	University of Arkansas for Medical Sciences/University of Arkansas at Little Rock
California	
San Diego State University	San Diego State University & University of California San Diego: AuD Joint Doctoral Program University of the Pacific–Audiology Program
Colorado	
University of Colorado, Boulder (SHS)	University of Colorado, Boulder University of Northern Colorado
Connecticut	
University of Connecticut (SLP and SHS)	University of Connecticut
District of Columbia	
Gallaudet University (SHS) Howard University (SLP)	Gallaudet University

continues

APPENDIX 12–3. *continued*

SLP/SHS PhD	*AuD*
Florida	
Florida State University (SLP) University of Central Florida University of Florida (SLP and SHS) University of Florida, Gainesville University of South Florida (SHS)	Nova Southeastern University–Audiology Program University of Florida University of Florida, Gainesville University of South Florida
Georgia	
Georgia State University University of Georgia (SLP)	
Illinois	
Northwestern University (SHS) University of Illinois, Urbana-Champaign (SHS)	Illinois State University Northern Illinois University Northwestern University University of Illinois, Urbana-Champaign Rush University
Indiana	
Purdue University (SLP and SHS)	Ball State University Purdue University Indiana State University Indiana University, Bloomington
Iowa	
University of Iowa (SHS)	University of Iowa
Kansas	
University of Kansas (SLP) Wichita State University (SLP and SHS)	University of Kansas Wichita State University
Kentucky	
University of Kentucky (SLP)	University of Louisville

SLP/SHS PhD	AuD
Louisiana	
Louisiana State University and A&M College (SLP) University of Louisiana, Lafayette (SLP)	Louisiana State University–Health Science Center, New Orleans Louisiana Technical University
Maryland	
University of Maryland, College Park (SHS)	Towson University University of Maryland, College Park
Massachusetts	
Boston University (SHS) Harvard Medical School (SHS) MGH Institute of Health Professions University of Massachusetts, Amherst (SLP and SHS)	Northeastern University University of Massachusetts, Amherst
Michigan	
Michigan State University (SLP) Wayne State University (SLP and SHS)	Central Michigan University Wayne State University
Minnesota	
University of Minnesota, Minneapolis (SLP and SHS)	University of Minnesota, Minneapolis
Missouri	
University of Missouri (SLP and SHS) Washington University (SHS)	Missouri State University Washington University
Montana	
University of Montana (SLP)	
Nebraska	
University of Nebraska, Lincoln (SLP)	University of Nebraska, Lincoln
Nevada	
University of Nevada, Reno (SLP)	
New Jersey	
Montclair State University (SHS) Seton Hall University	Montclair State University

continues

APPENDIX 12–3. *continued*

SLP/SHS PhD	*AuD*
New York	
Adelphi University (SLP) CUNY, The Graduate Center (PhD Program) (SHS) New York University (SLP) SUNY at Buffalo (SHS) Syracuse University (SLP) Teachers College, Columbia University (SLP)	CUNY, Brooklyn College/Hunter College–Graduate Center Long Island AuD Consortium: Adelphi/Hofstra/St. John's Universities SUNY at Buffalo Syracuse University
North Carolina	
East Carolina University (SHS) University of North Carolina, Chapel Hill (SHS) University of North Carolina, Greensboro (SHS)	East Carolina University University of North Carolina, Chapel Hill
Ohio	
Bowling Green State University (SLP and SHS) Case Western Reserve University (SLP) Kent State University (SLP) Ohio State University (SHS) Ohio University University of Cincinnati (SLP and SHS)	Northeast Ohio AuD Consortium (NOAC): Kent State/University of Akron Ohio State University Ohio University University of Cincinnati
Oklahoma	
University of Oklahoma–Health Sciences Center (SLP)	University of Oklahoma–Health Sciences Center
Oregon	
University of Oregon (SLP)	Pacific University–Audiology
Pennsylvania	
Pennsylvania State University (SLP) Temple University University of Pittsburgh (SHS)	Bloomsburg University of Pennsylvania Salus University–Audiology Program (AuD ONLY) University of Pittsburgh

SLP/SHS PhD	AuD
South Carolina	
Medical University of South Carolina (SLP) University of South Carolina (SLP)	
Tennessee	
University of Memphis (SLP) University of Tennessee Health Science Center (SHS) Vanderbilt University (SLP)	East Tennessee State University University of Memphis University of Tennessee Health Science Center Vanderbilt University
Texas	
Texas Christian University (SLP) Texas Tech–University Health Sciences Center (SHS) University of North Texas [Research Doctoral Degree in Speech-Language Pathology; Other (PhD in Health Services Research)] University of Texas at Dallas (SHS) University of Texas, Austin (SLP and SHS)	Lamar University Texas Tech University Health Sciences Center University of North Texas University of Texas at Dallas University of Texas, Austin
Utah	
University of Utah (SLP) Utah State University (SLP)	University of Utah Utah State University
Virginia	
James Madison University (SLP and SHS) University of Virginia (SLP)	James Madison University
Washington	
University of Washington (SLP and SHS)	University of Washington Western Washington University
West Virginia	
West Virginia University (SLP and SHS)	West Virginia University

continues

APPENDIX 12–3. *continued*

SLP/SHS PhD	*AuD*
Wisconsin	
University of Wisconsin, Madison (SLP and SHS)	AuD Consortium: University of Wisconsin–Madison & University of Wisconsin–Stevens Point

PART III

Disseminating Research in CSD

13

Dissemination by Publication

INTRODUCTION

With the explosion of Web-based content, much of which is unreliable, the clinical researcher can have a hard time keeping up with even a subspecialty, such as fluency disorders in children or aural rehabilitation in adults. The challenge to stay current in all the fields a generalist must know to study and treat a diverse population of individuals with communication disorders can be overwhelming. The late Dr. Sadanand Singh, founder and publisher of Plural Publishing as well as other scholarly imprints, used to bemoan all the "warp and weft" (it has to do with area rugs) in manuscripts that clouded the author's message. Nate Silver (2012) wrote about separating the signal from the noise by Bayesian statistical analysis (see Chapter 6).

Learning Objectives

After reading this chapter, the student will be able to

- identify aspects of peer review;
- identify the editorial process for acceptance or rejection of a manuscript; and
- identify how chapters are reviewed and edited differently from journal articles.

THE ARTICLE IN A PEER-REVIEWED JOURNAL

The title of the journal indicates the target audience that already knows basic information and wants in-depth content or the latest published research. Some journals are more broadly based than others, so the *Journal of Speech, Language, and Hearing Research* will publish in all areas of communication sciences and disorders (CSD) and *Brain and Language* will publish articles with many perspectives on neurogenic communication and its disorders, but the *Journal of Fluency Disorders* or *Aphasiology* will address only the communication disorders indicated in the title. Some journals, such as *Nature* will be the flagship journal in a publishing group with, for example, *Nature Reviews Neuroscience* publishing more focused research.

The audience for a peer-reviewed journal includes professors, students, and researchers. Published articles require an advanced reading level, as there will be technical language. Articles usually include relevant figures, tables, and statistics that illustrate and explain key concepts. The purpose of a peer-reviewed journal is to present reports of experimental studies, literature reviews with original syntheses, and sometimes lengthy reviews of scholarly books. CSD journals usually conform to the referencing style of American Psychological Association (APA) 2010. They may include many references (even 100 or more) that are cited in the body of the article and listed at the end, but few or no footnotes. CSD articles must show scientific rigor, novelty, and technical accuracy. The criterion for publication is usually approval from two to three peers, as well as approval from the associate editor or editor of the journal.

The best journals have a high impact factor. This means that articles published in a high-impact journal are cited in other published articles more than articles published in other, lower-impact journals. In a systematic review (Callaham, Wears, & Weber, 2002) of published research predicting citation in other journals, the impact factor of the original publishing journal was more important than any other variable. The impact factor, then, is a measure of a journal's importance. For example, *Nature* has a higher impact factor than *Brain and Language*, which has a higher impact factor than *Aphasiology*. Does that mean that you shouldn't bother to read articles in *Aphasiology*? Absolutely not, as articles in that journal are of consistently high quality. However, the focus of the journal is much narrower, and the likelihood is that broader-based journals of high quality will have more citations based on a wider range of areas of study. Be warned, though, that some open-access journals are reporting fake impact factors. When in doubt, check the Scopus indexed journals list that includes most of the journals that have true impact factors.

In general, a scholarly journal should not be in business to make a profit and should permit little or no advertising. Articles tend to be long, at least in comparison to those in newspapers and magazines, and the authors tend to have credentials in the areas related to the journal's title. Finally, articles published in scholarly journals are refereed (where a group decides that the article should be published), peer reviewed (a reviewer with in-depth expertise in the subject area decides), or both, in a process mentioned in Chapter 7 and elaborated on here. Peer review means that experts and scholars in the field have critiqued the manuscript and deemed it publishable in the journal in which it appears.

Advantages and Disadvantages of Peer Review

Spier (2002) offers a historical perspective of the peer-review process. Ancient scholars, such as Hippocrates and Aristotle, wrote manuscripts nearly 2,500 years ago that were untouched by reviewers and can still be found, in original form, on the island of Cos in Greece. However, the earliest biblical texts were amended and redacted until they were canonized around year 100 of the Common Era (CE). The invention of the printing press by Guttenberg permitted distribution of printed material, and regulations soon followed. The revolutionary idea of Copernicus that the Earth revolved around the Sun was published on the last day of Copernicus' life in 1543 CE, but it was retroactively rejected by the Spanish Inquisition. The review process could be cruel. In fact, it sometimes resulted in the author of writing deemed heretical to be burned at the stake. In the mid-18th century, the Royal Societies of Edinburgh and London asked their membership for help in selection of articles in their publication (Voight & Hoogenboom, 2012). Even as early as the 1700s, peer reviewers made an assumption of honesty; authors held responsibility for integrity (Rennie, 2003).

The use of outside peer reviewers began around 1940 by the *Journal of the American Medical Association*. The diversity and specialization in science overwhelmed the panel of experts in the sponsoring society, forcing them to recruit what is now known as ad hoc peer reviewers from the scientific community. Recently, a double-blind peer-review process has been used, only somewhat successfully, to prevent both authors and reviewers from knowing who wrote and who reviewed the work. I say somewhat successfully because it is often possible for an ad hoc reviewer to discern who wrote the article based on the content of the paper and the citations in the References section. Editors generally have a database of external reviewers that list their areas of expertise. Additional ad hoc reviewers may be recruited from editors' personal contacts, authors of articles previously published in the journal, authors of articles cited in the submitted manuscript, and searches of Medline or other electronic databases.

An advantage of the peer-review process is that it is a mechanism for self-regulation of scientific work (Thurner & Hanel, 2011). Clinical research contributes to the evidence required for evidence-based practice (EBP), and Justice (2008) notes that peer review promotes the best available evidence that is relevant and trustworthy. However, it is hard to evaluate the strengths and weaknesses of peer review as a selection mechanism. According to Smith (2016), its defects are easier to find than its attributes. For example, while peer review informs decisions about grant funding, academic publishing, and promotion of individual university scientists, it may be too narrowly scientific. Some pressing social challenges, including global environmental changes and the needs of aging populations, may be excluded because peer review does not address criteria relating to social relevance (Scott, 2007). It can be compared to democracy as a system full of problems but "the least worst we have" (Smith, 2016, p. 178). We must ask two questions about peer review: What is it for and does it work? The idealistic answer to the first question is that peer review results in the selection of the best grant applications to fund and the best journal articles to publish. The problem is that the scientific community varies in its definition of what constitutes a good research proposal or a good paper. A cynical colleague responded, "Perpetuating the garbage," when I asked what he was working on. To answer the question if peer review works, we need to compare it to something else. Two possible options are better than chance or better than a much simpler process. At present, the limited number of critical studies of the peer-review process does not permit systematic review or meta-analysis.

To summarize, peer reviewers must be dedicated to objectivity and must love high-quality science, with an absence of bias and selfishness. In CSD research, the presence of bias and selfishness leads to dominance in the professional literature of some experimental and clinical approaches to the exclusion of other legitimate pursuits, especially by novice investigators with new ideas (Pratt, 2010). Kreiman (2016) affirms that editorial filtering or gatekeeping in CSD journals allows established concepts to block publication of new ideas or clinical methods that contradict the orthodoxy of existing theory and practice. The process of peer review has been basically untested and its efficacy (efficiency and effectiveness) is pretty much unknown. In clinical neuroscience, the results of peer review were no different from chance in terms of acceptance of articles submitted to journals and abstracts submitted to scientific meetings (Rothwell & Martyn, 2000). Reproducibility may be poor because peer reviewers are uncertain about which aspects of the research to assess. The peer-review process may need to change from its present form to be more useful. However, at present, there are probably no alternatives to peer review to ensure quality control.

It is not easy for an author of a manuscript to accept peer review "as a beneficial activity rather than a painful nuisance" (Kreiman, 2016, p. 482). However, doing so can ensure that all aspects of the paper are accurate, written clearly, and easier to understand. Such a paper may be read and cited more often than it would have been in its original form. While authors, including the present one, resent the waiting period and may be annoyed by the comments that follow peer review, the process is meant to be helpful, not adversarial. Ad hoc reviewing of an article is hard work, it is unpaid, and it is rarely recognized. Why do reviewers spend so much time and effort on a task that yields virtually no personal gain? Admittedly, some reviewers pad the review with a demand for citations of their own work, but most, I hope, do not. Some may even sabotage work they perceive as competition. Just as reviewers are not rewarded for an honest and accurate job, they are not penalized for a sloppy and biased one (D'Andrea & O'Dwyer, 2017). A process of open review rather than masked review might result in greater accountability of reviewers as well as credit for the work they have done. The most compelling motivations to be an external reviewer have to be a desire to contribute more to the profession we love, to read cutting edge research before anyone else, and to include the service on your curriculum vitae. Those of us in academia are evaluated and need to excel in scholarship, teaching, and service. Providing service to one's national association as a peer reviewer is preferable, to many of us, to serving on a college's Committee on Committees.

How can a student find peer-reviewed articles? The best way to find an article in a peer-reviewed journal is to use a scholarly database, found in most university library online databases. There may even be an optional box to check that will list only peer-reviewed articles; otherwise, try the advanced search option. Synonyms that are sometimes substituted for *peer-reviewed* are *scholarly* and *academic* journal articles. In general, avoid self-published websites because they are not held to the same level of scrutiny as peer-reviewed journal articles. If you use your university library, there is even a second level of review by the librarians who decide whether the journal or book is appropriate for the collection.

Open Access Journals

As professional or student members of the American Speech-Language-Hearing Association (ASHA), we receive four peer-reviewed journals online: *Journal of Speech, Language, and Hearing Research; American Journal of Speech-Language Pathology; American Journal of Audiology;* and *Language, Speech, and Hearing Services in Schools.* We also receive electronic and hard copies of the *ASHA Leader*, a periodical that is not peer-reviewed but that includes interesting articles that are submitted by invitation. These are all called subscription journals, and they are paid for by our annual dues to ASHA (note that the *Leader* does accept advertisements). Only members and participating institutions such as your university library can access articles in the journals listed above. However, many articles in these journals acknowledge funding sources that may require release of the research online after a period of time. For example, the National Institutes of Health mandates free online access to NIH-funded research after an embargo period. In contrast are Open Access (OA) journals that are always freely available online.

More than 95% of scholars report knowing about one or more OA journals in their professional disciplines. The largest OA journal PLoS ONE, a highly respected journal, publishes thousands of articles a year, but more than half of the OA journals publish 25 or fewer. The average OA journal published 41 articles per year (Walters & Linvill, 2011). According to the Directory of Open Access Journals (DOAJ; http://www.doaj.org), an OA journal is defined as a journal that does not charge readers or their institutions for access. Another industry association that vets its members is the Open Access Scholarly Publishers Association (http://www.oaspa.org). Users have the right to read, copy, download, distribute, print, search, and link to full-texts of articles. Authors hold an unrestricted copyright to their work. The funding model varies, but it includes donations, advertisement, publication charges, and page charges. Journals listed with DOAJ must be peer reviewed with an editorial board or an editorial review that includes at least two reviewers. There are currently nearly 12,000 journals and more than 3,000,000 articles listed with DOAJ. Most journals listed with DOAJ are commercial or for-profit publications. However, other OA journals may be categorized as government, scholarly societies, and university or other nonprofit publishers. The impact factor of OA journals is usually low, and the vast majority of these journals do not provide citation data. Most journals that reported impact factors are in the biomedical fields and are comparable in quality with subscription journals reporting the same impact factor.

My colleagues and I receive a staggering number of e-mails and spam calls for papers to be published in OA journals we've never heard of that claim to be peer reviewed. We generally know which of the journals in our field are prestigious, midrank, or poor. It is no wonder that students and neophyte investigators who may not know the journals in their field can be duped into thinking that the solicitation is from a reputable journal. *Nature,* one of the most prestigious journals in the world, devoted an issue to this problem: How do you identify fake OA journals? Some predatory OA journals (Butler, 2013) exist not to disseminate new, verifiable, and useful information but to dupe researchers into wasting their money, sometimes a great deal of it. Aspiring authors and their mentors need to know how to evaluate journals to avoid predation by scammers (Mehrpour & Khajavi 2014). Some criteria include the following: layout and appearance of the website (amateurish or professional?), publisher associated with the journal (is the publisher well established?), indexing databases (e.g., Scopus), editorial board (names you know may not have given permission, so check with them), type and style of the peer-review report ("publication without modification" or "accept as is" should raise a red flag), length of the peer-review process (some fake journals guarantee a response within two weeks), scholars who publish in these journals (are there names of authors you know and respect?), selection of the referees (we are often e-mailed by scam OA journals asking us to review a paper in an area we have nothing to do with), copyediting and proofreading (look for poor quality), charging money (may be a sign of a for-profit business, not a scholarly journal), plagiarism (may be duplicates of articles previously published), and damaging the reputation of the OA system (check to see if the journal is listed with DOAJ).

So are OA journals a bane or a boon? Criticism of OA journals includes the following: fake peer review; sloppy editing; preying on inexperienced authors; and paying to publish. However, there may also be advantages of OA journals, at least according to the author of an article in an OA journal (Rohrer, 2014): making scholarship freely available may be in the public interest; OA journals may not limit publication pages as subscription journals do (of course, OA journals often have page charges paid by the authors); OA journals follow the NIH model of free online access to funded research, and do not even include an embargo period; and many subscription journals have already converted to the online format.

The print journals that also publish online still hold to the high standards of scientific rigor that they always did. However, some, but not all, Internet-only journals may have only the most cursory review process, and they tend to charge authors for online publication. (Box 13–1 indicates categories for evaluation of arti-

Box 13–1. Evaluating Articles on Websites

Author: Identification, credentials, affiliation, professional standing, contact information

Design: Easy to access and use, well organized, compatible search engine

Features: Not available in other formats, comprehensive coverage, needs of readership

Objectivity: Sponsorship or advertising, impartiality, purpose of site

Updates: Updates of site and links listed

Usefulness: Accuracy of information, reference list, types of research used (see Chapter 5)

cles appearing on websites.) University committees on retention, promotion, and tenure may take a dim view of articles published in such journals. Junior faculty should generally avoid publishing in them, and students should not cite them in research papers without their instructors' approval. As millions of pages of research ranging from outstanding to appalling are published daily, it is the job of student or faculty mentors to help new researchers in separating the wheat from the chaff.

The Editorial Process

This section will address frequently asked questions about the steps toward publishing an article in a refereed or peer-reviewed journal, securing grant funding, or presenting research at a scientific meeting (see Pearson, 2013, p. 147): How are reviewers or an editorial board chosen? How many people review a submitted manuscript? How do editors decide to publish a manuscript? Are there ever differences of opinion between reviewers?

The term *peer review* may be a bit of a misnomer. Authors of manuscripts for a journal article, proposals for grant funding, or presentation submissions for scientific meetings are not evaluated by individuals at the same stage of their careers. The editorial process usually involves a "top-down" procedure of a first review by subscription journal editors and associate editors as well as editorial boards for manuscripts. Another editorial process involves selection committees and senior colleagues for research proposals. Sometimes junior colleagues and professional technical editors are also involved. There may also be comments and criticism after the article is published (postpublication peer review). In high-impact subscription journals, the rejection rate may be as high as 80% to 90%. The inclusive philosophy of OA journals uses a "bottom-up" model of accepting everything that meets minimum standards and using peer review only to weed out research with methodological or ethical problems. Articles of interest only to a small audience may be published, and readers are not expected to be interested in everything published in the OA journal (Box 13–2).

There is also an editorial process for what may be called *pay journals* that includes both print and online publications. Funding comes from publication charges, page charges, or an agreement to buy reprints. This model refers mostly to pharmaceutical journals, where few subscribers are needed because their representatives distribute reprints. Companies can publish articles of routine or repeated studies that would be rejected by major journals but are needed for drug registration (Wager, Godlee, & Jefferson, 2002). A drug company that publishes in a peer-reviewed pay journal with an inclusive

Box 13–2. Editorial Processes

"Bottom-Up" (OA and pay journals)

- Advantages: likely acceptance, rapid decision making
- Disadvantages: less prestigious journal, cost

"Top-Down" (subscription journals)

- Advantages: more prestigious journal, detailed review
- Disadvantages: high rejection rate, slow decision making

model for acceptance still has more credibility than a company that self-publishes an article.

There are different editorial processes for review of journal articles, grant proposals, and conference presentations. Journals may use the following: single editor, all externally reviewed; editorial board with further review as needed; professional editor and staff with external review; editorial boards and committees; and statistical review (Wager et al., 2002). Journal submission instructions may require a disclosure of potential financial and nonfinancial conflicts of interest (peer reviewers must also indicate if there is a potential conflict of interest). Finally, high-quality journals will use copyeditors for accepted manuscripts to ensure that they conform to standards of accuracy, consistency, and house style. Grant proposals are generally sent to several external reviewers, but, in contrast to the blind review process for journals, the author of the grant is known. In fact, the grant applicant is usually required to submit full curriculum vitae (CV, or a detailed professional resumé) as part of the application to indicate requisite qualifications and experience needed to do the work. Scientific meetings often have a selection committee functioning as an editorial board. The author may submit work in progress that should be completed at the time of the presentation, and the abstract of the accepted presentation is usually published in the conference booklet without revision.

The publication process begins with an author submitting a manuscript to a journal. Assuming you are submitting a clinical research manuscript to a high-quality scholarly journal, you can expect the following editorial process, or something very similar to it.

The editor will look for evidence that the manuscript meets the selection criteria for the particular publication. There may be an editorial assistant who will check for similarity to other sources using similarity detection software such as iThenticate (Ali & Watson, 2016, p. 193). If there is not sufficient evidence for publication, the editor will quickly reject the submission outright. As many as half of the submissions to the most competitive subscription journals are rejected at this stage. If there is sufficient evidence for publication, the associate editor in charge of the area (say language, speech, or hearing) will take over.

The associate editor will contact two or three ad hoc peer reviewers, probably from a database listing the reviewers' areas of expertise. Peer reviewers will be given a deadline of a few weeks to produce a detailed report, according to the style of the journal.

The ad hoc peer reviewers will carefully review the manuscripts to filter out research that has been poorly conceived, designed, and executed. Articles selected for publication will have scientific merit, validity, novelty, and appropriate methodology. They will be relevant to the goals of the publication, understandable, and readable. Reviewers send detailed comments to the associate editor who will make a recommendation to the editor to publish without revisions, with minor revisions, with major revisions, or not to publish. Authors will not see the comments sent to the editor, but most journals give reviewers the option of addressing additional comments to authors.

The critique of the manuscript focuses on the nine aspects of a journal article:

- *Title:* In 10 words or so, the author told the reader about the classification variables and the target population being studied, and also tried to attract the reader's interest.
- *Abstract:* In about 150 words, the author reported the purpose of the study, the important results, and implications of the research. Pertinent characteristics of participants might include number, age, gender, and type of communication disorder. The experimental method might include the apparatus and data-gathering procedures. Findings might include statistical significance levels. Authors should have added keywords and learner outcomes if required by the journal.
- *Introduction:* The author started with a clear statement of the general problem; presented operational definitions; provided an original synthesis of a large body of information; indicated what is valuable as well as weak or erroneous in these studies; presented alternative theories on the specific or a related subject; all roads led, logically and convincingly, to hypotheses. Reviewers determine if the research in the literature review is reported correctly and that previous relevant work is acknowledged.
- *Method—Participants:* The author presented an adequate description of the proposed population, such as treatment group and control group (with inclusionary and exclusionary criteria); author used adequate sample size to permit statistical analysis and generalization; described methods of assessment, including type and severity of disorder; controlled relevant participant variables.
- *Method—Materials:* The author described standardization and calibration of instrumentation, including human instruments; described novel materials in sufficient detail to permit replication of the study.
- *Method—Procedure:* The description of how the study was done was sufficiently detailed to permit replication of the study; author controlled variables, such as practice effect, order of presentation, randomization of stimuli, recording of responses, and reliability of and correlation between scorers to limit threats to internal validity; described baseline and baseline recovery procedures.
- *Results:* Key findings were reported, but not interpreted; summary of data was presented in table or figure format according to the style (e.g., APA 2010) of the journal; all findings were reported, even those that did not support the hypotheses; there was an adequate description of statistical analyses with visual displays used as needed.
- *Conclusion and Discussion:* Results presented were interpreted correctly and all possible interpretations were considered; author showed evidence of new research and theories; compared a summary of key findings to research reported in the Introduction section; described how results supported or refuted research hypotheses; included clinical implications if appropriate.

- *References:* Works cited were reported according to the style of the journal (e.g., alphabetically in APA 2010 style); the author avoided abstracts and Internet sites that were not peer reviewed; all references and only the references cited in the body of the paper were listed.

For specific information about publishing an article in a peer-reviewed journal, see articles about analyzing the structure of your research paper (Skelton, 1994), the editor's perspective (Samet, 1999), adapting a course paper to become a publishable manuscript (Rew, 2012), understanding what a reasonable topic and scope is for a particular journal (Pierce, 2009), publishing in an international journal (Tress, Tress, & Saunders, 2014), where to submit if a paper is rejected (Have & Gordijn, 2015), dealing with the publishing delay (Björk & Solomon, 2013), and general suggestions about navigating the peer-review process (Constantinescu, 2009; Dimitroulis, 2011; Jha, 2014; Mueller, 2001).

Readers are encouraged to download the PowerPoint, "From Adelphi University: Syntax Training" (FAUST) from the companion website associated with this book and follow the template for writing an original clinical research experiment.

Submission Decisions

Authors have several goals in publishing an article in a peer-reviewed journal that may be in tension when they decide how and where to submit their manuscripts. They may want to share their findings as widely as possible, and citation counts can serve as a proxy for this goal. They may want to minimize the time between initial submission and final decision. Finally, they may want to minimize the likelihood of rejections and resubmissions. Authors may have different objectives at different stages of their careers.

For some institutions and authors working at them, the impact factor of a journal is of utmost importance. Publication in a high-impact journal is more likely to land you an academic job and will help in retention, promotion, and tenure. Recall that impact factor refers to the number of times per year a given article in a journal is cited in other work. The impact factor refers to the journal and not to the author, so it is not especially useful in evaluating the productivity or potential of an individual researcher. It also does not record the number of page or article views, a metric of increasing interest to consumers of online publications. Still, impact factor is positively associated with how influential a paper is likely to be.

For some researchers, it is more important to limit the time length of the review process. The article may garner fewer citations in other research articles over time, but there may be a smaller likelihood of required resubmission, so the new knowledge reaches its intended readership sooner. The target journal may also have a policy of reduced time from submission to decision and a higher rate of acceptance. There is a method for ranking journals that seek to minimize effort objectives while maximizing citation count. This is the *conditional impact factor* (Wong, Srikrishnan, Hadka, & Keller, 2017) that multiplies impact factor by acceptance rate.

One motivation for getting your work out sooner is the consequence of "scooping," where another research team publishes a similar article first, thereby reducing the novelty and impact of your manuscript. Another reason to opt for reduced time to publication and higher rate of acceptance has to do with multiple authors who may have different goals for publication. There may need to be compromises when there are different decision makers who have different career concerns and who will be affected differently by such uncertain factors as scooping.

Wong et al. (2017) focus on three objectives, using mathematical models and key equations to resolve seemingly conflicting goals. Authors want to maximize the expected number of times the paper will be cited; they want to minimize the likelihood of manuscript rejections, revisions, and resubmissions; and they want to minimize the expected time from initial submission to final acceptance (or rejection). These multiple objectives may require trade-offs, especially if one decision does not dominate the others. If you think this decision will be easy, consider that there will be more than 700 million permutations of five journals out of a total set of 61 journals (Wong et al., 2017).

Here is a simple scenario with two authors who have a conflict. The junior author is a graduate student who wants to publish a portion of her doctoral dissertation as soon as possible with the motivation of strengthening her position in the job market. Her faculty advisor, a tenured faculty member with many years of experience, wants to maximize the likelihood of citations of the work by publishing it in a high-impact journal. The junior author's model will probably result in a faster review and more likely acceptance of the manuscript, while the senior author's model will probably result in a publication that is more widely read, cited, and respected. They reach a compromise to submit only to high impact journals that have a turnaround time of five months or less.

Electronic submission of manuscripts has resulted in reduced time to decision. For example, the *American Journal of Speech-Language Pathology* (AJSLP) moved from a paper-based submission and peer-review process to Manuscript Central (a Web-based system; link is http://asha.manuscriptcentral.com/) in 2002 (Lockney, 2002). The author who uploads a manuscript online receives an instant confirmation of receipt. The editor can access the manuscript immediately and assign it electronically to the appropriate associate editor and ad hoc peer reviewers. Turnaround time has been reduced by half, and readers have access to more current research. Authors can track the status of the review anytime, anywhere online. The system tracks late reviews so that the process does not get stalled. There are no postal delays that had previously exasperated international authors.

Responding to Ad Hoc Peer Reviewers

The Instructions for Authors link in most CSD online and print journals has surprisingly little information about how to respond to the comments from ad hoc peer reviewers. Science writing manuals are not much help either. An effective response to reviews has four likely outcomes (Taylor, 2016): it affects whether the manuscript will be accepted or rejected; it increases the speed at which the response to reviews moves through the editorial process, provided it is well-organized and concise; it helps journals work with the volunteers (ad hoc reviewers) who must rereview the manuscript while attending to competing demands; and it includes the revisions from reviews that improve the quality and clarity of the manuscript, as well as the likelihood that the published article will be cited by others.

Who reads the revised manuscript? The response to reviewers will probably be submitted electronically and will probably be downloaded by an editorial assistant. Depending on the journal, the revised manuscript will immediately or eventually end up with the associate editor with expertise in the area of the submission. Since the associate editor has probably not corresponded with the authors and may not even be known to them, the response letter should be addressed to the person who signed the decision letter. However, it will likely be the associate editor who reads the revised manuscript carefully and makes the following recommendations to the editor: accept the manuscript in the current form without resending it to referees; decline to publish the manuscript; send the manuscript back to the original reviewers or new reviewers for further reviews; or accept without further review but with major or minor revisions. The authors' concise and well-organized response to reviewers may save time because the associate editor can make a determination (one of the previously mentioned four options) without requesting additional input from reviewers. Finally, the editor will review the recommendation by the associate editor and will contact the authors with an official decision.

There are strategies that authors can use to speed up the publication process. There will be two or three sets of comments from the reviewers, some similar and sometimes some quite different. It is important that an associate editor can easily find the responses to comments and related changes in the manuscript. In cases of papers with multiple authors, the corresponding author who is often the director of the laboratory will handle correspondence to the person who signed the decision letter. The first author should write the response to reviewers, share it with the other authors, and make any revisions before sending it to the corresponding author for submission. Organize the responses to the comments from the two or three reviewers unambiguously to minimize time-consuming confusion and frustration for the associate editor. If there is a list of comments, organize the responses numerically to match that of the reviewers. If there are general comments, reply in paragraph form. Keep the exact text of the reviewer when possible. Taylor (2016) recommends using a table style of rows and columns to make the associate editor's job easier, but this strategy is rarely used by authors.

Noble (2017) is more specific, offering 10 rules for writing responses to reviewers:

Rule 1: Provide an overview and then quote the full set of reviews.

Rule 2: Be polite and respectful of all reviewers.

Rule 3: Accept the blame.

Rule 4: Make the response self-contained by quoting the changes directly in the response.

Rule 5: Respond to every point raised by the reviewer.

Rule 6: Use typography, such as changes in typeface, color, or indenting to help the reviewer navigate your response.

Rule 7: Whenever possible, begin your response to each comment with a direct answer to the point being raised.

Rule 8: When possible, do what the reviewer asks.

Rule 9: Be clear about what changed relative to the previous version.

Rule 10: If necessary, write the response twice.

Remember that authors do not have to agree with all the ad hoc reviewers' comments. Indeed, the authors should be considered the experts regarding the work in the manuscript. However, all comments must be addressed, even if there is disagreement. Do not assume that the reviewer is biased or is trying to sabotage the authors' work; for the most part, the reviewers' motivation is to improve the quality, clarity, and readability of the authors' work. Authors will, at minimum, have to convince the associate editor that requested changes do not need to be made. Rather than simply asserting disagreement, present a well-reasoned and detailed justification to help reviewers and associate editors understand why the requested change is either unnecessary or unjustifiable. Feel free to disagree, but the burden is on the authors (who most want the article to be published) and not on the reviewers or the associate editor.

Sometimes, indirect requests for revisions can be difficult to decode, especially for the researcher who is newer to the peer-review process. A study of 95 reviewers' reports revealed that many changes were requested directly, but many were not (Paltridge, 2015), and that such terms as directions, clarification requests, suggestions, and recommendations confused the authors, whether they were native or nonnative speakers. For example, if a British reviewer writes, "I would suggest . . . " the author should interpret this as a requirement, but many non-British authors interpret the terminology as indicating an option. Similarly, "please consider . . . " should be interpreted as a required change. A request for major revisions may discourage authors to the extent that they do not resubmit the manuscript, but surveys (Paltridge, 2013, 2015) revealed that many were ultimately published in the journal requesting the revisions. My own strategy as a peer reviewer is to begin with some good news, that is, to highlight positive aspects of the manuscript before offering critical comments and suggestions for revisions.

Following are examples of requests for revisions in my own ad hoc peer review, for an article that was ultimately accepted, according to Paltridge's (2015) speech act categories. My questions (Q) are in italics.

Direction

Q. There were a small number of participants (17), which, although acknowledged in this section, did not stop the authors from making claims in the conclusion and discussion sections that are too broad for the data collected.

R. We have now reworked the discussion section, introducing the small number of participants as one of the principal limitations of our study and scaling back our general conclusion.

Suggestion

Q. The second paragraph reviews literature that is 20 to 30 years old, and begins with "more recently"—certainly more recent than the 100-year-old references that were cited in the preceding paragraph, but not current. The authors also neglected the discussion of "schizophrenic" language by linguistics in one journal in the 1970s (Chaika, 1974; Fromkin, 1975; Lecours & Vanier-Clement, 1976). They do not mention the notion of "schizophasia," although they use tests for aphasia in identifying language disorders in their participants.

R. We have now added the literature suggested by the two referees and mentioned the notion of schizophasia, as requested. We also made clearer that our communicative assessment is focused less on language abilities than on pragmatic abilities, expressed not only by language but also through gestures, prosody, and so on. Therefore the references to the wide literature on linguistic or aphasic deficit in schizophrenia were necessarily reduced.

Clarification Request

Q. The authors claim that "the current literature on communicative impairments in patients with schizophrenia mainly focuses on linguistic abilities for communicative purposes." There is a substantial literature in neurolinguistics that addresses language deficits in schizophrenia resulting from functional frontal lobe deficits and temporal lobe overactivation.

R. We have now clarified that the area of interest of our study was neither language dysfunction nor neurolinguistic dysfunctions in schizophrenia, but the pragmatic communicative domain expressed by different means. We are aware that the current literature addresses different brain areas as responsible for language deficit in schizophrenia, but we believe that this interesting domain of research was not so central for our paper.

Recommendation

Q. Uncorrected vision or hearing impairments should also be cited as exclusionary criteria.

R. We now explicitly cite the presence of vision or hearing impairments as exclusionary criteria.

BOOKS AND PORTIONS OF BOOKS

When I first approached Plural Publishing to consider my idea for this book, there were specific proposal submission requirements that can be found on the Plural website. In addition to their editorial and marketing questionnaire, authors are instructed to submit an abbreviated CV and a draft manuscript or two sample chapters. The purpose was to give Plural an idea about the themes, style, and content of the proposed book.

The proposal was then evaluated by Plural's marketing director and editorial board to evaluate the content, quality, and potential demand for the proposed book. I was contacted about a month later by the acquisitions editor who wrote that the proposal was accepted and included comments from 14 anonymous peer reviewers. Most but not all reviewers recommended acceptance of the proposal, and all had valuable suggestions for the book that are incorporated in the final version that you are reading today. After I finished a preliminary manuscript version of the book, Plural editors sent it to five anonymous peer reviewers, all of whom provided comments and three of whom sent very detailed notes. The Plural editor working with me on the current book indicated that I was free to include or exclude any of the requested revisions. I have addressed all comments and notes that I determined would improve the quality of the final manuscript.

How Do You Know If a Book Has Been Peer Reviewed?

To find out if a book is likely to have been peer reviewed, it is helpful to consider the following questions about the author, publisher, content, and citations:

- *Author:* Does the author have an advanced degree and an appropriate professional affiliation? The author's degree will generally be PhD, EdD, AuD, or MD and the affiliation will likely be a college or university, hospital or medical center, or research laboratory. A scholarly publication will also list the author's title at the institution, such as assistant professor, associate professor. or professor; research scientist; or section or service chief at a medical center.
- *Publisher:* If the book is published by a university press or a scholarly society, it is likely to be peer reviewed. You can find out from your library if your college or university publishes manuscripts from faculty and others and what the criteria are for acceptance of a proposal. An example of a scholarly association that publishes peer-reviewed books is the American Academy of Sciences. If the publisher is a for-profit enterprise, go to the website and check information for authors.
- *Content:* Consider accuracy, bias, and audience appropriateness. Be wary of political and religious affiliations that may have a particular mission in addition to or instead of objective presentation of content. Look for technical information that indicates the book was written for an academic audience. The title should be straightforward and not promise outrageous results. Books called *Curing Stuttering* or *Hearing without Ears* should be avoided.
- *Citations:* Unless it is a workbook, and even then, peer-reviewed books should have extensive citations, as well as a bibliography. Works cited should include a great preponderance of primary sources, such as articles in peer-reviewed journals, and a much smaller number of books. The reason is that books, even the present one, are secondary sources that synthesize a great deal of information from other literature. If the book by Smith cites the journal article written by Jones, the information included may or may not be of as much interest to you as the primary source—the article by Jones. Good scholarship requires that you read the original source, and not only books or other articles where the primary source is cited. If you are still not sure if the book is scholarly, ask your librarian.

Another way of evaluating the information in books is to apply the CRAAP test, developed by the Meriam Library at California State University, Chico in 2010 (http://www.csuchico.edu/lins/handouts/eval_websites.pdf). Some of the information is a variation of what was described previously.

- *Currency:* This refers to timeliness of information, as well as information that has been updated, revised, or amended as needed. For example, the ASHA Code of Ethics is revised periodically, and practitioners are professionally bound to follow the most recent code.

- *Relevance:* The information should be important to your needs, relate to your topic, and answer your questions. For example, a general text on audiology may not be as useful as one on cochlear implantation, if that is your topic.
- *Authority:* This refers to the source of the information. The author should have appropriate credentials, experience, and affiliations.
- *Accuracy:* The information should be truthful, supported by evidence, and refereed or peer reviewed. For example, while the cause of autism is not currently known, there is extensive evidence that preservatives in vaccinations do not cause autism, even though some celebrities and even physicians may make that claim.
- *Purpose:* The information may be presented to educate, inform, sell, entertain, or persuade. Good scholarship requires that authors disclose financial and nonfinancial conflicts of interest. Many diagnostic tests have been peer reviewed, but the authors are also paid when more practitioners buy the test.

Writing Style

The style of writing and structure of an article for publication in a scientific journal is generally universal across different journals, languages, and countries. A mock study on the companion website for this book called FAUST (From Adelphi University: Syntax Training) is a template for writing a CSD experiment and structuring it as a journal article. Books allow considerable variations in scholarly writing style, and readers may be drawn in by the "voice" of some writers and discouraged by others. However, professional writing style has abundant rules, and there are many guides to assist the speech-language pathologist and audiologist, including our own (Goldfarb & Serpanos, 2020). Box 13–3 provides a comparison of writing style in books and journal articles.

There are also fairly consistent rules that publishers use to determine whether or not to accept a proposal for a new book. Most editors will want answers to the following five questions (Rabiner & Fortunato, 2002, p. 38):

- What is this book about?
- What is the book's thesis (many in publishing refer to it as the book's argument), and what's new about it?
- Why are you the person to write this book?
- Why is now the time to publish this book?
- Who makes up the core audience for the proposed book, and why will they find it appealing?

The book proposal should tell a short story in about 10 to 20 pages. Many scholarly book publishers will require completion of some kind of marketing form, a detailed outline of the proposed book, and

Box 13–3. A Comparison of Writing Style in Scholarly Books and Academic Journal Articles

	Books	*Articles in Journals*
Evaluators	Marketing director; editorial board	Editor; associate editor; ad hoc peer reviewers
Form	Chapters	Sections
Beginning	Preface, introduction	Abstract
Literature review	Throughout	Introduction section; conclusion
Main ideas	Thesis or argument	Hypotheses
Summary	End of each chapter	End of article
Visuals	Figures and tables	Figures, tables, statistics
Extras	Dedicated website	Appendices

a CV, as well as a sample chapter or two. As Rabiner and Fortunato (2002) indicate, your proposal is offering a publisher the following two commodities: your proposed book and you. The short story the author tells about the proposed book will reveal the following:

- The author has command of the material and is not afraid to make inferences, but is respectful of and includes alternative points of view.
- The literature review is wide-ranging and comprehensive.
- The author knows what to include and what to leave out. Just as a doctoral dissertation must be streamlined to be suitable as a journal article, a scholarly book should not include everything in the course syllabus and education platform associated with the course.
- The author, as a professional writer, knows the rules of good professional writing overall and in the subject matter. There is limited use of professional jargon that is explained after the first usage. Follow a diagnostic label with the words *characterized by*, as in "The patient had Broca's aphasia, characterized by effortful speech, nonfluency, reduced available vocabulary, and impaired expressive syntax." Operational definitions (see Chapters 4 and 7) should be identified as such.
- The author should have a consistent voice. While the passive voice is used in journal articles (and in the first part of this sentence), use the active voice

primarily in books (and in the second part of this sentence). Use the greater length permitted in books to give plenty of examples that reflect your expertise and experience.

- The author raises controversies, but does not have to be neutral to be fair.

Publishing a Contribution to a Book

Authors can contribute to a book by writing a chapter or an essay, producing a written version of a presentation at a scientific meeting that is organized in a volume of conference proceedings, giving an editor permission to publish a paper presented at a symposium or given as a lecture, and giving permission to have an article reprinted.

The peer-review process is different from that required for publishing an article in a scholarly journal or authoring a book. A book editor approaches a publisher's marketing director in the same way a book author would. If a marketing director identifies a potential readership for the edited book, the editorial board reviews the proposal and recommends acceptance or rejection, along with suggestions for improvement. If the proposal is accepted, the book editor functions as the editorial board regarding individuals who contribute to the book.

Following are two examples of books I edited that followed different main ideas (see "thesis" or "argument" in Box 13–3). The first book (Goldfarb, 2006) resulted from an all-day symposium where speakers responded to ethical consequences of a study on stuttering done in 1939. You may think that the thesis would be hard to sell to a marketing director and that the book would probably not be a best seller. It was fortuitous that Dr. Sadanand Singh was just starting the Plural imprint and was glad to publish a book addressing an important topic with some of the best-known scholars in CSD contributing chapters. I think a marketing director would probably have rejected the proposal. The book did not sell well although it did receive generally good reviews. The second book (Goldfarb, 2012), the first of its kind addressing translational research in SLP/A, was a labor of love for all involved. Dr. Singh had recently died and all royalties from the editor and contributors were assigned to the Sadanand Singh Foundation in San Diego, California.

How did I decide whom to invite to contribute to the books? For the ethics book, the decisions had to do with the speakers at the symposium. It started with the coordinator of the symposium, who later became editor of the book, inviting some well-known colleagues (ASHA Fellows and Honorees) who published articles related to the thesis of the symposium. Some of these colleagues suggested that I contact additional individuals with high qualifications, and one asked if she could recruit two doctoral students to assist. Often, the first book contribution by a newer scholar comes at the invitation of a senior colleague or mentor to cowrite a chapter.

For the translational research book, once the proposal was accepted, I asked Angie Singh, Dr. Singh's widow and current president of Plural Publishing, for a list of Plural authors who remembered her husband fondly and might be willing to work for free (royalties going to the Singh Foundation). Many boldface names in our field responded affirmatively, and most of them were able to provide an essay within the allotted time. I also contacted several junior colleagues who would benefit from a publication and who knew of Dr. Singh, even if they did not know him personally. This is another way that newer scholars get to contribute to a book; the editor reaches out to them, motivated by their previous work.

ADVANCED STUDY

The author proposes that dissemination by publication skills are necessary for an individual to be granted power of professor. With new generations of scholars and researchers needed every 10 years, professors and master clinicians have an obligation to prepare individuals with adequate knowledge and skills to undertake the tasks of scholarship and research, and dissemination by publication is a key component. For evidence of the requisite dissemination by publication skills, complete the following and have your instructor, academic adviser, mentor, or CSD department chair review that you have completed the requirements and sign and date where indicated.

Student's Name: ______________________________

1. What does the term "impact factor" tell you about a journal? Why is it important?
2. Describe three advantages and three disadvantages of peer review.
3. Describe three similarities and three differences between subscription journals and open access journals.
4. Describe the editorial process for accepting or rejecting a manuscript in a peer-reviewed journal.
5. Describe the nine aspects of a journal article.
6. How do peer reviewers evaluate the information in books?
7. What are the best strategies to use if you want to publish a contribution to a book?

Date of Completion: ______________________________

Faculty/Supervisor Signature: ______________________________

REFERENCES

Ali, P. A., & Watson, R. (2016). Peer review and the publication process. *Nursing Open, 3*, 193–202. doi:10.1002/nop2.51

Björk, B., & Solomon, D. (2013). The publishing delay in scholarly peer-review journals. *Journal of Informetrics, 7*, 914–923.

Butler, D. (2013). Investigating journals: The dark side of publishing. *Nature, 495*, 433–435.

Callaham, M., Wears, R. L., & Weber, E. (2002). Journal prestige, publication bias, and other characteristics associated with citation of published studies in peer-reviewed journals. *Journal of the American Medical Association, 287*, 2847–2850.

Constantinescu, A. (2009). Publishing in peer-reviewed journals as the major mechanism for the dissemination of scientific knowledge. *Review of Contemporary Philosophy, 8*, 124–128.

D'Andrea, R., & O'Dwyer, J. P. (2017). Can editors save peer review from peer reviewers? *PLoS One, 12*, 1–14.

Dimitroulis, G. (2011). Getting published in peer-reviewed journals. *International Journal of Oral and Maxillofacial Surgery, 40*, 1342–1345.

Goldfarb, R. (Ed.). (2006). *Ethics: A case study from fluency*. San Diego, CA: Plural.

Goldfarb, R. (Ed.). (2012). *Translational speech-language pathology and audiology*. San Diego, CA: Plural.

Goldfarb, R., & Serpanos, Y. (2020). *Professional writing in speech-language pathology and audiology* (3rd ed.). San Diego, CA: Plural.

Have, H. T., & Gordijn, B. (2015). Publications and rejections. *Medicine, Health Care, and Philosophy, 18*, 167–170.

Jha, K. N. (2014). How to write articles that get published. *Journal of Clinical & Diagnostic Research, 8*, 1–3.

Justice, L. (2008). The *peer* in *peer review*. *American Journal of Speech-Language Pathology, 17*, 106.

Kreiman, J. (2016). On peer review. *Journal of Speech, Language, and Hearing Research, 59*, 480–483.

Lockney, E. B. (2002, March). AJSLP moves to Web-based system. *The ASHA Leader, 7*, 3–5.

Mehrpour, S., & Khajavi, Y. (2014). How to spot fake open access journals. *Learned Publishing, 27*, 269–274.

Mueller, M. J. (2001). The publication process for peer-reviewed journals. *Cardiopulmonary Physical Therapy Journal, 12*, 17.

Noble, W. S. (2017). Ten simple rules for writing a response to reviewers. *PLoS Computational Biology, 13*, e1005730.

Paltridge, B. (2013). Learning to review submissions to peer reviewed journals: How do they do it? *International Journal for Researcher Development, 4*, 6–18.

Paltridge, B. (2015). Referees' comments on submissions to peer-reviewed journals: When is a suggestion not a suggestion? *Studies in Higher Education, 40*, 106–122.

Pearson, G. S. (2013). The process of a peer-reviewed journal. *Perspectives in Psychiatric Care, 49*, 147–148.

Pierce, A. (2009). Realities of publishing in a journal: Why should you submit, what should you submit, and what problems might you encounter. *Proceedings of Meetings on Acoustics, 6*, 1–14.

Pratt, S. R. (2010). Reviewers are critical to the peer review process. *American Journal of Audiology, 19*, 85.

Rabiner, S., & Fortunato, A. (2002). *Thinking like your editor: How to write great serious nonfiction—and get it published*. New York, NY: W.W. Norton.

Rennie, R. (2003). Editorial peer review: Its development and rationale. In F. Godlee & T. Jefferson (Eds.), *Peer review in health sciences* (2nd ed., pp. 1–13). London, UK: BMJ Books.

Rew, L. (2012). From course assignment paper to publishable manuscript. *Journal of Holistic Nursing, 30*, 270–276.

Rohrer, J. E. (2014). Open-access journals: Bane or boon? *Inquiry-Excellus Health Plan, 51*, 1–2.

Rothwell, P. M., & Martyn, C. N. (2000). Reproducibility of peer review in clinical neuroscience: Is agreement between reviewers any greater than would be expected by chance alone? *Brain, 123*(9), 1964–1969.

Samet, J. M. (1999). Dear author—advice from a retiring editor. *American Journal of Epidemiology, 150*, 433–436.

Scott, A. (2007). Peer review and the relevance of science. *Futures, 39*, 827–845.

Silver, N. (2012). *The signal and the noise: Why so many predictions fail—but some don't*. New York, NY: Penguin.

Skelton, J. (1994). Analysis of the structure of original research papers: An aid to writing original papers for publication. *The British Journal of General Practice: The Journal of the Royal College of General Practitioners, 44*, 455–459.

Smith, R. (2016). Peer review: A flawed process at the heart of science and journals. *Journal of the Royal Society of Medicine, 99*, 178–182.

Spier, R. (2002). The history of the peer-review process. *Trends in Biotechnology, 20*, 357–358.

Taylor, B. W. (2016). Writing an effective response to a manuscript review. *Freshwater Science, 35*, 1082–1087.

Thurner, S., & Hanel, R. (2011). Peer-review in a world with rational scientists: Toward selection of the average. *The European Physical Journal B, 84*, 707–711.

Tress, G., Tress, B., & Saunders, D. A. (2014). How to write a paper for successful publication in an international peer-reviewed journal. *Pacific Conservation Biology, 20*, 17–24.

Voight, M. L., & Hoogenboom, B. J. (2012). Publishing your work in a journal: Understanding the peer review process. *International Journal of Sports Physical Therapy, 7*, 452–460.

Wager, E., Godlee, F., & Jefferson T. (2002). *How to survive peer review.* London, UK: BMJ Books.

Walters, W. H., & Linvill, A. C. (2011). Characteristics of open access journals in six subject areas. *College & Research Libraries, 72*, 372–392.

Wong, T. E., Srikrishnan, V., Hadka, D., & Keller, K. (2017) A multi-objective decision-making approach to the journal submission problem. *PLoS ONE, 12*(6), e0178874. doi:10.1371/ journal.pone.0178874

14

Oral Presentation of Research

INTRODUCTION

Authors may submit abstracts for poster or paper consideration. Depending on the meeting, a paper presentation may be a short platform presentation of about 15 min, a miniseminar of about one hr, a short course of two hr or longer, or a complete symposium proposal. Poster sessions are effective and popular methods for communicating information. They provide a more personal forum for informal discussion than is permitted by regular platform presentations. Poster presenters stay with their poster for the duration of the poster session (90 min for ASHA) and are encouraged to upload a PDF handout to the meeting app.

Paper sessions are presented orally, usually in the context of a single topic with four to six in a session. There may be a moderator who will introduce the speakers, keep track of time limits, and field questions at the end when there is audience discussion. Symposia are topical platform sessions of 60 to 90 min that are submitted as integrated session proposals with an overall proposal and four to five abstracts. This format is more popular at regional and state association meetings than at national and international meetings. Symposia address clinical or professional topics rather than new scientific research. For example, a fascinating symposium at a state association many years ago addressed diagnostic testing, with the four presenters claiming, respectively, that tests were crucial, important, useless, or dangerous.

Hour-long or 90-min platform presentations, sometimes called miniseminars can address scientific research, case studies, topical areas, or professional issues. They are organized in the convention program under disorder type (e.g., adult language disorders, audiological evaluations, or autism spectrum disorders) or professional areas (e.g., private practice, state licensure requirements, or association updates). I recommend that you get out of your comfort zone and attend, for example, presentations on hearing aids or speech science if you are a speech-language pathologist (SLP) with an interest in specific language impairments in children. A broader exposure to research may result in your consideration of questions that had not occurred to you previously.

Long-format presentations of 2 hr or more tend to include experiential learning, where the audience has time to view and react to videos of individuals with communication disorders and responses to treatment; to break up into small groups to consider subareas of the main issue; or to engage with new instrumentation, depending on the topic and the size of the audience. Often, speakers are renowned in their areas of expertise and are even paid to present at the convention.

Learning Objectives

After reading this chapter, the student will be able to

- write an abstract for a platform or poster presentation;
- prepare and rehearse the presentation;
- present the poster or platform information orally; and
- use educational technology to support the presentation.

CONFERENCE PRESENTATIONS

Submitting an Abstract

Abstracts for regional, state, national, and international conventions and scientific meetings are submitted online no later than the abstract submission deadline (e.g., Friday, August 10, 2018, at exactly 11:59 PM eastern standard time for the annual meeting of the International Neuropsychological Society in 2019). Submissions that are not completed are considered to be in draft status and will not be considered unless they are completed by the deadline. By submitting, authors commit to be available to present on the date and time they are assigned. Accepted abstracts may be scheduled at any time during the meeting at the discretion of the program chair.

The body of submitted abstracts may not exceed a certain number of characters; for example, 2,000 characters including spaces. Paper or poster submissions are usually organized under these or similar headings: purpose or objective, participants and methods, results, and conclusions. All submissions must consist of original work. Abstracts submitted to other meetings or that have been previously published should not be submitted. Box 14–1 provides an example of an accepted abstract for a poster presentation.

Some meetings permit submission of research in progress, but for others, all research, results, and conclusions must be final at the time of submission. Case reports may be submitted, but the abstract should clearly describe the uniqueness of the case and how it addresses critical knowledge gaps in the field. Submissions are often published in the conference booklet or in a supplementary issue of a journal (e.g., Academy of Aphasia abstracts are published in *Brain and Language*) exactly as received, so proofread carefully before finalizing your submission. All submissions should be peer reviewed by the conference program committee with the

Box 14–1. Sample Poster Presentation Abstract

Title: Semantic Memory Processing in Early-Stage Alzheimer Disease: Behavioral and Electrophysiology Evidence

Purpose: The purpose of this study is to investigate the semantic breakdown at the word-class level (nouns, verbs, adjectives) in the early-stage of Alzheimer disease (AD) using both behavioral and electrophysiological (EEG) measures.

Method: Cognitive and language skills were examined with the standardized tests of the Arizona Battery of Communication in Dementia (ABCD), and semantic memory skills in pictures versus words with the Pyramids and Palm Tree (PPT) test were also examined. The EEG testing examined word associations of a picture (i.e., object versus action) and auditory word (i.e., adjective, noun, verb) in a semantic priming paradigm to show whether the degree of the deficit depended on word class and modality. High-density EEG results from a group of adults who have a diagnosis of early-stage (i.e., mild) AD were recorded and the results were compared to recordings from a comparison group of adults who had typical language and cognitive skills.

Results: The participants with AD performed significantly poorer on the subtests of the ABCD of mental status, linguistic expression, linguistic comprehension, and visuospatial skills as compared to the comparison group. The individuals with AD performed poorer on the picture condition of the PPT versus the word condition. Accuracies for the EEG experiment revealed that the AD group was significantly less accurate than the comparison group with a significant main effect for word classes and the descriptive level being less accurate than category and function levels. Response time with and without the outliers showed similar patterns with the congruency effect being significantly larger in the verb condition than in the category condition. The EEG results revealed an N400 for congruency for the comparison group and a reduced N400 for the AD group. There is a late positivity component (LPC) seen predominantly in the AD group with a sensitivity for category and function and a negativity for the descriptive level in the incongruent condition.

Conclusion: These behavioral and EEG findings reveal a breakdown in the attribute level in the early stage of the disease. The response time data did not align with this finding. There was also a LPC seen in the AD group that should be further explored in future studies.

committee chair making the final decision. Accepted abstracts must be presented by the presenting author or an officially designated representative. Box 14–2 provides an example of a letter of acceptance for a poster presentation at ASHA.

Box 14–2. Example of a Lightly Edited ASHA Acceptance Letter

On behalf of the 2018 Convention Program Committee, we are pleased to inform you that the submission listed below has been accepted for presentation as a poster session at the ASHA Annual Convention, November 15 to 17, 2018, at the Boston Convention & Exhibition Center (BCEC) in Boston, Massachusetts.

Don't forget about the Speaker/Presenter Management Center! This center will give you access to all your submitted proposals, e-mail notifications, and disclosure form links throughout the Call for Papers process. All proposals and e-mail notifications will be in viewable format only.

The selection process was extremely competitive this year. All submissions were reviewed by the program committee and accepted and scheduled with consideration to educational content, presentation format, scheduling requests, possible conflicts, and the overall flow of the meeting. All sessions are final as scheduled and we are unable to honor requests for changes to time and/or date. Please carefully review the session information below. This is your last opportunity to correct any minor errors and/or typographical errors (e.g., author order or who is actually presenting versus author only) before your session information is made public.

Your presentation has been scheduled as follows:

Topic Area: Language Disorders in Adults

Session Number: 8277 Poster Board 691

Title: Word Associations in Early-Stage Alzheimer Disease: Behavioral & EEG Evidence

Session Format: Poster

Day: Saturday, November 17, 2018

Time: 2:30 p.m.–4:00 p.m.

Authors: Susan DeMetropolis (PRESENTING AUTHOR: Author who will be presenting), Melissa Randazzo (PRESENTING AUTHOR: Author who will be presenting), Laura Koenig (AUTHOR ONLY: Author, but will NOT be presenting), Robert Goldfarb (AUTHOR ONLY: Author, but will NOT be presenting), Reem Khamis-Dakwar (AUTHOR ONLY: Author, but will NOT be presenting)

We look forward to your participation at the ASHA Convention.

Sincerely,
2018 Convention Program Committee Co-Chairs

Preparing the Presentation

We have discussed elsewhere (Goldfarb & Serpanos, 2020, Chapter 7) about writing for oral presentation. It is important to remember that the same ethical concerns and plagiarism constraints that bind writing also apply to oral presentations. That is, orally presented research follows the same guidelines that you would use in a written research paper. A speaker's presentation must be supported by evidence, and there should be a written or uploaded reference list. In preparing a speech, create a set of index cards called a speaker's outline with key words or phrases, rather than full sentences, to guide you. Begin with a statement of purpose and organize your presentation as introduction, body, and conclusion.

Oral Presentation

When delivering an oral presentation, use computer-generated visual support in the form of graphs, charts, tables, diagrams, photographs, as well as tangible items such as models, objects, and instruments to relate to your text. Be sure that objects and computer-generated images are large enough to be seen in the back of the presentation room. Links to audio and video clips can be embedded in the slides accompanying your talk. At the same time, avoid overreliance on animation and sound effects as the equipment at the convention may not be completely compatible with the computer-generated slideshow you created. Never read the slides to your audience, but comment on them using your speaker's outline. Limit the number of words in a single slide; a good rule of thumb is a 25 to 50 word maximum with no more than 7 words on a line and 7 lines. Remember that some people in the audience may be sitting far away, but they should still easily see your images or text.

An effective presentation requires the skills you learned in a voice and diction class. That is, vary vocal pitch, volume, and intensity as appropriate; make sure your articulation is intelligible; and use professional grammar while avoiding colloquial language and fillers ("um," "you know," "like"). Show self-confidence while indicating interest in the audience. While eye contact is probably the most important nonverbal aspect for a speaker, don't forget about facial expressions and gestures. Professional attire and grooming show respect for the venue and the circumstance of your presentation. Finally, it is expected that there might be some speech anxiety, but solid preparation and practice will likely ease the "butterflies" that come with public speaking.

Poster Presentation

Many student researchers, as well as their mentors, prefer submitting their work as part of a poster session, rather than as a traditional platform presentation. You will remain with your poster for an hour or longer, so plan answers to questions that you anticipate visitors will ask. Include a handout on the convention app if it is available, so you can refer to it for additional information. Convention instructions for submitting an abstract for a poster will indicate size limits. Remember that visitors will tend to stand about six feet away from the poster, so make sure your type font is large enough to be seen. Use larger fonts, graphics, and highlighting to emphasize the most important information. Prepare your poster as you would a research article and include an introduction, methods, results, and conclusions, together with a reference list. Now shorten the research paper severely, add graphs, tables, or figures for visual interest, and prepare to copy and paste onto the poster (follow the template for a poster included in the companion website for this book). Refer to the sample posters for a state and a national convention (Figures 14–1 and 14–2, respectively) in the following instructions. Note that the poster for a national convention based on a PhD dissertation (DeMetropolis, Randazzo, Koenig, Goldfarb, & Khamis-Dakwar, 2018) is more elaborate than the "brown bag" study presented at a state association convention (Abramowitz & Goldfarb, 2018).

The very top left, right, or both sides of the poster should include the logo of your university or place where you did your research (or both). Centered at the top of the page is the title of the presentation, authors' names and credentials on the next line, and affiliations of the authors on the following line. If there are authors with different affiliations, use a superscript letter or number to identify the author with the affiliation. On the last line centered on top, write the name of the professional association, location, and date of the presentation.

On the top left side of your poster, write your shortened introduction and include the purpose of the study in the first sentence. Briefly provide enough literature to motivate your hypotheses that you will list last in this section. On the bottom left, describe your participants, materials, methods, and results. You can extend this section to the center and top right if you have room. However, be sure to leave room for items of visual interest. It is best to center these items if possible. On the right side of your poster, write your conclusions, discussion, and clinical implications. On the bottom left or right, list your references and email contact for the corresponding author.

ePosters

Some scientific meetings now invite participants to submit abstracts for an electronic poster or ePoster. In this format, a large monitor and computer display multimedia versions of a poster. Some ePoster presentations include two or three posters from the same authors that rotate according to a time lag. As ePosters may involve animation, they enhance visualization and engage the interest of attendees.

Prepare your ePoster with the intent to display your information in a way that is not possible with a traditional poster, so do not have a static ePoster. Dynamic elements in an ePoster include multimedia content. For example, use such dynamic visual elements as videos, slideshows, animated charts or graphs, scrolling text, or 3D rotation of a model.

Rehearsing the Presentation

Whether the presentation is platform or poster, you need to rehearse before you present at a professional meeting. One effective way to rehearse is through a simulation. If you are a member of a lab, ask your mentor or lab manager if you can use part of a lab meeting to practice your presentation. Otherwise, ask a faculty mentor to help you arrange for a group to give you feedback. The audience should have some expertise or at least familiarity with the topic you will address; the

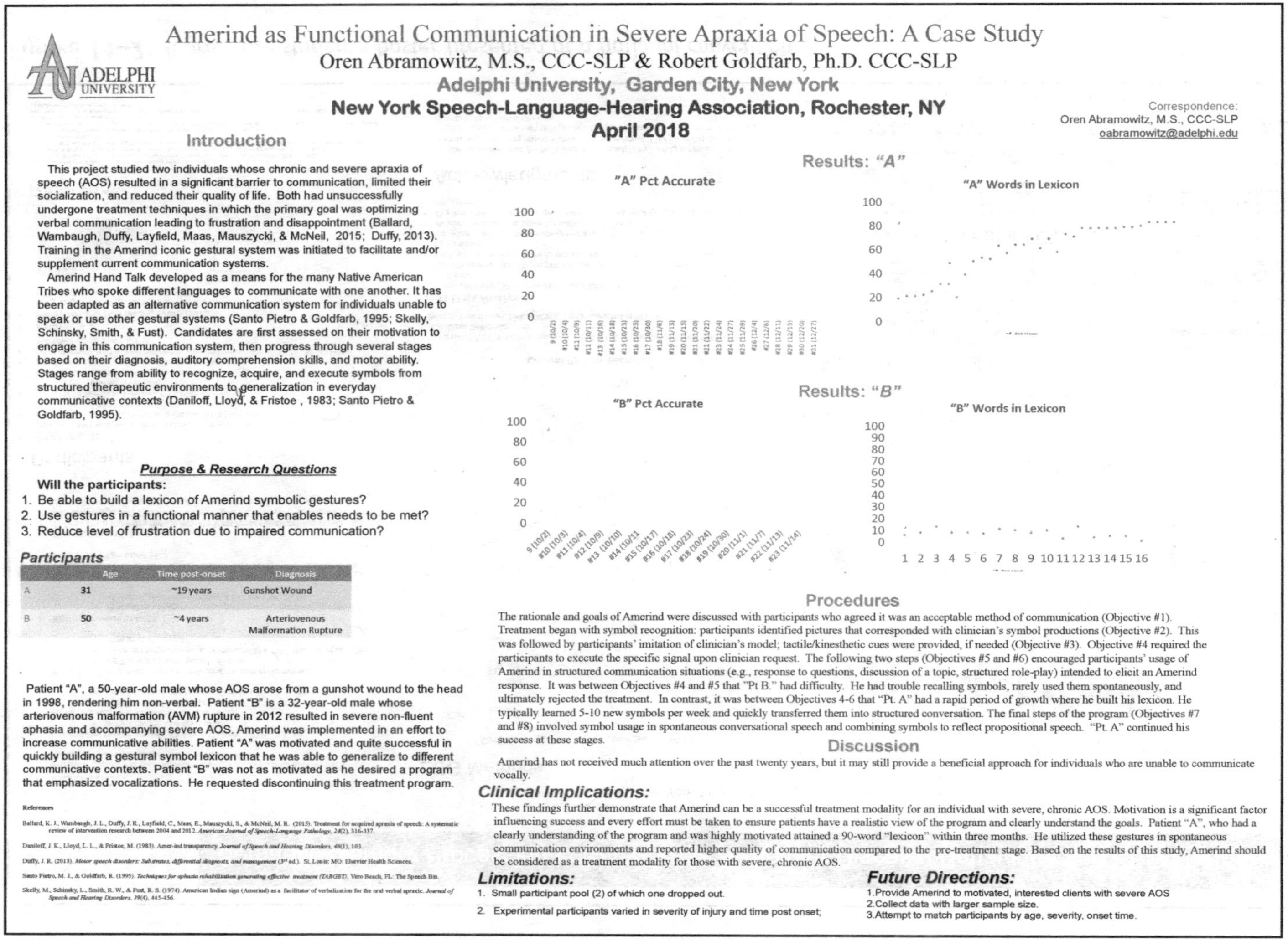

Figure 14–1. *A graduate student's poster presented at a state convention.*

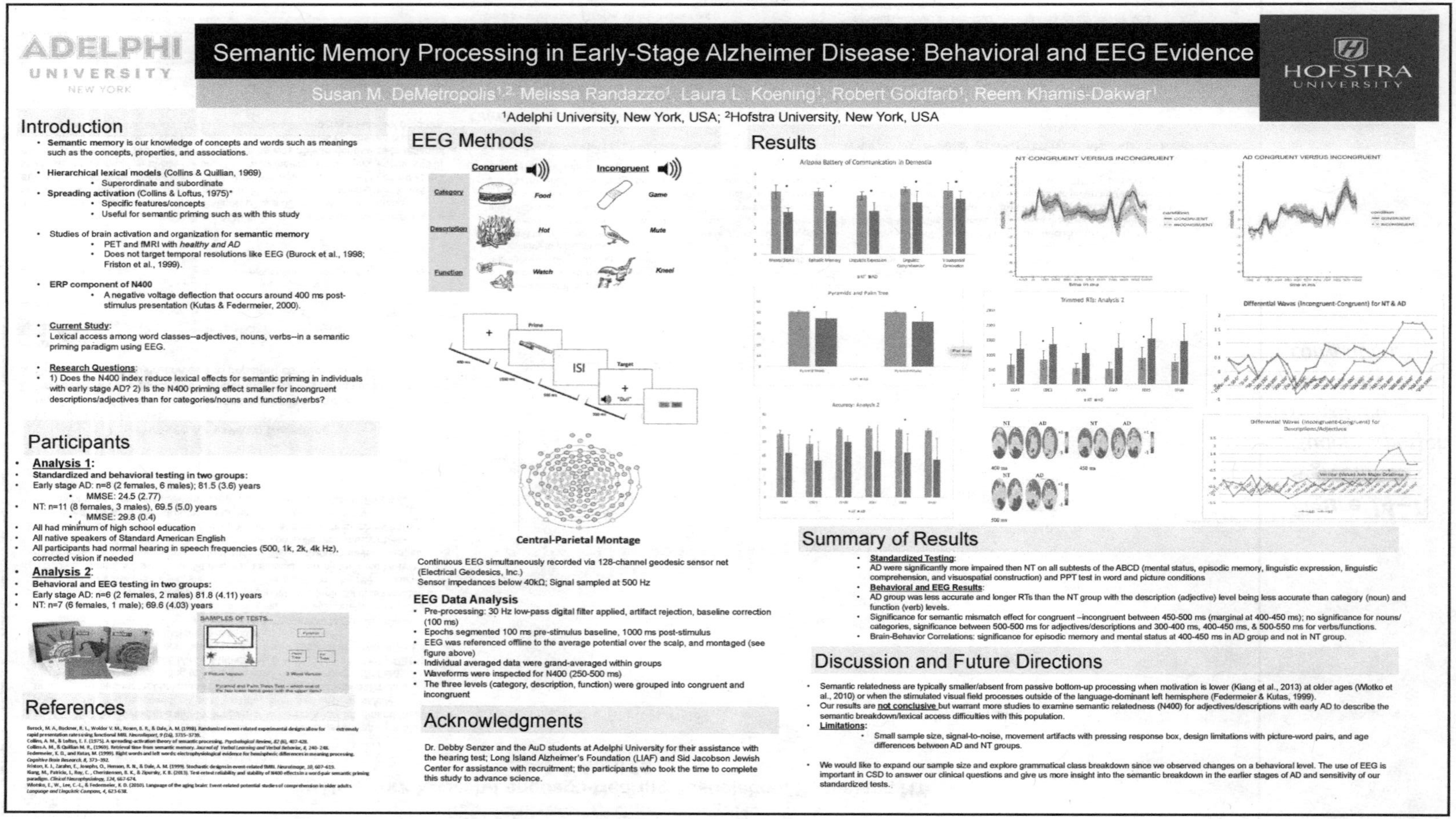

Figure 14–2. *A graduate student's poster presented at a national convention.*

faculty member or mentor may choose to assign a reading or two in advance of your practice session.

For a platform presentation, it is crucial that you observe the time limit; the moderator at the conference may cue you if your presentation seems to be running long, but may also just cut you off when your time is up. For the practice presentation, ask a friend to time you and also take notes about the questions asked and your responses to them. Present from a standing position and present your slides as you would at the conference. Prepare a list of questions for the lab members or other group to complete, including those listed in Box 14–3.

For a poster presentation, have the audience at your practice session stand six feet away from your poster. This means that you will have to project your PowerPoint poster slide at the correct size (preferred, because you can make changes to it if necessary) or show your printed poster. Make sure the key information on your poster is visible from that distance. Ask a friend to take notes and also record the questions and your answers. Remember that you know the information on your poster better than anyone, so answer directly and with confidence. Review the recording and the notes from your friend, and address any areas of concern before the conference presentation.

PRACTICE-BASED NETWORKS

An informal way of disseminating research findings is through communities of practice where the goal is to share knowledge. Guest speakers may present recent research or the group can collaborate on

Box 14–3. Questions for the Audience at the Presentation Rehearsal

Did the speaker

- Read from the slides?
- Show familiarity and confidence with the material presented?
- Gain the audience's attention at the beginning and maintain it?
- Make eye contact with attendees?
- Vary vocal pitch, volume, and voice quality to keep the presentation interesting?
- Speak slowly and clearly?

Were the slides

- Working as planned?
- Enhancing the oral presentation or distracting from it? Which slides did the audience (not) like?
- Visible from a distance?

Was the presentation

- Appropriate for the level of expertise indicated on the abstract (beginner, intermediate, or advanced)?
- Accurate?
- Fair to different points of view?
- Overly critical or completely uncritical of the literature?

collecting and reporting data. Practice research networks (PRNs) are defined (Papir-Bernstein, 2018) as a large number of practitioners who agree to collaborate in order to collect and report data. I have served on executive boards of the Aphasia Study Group of New York and the New York Neuropsychology Group, but there are many PRNs linked to academic centers, professional study groups, and university programs. Depending on the focus of the group, both evidence-based practice and practice-based evidence can control the research agenda.

EDUCATIONAL TECHNOLOGY

Use Your Computer to Record a Research Presentation to YouTube

YouTube can be a familiar and easy tool for presentation of research. Record and upload videos in advance of a conference presentation and embed a link to the video in your slideshow. You can also embed the link in the PDF handout that will appear in the meeting app for the conference. Embedded YouTube videos are helpful to show and comment on clinical interactions with clients who have communication disorders, model use of AAC devices, and demonstrate speech and hearing science instrumentation. Conference attendees can also view the video at their own pace from the PDF link, take notes, and catch up on something they might have missed.

Before You Start to Record

Create a set of index cards or a speaker's outline (see previous section, "Preparing the Presentation") to provide a script or a series of talking points. Have all your visual aids, such as a portable audiometer, anatomy model, or AAC device within easy grasp. Rehearse your presentation multiple times. If your university or work setting is a center that produces TEDx talks, attend some presentations to give you an idea of an effective 18-min presentation.

Hardware That You Will Need

You will need a computer and a webcam. Most of the newer laptop computers have built-in webcams for audio and video recording. If you have an older model or if you are using a desktop, you can purchase a USB webcam or see if one is available to borrow from your library. Some retailers that sell USB webcams are Staples and Best Buy, as well as multiple sources on the Internet.

Recording Your Presentation

Sign in to YouTube or enter the requested information following the prompts if this is your first time. After successfully signing in, click "Upload" and click at the bottom of the page to increase your limit. Click on https://support.google.com/youtube/bin/static.py?hl=en&topic=1719825&guide=1719823&page=guide.cs&answer=71673 and follow the steps to allow for a longer presentation by verifying your account with a mobile phone. You are ready to begin recording with a longer limit for the video. If you have a USB webcam, connect it now.

It's time to record your video. On the upload page, click "Start Recording" then "Stop Recording" when you are finished. You can repeat the procedure if you need to re-record. When you are satisfied with the recording, click "Upload" and wait a few minutes for your recording to become available. You now have to decide on a title and a description, as well as select your privacy settings. While there are far too many public YouTube videos of therapy demonstrations that are done poorly, remember that if you select "Privacy," you will have to provide the email addresses of those who are permitted to see your video.

Once you have entered the identification information and privacy settings, click "Save Changes." To view your video and find your link, click "Video Manager" in the upper, right-hand corner. When you click on the title, your video will appear. To save the link, click the "Share" button below your video. Right-click and select "Copy" or select "Copy" from the "Edit" pull-down menu. You may choose to paste the link on your slideshow, on the PDF for the conference app, or on such educational platforms as Blackboard and Moodle. If you have made more than a few videos, organize your links with titles and descriptions as a Word document labeled "YouTube Videos" and keep it on your desktop or in an e-file.

Use Your iPad or iPhone to Make a YouTube Recording

Instructions are similar to those for recording on a computer, but your maximum limit for these mobile devices is 15 min. Position your iPad in landscape position in a well-lit and quiet place. I like to use a music stand, but a stack of books will also serve you well. Touch and open your camera app and use the slider to select the video camera icon. After you have prepared your presentation (see previous sections), touch the record button. When you are finished, touch the record button again. Open your video by touching the icon in the lower, left-hand corner. Touch the share button and then touch the YouTube app. Enter a title, a description, and a tag (required fields) and then select your privacy settings. When you are finished, touch "Publish." Wait for the video to upload and then touch "View" on YouTube.

Now your video is available on the YouTube channel on your mobile device or computer. Touch the video to open it; touch "Share"; and finally touch "Email" to send the link to yourself. Follow the instructions for creating YouTube videos on your computer above to save and distribute the link as you wish.

Narrating PowerPoint Presentations

Classroom and convention presentations using Microsoft PowerPoint are virtually ubiquitous, even though there are problems with compatibility of different versions with different computers, and other software can be at least as effective. Follow the rules for effective use of computer-generated visual support described above and in detail elsewhere (Goldfarb & Serpanos, 2020). You will need a laptop computer with a built-in microphone, as well as an existing PowerPoint presentation.

Begin by rehearsing your narration. Continue by opening the PowerPoint presentation and selecting a slide for narration. Click on the "Insert" ribbon; then click on the drop-down arrow under "Audio"; then select "Record Audio." Enter a short name for the audio (e.g., Slide 2). Press "Record" and "Stop" as needed. Review your recording with the "Play" button and select "OK" when you have finished the narration for the current slide. You will see that an audio icon of a megaphone has appeared on your slide. Repeat these steps until you have finished narrating all your slides.

SECURING FUNDING FOR TRAVEL AND EXPENSES

Chapter 12 includes a detailed section on funding for students from undergraduate to postdoctoral levels. In this section, I assume that you have completed a research project and that the abstract has been accepted for presentation at a scientific meeting or convention. There are several sources of support for your travel, registration at the convention, and per diem expenses.

Government Support

As described in Chapter 12, undergraduate students who have collaborative student–faculty projects accepted for a poster presentation at The Council on Undergraduate Research (CUR) (https://www.cur.org/) annual conference will have all travel and poster costs covered. Bridges-to-the-Doctorate is a program through the National Institutes of Health (R25) to help students in biomedical sciences make the transition from a master's to a doctoral degree program. The grant I was affiliated with targeted underrepresented minority groups, as do minority biomedical research support (MBRS) and maximizing access to research careers (MARC) grants (see Chapter 12). Finally, the Ruth L. Kirschstein Predoctoral Individual National Research Service Awards (NRSA) (F30 and F31) and postdoctoral NRSA (F32) can include funding for presentation of research at scientific meetings.

Support from CSD Faculty Members

If you are fortunate enough to have a mentor who is a top-tier researcher with multiyear, renewable NIH funding (e.g., RO1), then that individual might be able to use RO1 funding to pay for your expenses; you also may be engaged in research beyond the scope of this book. For the rest of us, for whom this book is intended, support for research-related travel may be included in start-up funding for new faculty, in university faculty development awards, or in small local research awards to faculty.

Support from the University Administration

Most communication sciences and disorders (CSD) programs have a student club affiliated with the National Student Speech, Language, and Hearing Association (NSSLHA). Minimal student dues are supplemented by support from the Student Life division of the university. Academic clubs such as NSSLHA may be supported by your Center for Student Involvement, although titles vary, so check the links on your university's intranet. There may also be student research travel funding available through the CSD Department or through the office of your divisional dean. Finally, alumni support may be targeted to fund student research travel.

ADVANCED STUDY

The author proposes that oral presentation of research skills are necessary for an individual to be granted power of professor. With new generations of scholars and researchers needed every 10 years, professors and master clinicians have an obligation to prepare individuals with adequate knowledge and skills to undertake the tasks of scholarship and research, and oral presentation of research is a key component. For evidence of the requisite oral presentation of research skills, complete the following and have your instructor, academic adviser, mentor, or CSD department chair review that you have completed the requirements and sign and date where indicated.

Student's Name: ______________________________

1. Write a 75 to 150 word abstract for a proposed conference presentation on a CSD topic of your choice.
2. Write two ways that posters and platform presentations are similar and two ways that they are different.
3. Write two paragraphs describing how you prepare to present a poster.
4. Write two paragraphs describing how you prepare a platform presentation.
5. Describe how to record a YouTube video.
6. Describe how to narrate a PowerPoint presentation.

Date of Completion: ______________________________

Faculty/Supervisor Signature: ______________________________

REFERENCES

Abramowitz, O., & Goldfarb, R. (2018, April). *Amerind as functional communication in severe apraxia of speech: A case study.* Poster presentation at the New York State Speech, Language, and Hearing Association, Rochester, NY.

DeMetropolis, S. M., Randazzo, M., Koenig, L., Goldfarb, R., & Khamis-Dakwar, R. (2018, November). *Word associations in early-stage Alzheimer disease: Behavioral and EEG evidence.* Poster presentation at the American Speech-Language-Hearing Association, Boston, MA.

Goldfarb, R., & Serpanos, Y. (2020). *Professional writing in speech-language pathology and audiology* (3rd ed.). San Diego, CA: Plural Publishing.

Papir-Bernstein, W. (2018). *The practitioner's path in speech-language pathology: The art of school-based practice.* San Diego, CA: Plural Publishing.

15

Nontraditional Dissemination of Research

INTRODUCTION

Rosenbek (2012, p. 37) considered dissemination to require "building a bridge of data and action between laboratory and clinic." He and many others were concerned that empirically based treatments were slow to diffuse into professional practice, while treatments that lack empirical support were diffused more rapidly, resulting in a quality gap in the care of individuals with communication disorders. Our mutual friend, the late Dr. Sadanand Singh (Plural Publishing's founder), was concerned that clinical activity was motivated more by belief, tradition, and habit than by data.

The gap between knowing and doing is only partially spanned through a clinician's consumption of the latest research from publications, continuing education, and professional meetings. Providing effective and efficient care to individuals with communication impairments requires clinicians and clinical researchers to study the science of dissemination. Translational research (see Chapter 5) includes models of bench-to-bedside, bedside-to-community, and back again, as well as the concepts of evidence-based practice (EBP) and practice-based evidence (PBE). This may also be called implementation research (Feuerstein et al., 2018) that highlights the value and partnership between researchers and practitioners.

Learning Objectives

After reading this chapter, the student will be able to

- describe a marketing strategy for a device, instrument, therapy, or test you have developed;
- describe differences between Web 1.0 and Web 2.0 technologies; and
- describe how to disseminate research through social media.

CHALLENGES TO DISSEMINATION

Marketing and Distribution

There is an enormous infrastructure in place to support research. Notwithstanding stiff competition, there are almost too many funders and funding mechanisms to count in health-related fields with highly coordinated systems that solicit, review, score, and process research grant applications. Extensive peer-review systems evaluate research findings from individual studies, and systematic reviews and meta-analyses review the evidence from multiple investigations. Extensive data from demographic studies direct our focus, provide a rationale for research, and help us to form hypotheses. In other words, researchers are well supported, well trained, well supervised, and well directed to collect the evidence basis for efficacious (effective and efficient) treatment of communication disorders. Now contrast this vast support with the meager efforts our professions have made or the limited systems put in place to help with distribution or even marketing the remarkable evidence that clinicians in the field and scientists in the laboratories have collected.

Writing from their perspective as public health professionals, Kreuter and Bernhardt (2009) identified a system of links in a marketing and distribution chain that is necessary to disseminate public health information. They hold up the National Vaccine Plan as a system that works, but note the lack of other coordinated health care systems. There are far more gaps in the dissemination chain than links. Marketing and distribution functions are needed, but we don't know who will perform these functions.

Here is a hypothetical example. You have read research (see, e.g., Baylow, Goldfarb, & Steinberg, 2014) that evaluated both pharyngeal transit times and pharyngeal delay times for swallowing in adults with acute stroke. Results demonstrated that for adults with acute stroke and dysphagia, swallows were significantly longer for a 1-ml liquid bolus immediately after compared to immediately before a videofluoroscopic swallowing evaluation (VFSE). Based on this evidence, you have developed a handheld device to measure pharyngeal transit and delay times. Recall that research and development (R & D, or research designed to justify marketing a product) requires that you include a disclosure of a financial interest when you submit your results for publication. You have done a proof-of-concept study as well as Phase I and Phase II trials (see Chapter 5) that supported the conclusion that you have an effective device. Using this device would be much cheaper and safer than VFSE for adults with acute stroke who have suspected dysphagia. It would also benefit homebound adults with strokes who cannot get to a hospital for a VFSE. How do you get your device into the hands of the people who can use it? Box 15–1 shows the links in the dissemination chain that we currently can do and cannot do, or cannot do well (Bernhardt, Mays, & Kreuter, 2011; Kreuter & Bernhardt, 2009).

Of the 14 links in the dissemination chain noted, most of them are broken. Putting them in place would be time consuming and expensive, and most researchers are ill equipped to commit either the time or the money.

Box 15–1. Links in the Marketing Chain for Dissemination

Client research and segmentation: We have some good information about the target population as well as connections to some potential adopting organizations.

Packaging: We can probably do a good job of including all information required for use, making the product easy to set up and operate, and even put it in an attractive package.

Promotion: We may be able to disseminate the device one by one, but we do not have good ways of increasing awareness and demand for the device, much less knowing how to segment potential adopters into homogeneous groups on the basis of needs.

Transfer: Our professions do not have much experience in moving a product from a producer to a distributor.

Distribution: We do not have a network that offers potential consumers convenience and access in acquiring your device. There is no efficient distribution infrastructure to enhance translation of research evidence to clinical practice (Bernhardt et al., 2011).

Inventory management: You will have to find someone to perform this task.

Sales: Some person or persons will have to determine and negotiate pricing, process payments, and evaluate sales.

Communication: You or your designees will have to ensure that appropriate information is delivered before, during, and after a user gets the device.

Training: Will the device be appropriate for self-guided use? Will clinicians need training?

Technical assistance: Implementation support may require availability of local agents.

Customer service: There must be a rapid response to user needs and questions.

Product service: You must repair broken devices and honor warrantees.

Coordination: All intermediaries must work seamlessly together.

Evaluation and data analysis: You must assess all aspects of marketing and distribution.

Web 2.0 Technologies

Dissemination of information through publication in peer-reviewed journals, presentation of research at professional meetings, academic syntheses of research in university and continuing education, and other traditional strategies will always remain important. Similarly, researchers will continue to synthesize literature, develop hypotheses, and secure funding. At present, it is mainly up to professors, medical center and laboratory researchers, and others with ties to academic domains to carry out the research that generates evidence while clinicians and other practitioners incorporate and implement the evidence into everyday practice. However, Bernhardt et al. (2011) advocate for leveraging Web 2.0 technologies to enhance dissemination of research and implementation of evidence-based practices. Web 1.0 refers to Internet-based technologies that limit users to the passive viewing of content created by others. A general understanding of the term *Web 2.0* is that electronic, Web-based applications and technologies can be harnessed to improve interactive collaboration, user-friendly design, and interoperability.

In traditional media, information is passed down from a source to an audience. In a Web 2.0 application for communication sciences and disorders (CSD), the orientation will be client-centered with a major focus on sharing information interactively. Users of Web 2.0 applications will interact with other users, application developers, and laboratory researchers; all will be able to create and have control over content. Applications will be available via wireless devices, such as smart phones and watches (and who knows what else). Some commonly used Web 2.0 examples at present include social networking, wikis, blogs and microblogs, educational platforms, and other sharing sites. No doubt, when this book is published, there will be additional means of improving interactivity, user engagement, and multidirectional information exchange. The hope is for translational speech-language pathology and audiology research (see Chapter 5) to be disseminated seamlessly, either as EBP or as PBE. In other words, we need dissemination 2.0 to correspond with and take advantage of Web 2.0, bearing in mind that dissemination overload can lead to message fatigue in potential recipients.

Most scientists and clinicians agree that new developments often fail to pass from academic to treatment environments. As Rosenbek (2012, p. 39) says, "Gown and town are different, not in value but in values, and the differences matter." He continues that most research studies are done with validity, not translation in mind, and finds it ironic that the studies with the greatest validity may be the least likely to be implemented in clinical practice. That is, studies with strong validity have rigid participant criteria and protocols that must be administered in specific ways. Compare this to the typical clients in a caseload who may bear only a resemblance to the study participants and to the clinicians who may not have the time, tools, or motivation to match the implementation procedures of the protocol.

Rather than requiring a clinician to follow the exact recipe (protocol) of a study that provides the evidence basis for treatment, Rosenbek (2012) recommends that researchers identify the active ingredients, or the parts of the treatment that are critical to its effects. Clinicians who provide these active ingredients would ensure fidelity to the treatment protocol. Treatment fidelity (Hinckley & Douglas, 2013) measures the reliability of the administration of an intervention in a treatment study; it has implications for implementation in clinical practice. This seems to be a crucial measure, but only a small fraction of the aphasia studies reviewed explicitly reported treatment fidelity.

Disseminating Research Through Social Media

What are you trying to achieve when you use social media for dissemination of research? There are many benefits, but also some disadvantages (Devitt, 2016). The main advantage is that social media has the potential of reaching vast numbers of people. There is also a minimal amount of time between writing and publishing. However, remember that once an article is published on the Internet, it is there to stay and it prevents you from submitting the work to peer-reviewed journals that accept only unpublished manuscripts. When consuming nontraditional information on social media, remember that it has not been peer reviewed, so be skeptical, especially of grandiose claims. As the U.S. dollar indicates, "In God we trust," but we might add, "All others show data." Finally, you need to check if the university, agency, or other institution where you study or work has a policy about social media.

Social media such as Facebook and microblogging sites such as Twitter can be very effective in publicizing work that has been published in a traditional format. In fact, some journals even have shortened URLs that can be included as hyperlinks without using up too much of your 280-character limit on Twitter. This click-through function of embedded hyperlinks is also available on Facebook. Use of hashtags not only allows you to widen the distribution of your messages, but it also enables you to measure how often people are tweeting about the work. If you have followers, you can encourage them to retweet your messages. Notwithstanding all the warnings about self-publishing, the easiest way to get your work out is through a blog covering your research. There is no way to predict which sites will be available at the time this book is published to host your blog at no charge. Upgrades and premium services will likely come at a cost. Social media resources for scientists (Bik & Goldstein, 2013) can be informative and rewarding and can enhance professional networking. A list of them appears in Box 15–2.

There is an ASHA social media blog called ASHAsphere (https://blog.asha.org) that started August 31, 2010. Bloggers share clinical insights and are occasionally invited by the *ASHA Leader* to submit a post on the blog. For example, my colleague and I were asked to write about the ups and downs of working as Fulbright Specialists (http://blog.asha.org/2013/07/30/what-does-a-fulbright-specialist-do/?utm_source=feedburner&utm_medium=feed&utm_campaign=Feed%3A+ASHAsphere+%28ASHAsphere%29) after we returned from our overseas posts.

Social media is also an excellent way to connect with like-minded individuals when looking for a graduate school, an internship, a fellowship, or a job. It is helpful to have an online description of your professional background. Setting up an academic profile is easy, and you may already have one where you work or study. For example, my faculty profile is found at https://www.adelphi.edu/faculty/profiles/profile.php?PID=0020 and you can use it as a guide to set up yours. If you have a Google account, you can generate or activate an academic profile on Google Scholar. Finally, researchers and academics have their own social networks. With the most prominent of these, ResearchGate and Academia, you can develop an online profile that will allow you to post your published research as well as works in progress. LinkedIn, with its legions of members, does not yet have a mechanism to publicize or develop clinical research.

Box 15–2. Social Media Resources for Scientists

Type	*Description*	*Examples*
Aggregate media	Organize tweets, videos, blog posts	Storify
AAC apps	Software used on mobile devices	Visual Talker, My Talker
Blogs	Traditional, long-form, online narrative	Wordpress, Blogger
Linking communities	Content aggregation sites	Digg, MetaFilter
Microblogging	A. Hashtags let users aggregate tweets	Twitter
	B. Publish any type of media quickly	Tumblr
Photo-only microblogging	Themed "boards" for posting content	Pinterest
RSS Feeds	Mine blog/website updates without a Web browser	Google Reader
Social profiles	May reach a different audience; can be private	Facebook

Disseminating Research to Communities

A systematic review of outpatient and community-based interventions for aphasia (Lanyon, Rose, & Worrall, 2013) raised three broad questions: Will participation in these groups help adults with chronic aphasia communicate better? Will participation improve quality of life and psychosocial well-being for these people? Will both improvements occur? Results showed that community-based participation can result in improvement of specific linguistic processes. There was also a trend toward a benefit in establishing social networks and community access, but little evidence for improvement in functional communication. The 29 studies that met the criteria for inclusion were Level II and Level III studies that showed medium to large effect sizes.

Systems for appraising research evidence usually place qualitative evidence at lower levels, but strategies to disseminate research to communities should consider qualitative as well as quantitative findings. The definition of EBP is broad enough to include qualitative inquiry and recognize it as an important and even unique source of information. This expanding view of evidence led to three hypotheses about clinical intervention in CSD (Mastergeorge, 2007): qualitative interviews can be an EBP; maternal beliefs are relevant evidence; and both are needed to inform clinical decision making. Mothers of children with developmental delay (DD) were matched with an equal number of mothers of typically developing children. There was a special learning environment for the DD group as their skills were highly variable with resultant difficulty in establishing daily routines. These trends were observed in descriptive analyses of discourse data. The data from these analyses and interviews showed similarities in beliefs and goals of the mothers of the children in the DD group. Maternal belief systems affect parent–child interactions, can be linked to clinical interventions, and may be dependent on context and cultural practices.

Levels of evidence also differ according to the audience addressed. For example, a successful protocol for implementing newborn hearing screening must satisfy quite a few stakeholders: families of children who are deaf or hard of hearing, the general public, the Deaf communities, health care administrators, physicians of a number of different specialties, private and governmental insurance providers, managed care, and politicians (Yoshinaga-Itano, 2004). There is a robust and repeatable positive effect of screening on early identification and intervention in the first 6 months of life. However, the skill set that produces the scientific rigor of a screening study is not the same as that required to bring all the stakeholders on board to establish health care policies. We find an example in a study of resilience in children with communication disorders (Nelson, 2012). Early intervention and prevention programs typically start in pre-K or kindergarten and can run through middle school to help children with language and learning disabilities develop resilience. CSD professionals need to develop both EBP and PBE to examine causal relationships between resilience intervention and developmental outcomes, relationships between prevention efforts and effects outside of the immediate domain of treatment, changes that persist over time through longitudinal studies, collaboration between researchers and clinicians, and cost–benefit analyses (Nelson, 2012).

As noted above, collaboration among such stakeholders as clinicians, families, researchers, and funders is essential but challenging. Theoretical rationales supporting such collaboration are helpful and include translational research, the bidirectional exchange of information between researchers and practitioners, and community-based participatory research that supports implementation of evidence-based practices in community-based settings and maximizes interactions between and among researchers, therapists, and parents (Searcy, Stahmer, & Brookman-Frazee, 2012). An early-intervention effort for children with autism spectrum disorders called the BRIDGE Collaborative (Searcy et al., 2012) brought together a transdisciplinary team that is currently working with new funding agencies, developing new training methods, and expanding to new communities.

The harmful effect on hearing of excessive noise has led to the U.S. Environmental Protection Agency Noise Control Act, 42 U.S.C. §4901 (1972) that alerts the public to potentially hazardous noise-emitting products. Manufacturers are required to include a decibel level in the noise rating of the product. Serpanos and Berg (2012) identified ways for health care professionals to disseminate findings about research related to noise-induced hearing loss. These include regular and periodic education of NICU personnel; guidelines from AAA and ASHA to reflect current knowledge about hearing screening protocols to identify high-frequency hearing loss; public health campaigns to specify guidelines for safe operation of personal listening devices (PLDs), toys, and other noise-emitting devices; research and development for sound-isolation and noise-cancelling functions of PLDs and the other devices mentioned previously; local legislation to limit noise levels and national legislation to require disclaimers on noise-emitting products; and hearing conservation programs that target vulnerable populations such as children and adolescents.

Hapner (2012) reported that large-scale, community-based oral cancer screenings were reported in Japan and some European countries, but they were rare in the United States. In an earlier study, she and a colleague (Hapner & Wise, 2011) found that a large-scale, community-based screening that targeted an at-risk population could be effective. In the Hapner & Wise study, the at-risk population included NASCAR (auto racing) fans, who were identified by the researchers as more likely to smoke and use alcohol. SLPs provide treatment for the communication and swallowing problems that accompany head and neck cancer and are well positioned to assist otolaryngologists in developing and applying prevention strategies, as well as in educating colleagues and the general public about personal wellness strategies. The SLP who wants to implement and disseminate a head and neck cancer prevention and wellness program has access to the following resources (Hapner, 2012, p. 73): an oral cancer screening tool (http://www.mouthandthroatcancer.org) from the nonprofit organization Voices of Hope; training and interpretation of FEES in adults (http://www.pluralpublishing.com/publication_tif.htm); and interpretation of videostroboscopy (https://pluralpublishing.com/publication_rlvc.htm and http://www.emoryvoicecenter.org).

Summary

Implementation research requires researchers to embrace practitioners' views. A study of a treatment protocol for intentional communication (Feuerstein et al., 2018) used qualitative methods to explore practitioners' perceptions about the following: early intervention, assessment, and treatment of intentional communication; training for the evidence-based protocol; and use of the protocol in clinical practice. Regardless of the strength of research findings, it is up to practitioners to implement the treatment protocol. There is always a tension between theory and practice, and collaboration must recognize differences in knowledge (scientific rigor of researchers and in-depth understanding of applications of practitioners) and beliefs (active ingredients of the intervention, dosage, outcomes, and treatment fidelity for the researchers; variables associated with service delivery, such as client, practitioner, and practice setting characteristics for the practitioners). In a traditional approach, the one that seems to be in operation at present, researchers seem to be driving the implementation process, and practitioners may offer advice but have minimal involvement in designing the protocol. The skewed investment in the treatment approach may adversely affect its success.

SUPPORT GROUPS FOR COMMUNICATION DISORDERS

Individuals with communication disorders and their caregivers are often exposed to new research in causes, treatments, and prevention of their individual speech, language, or hearing disability through an advocacy or support group. Professionals can find support in a variety of areas through the ASHA Special Interest Groups (SIGs). SIG publications, which are considered peer-reviewed starting in 2018, offer opportunities for the continuing education hours required for speech-language pathologists (SLPs) and audiologists (As) to maintain their Certificate of Clinical Competence from ASHA as well as state licensure. While the following discipline-related list is hardly comprehensive, it represents an array of support groups for individuals we serve. There are also support groups identified with an overall disorder, such as Alzheimer, amyotrophic lateral sclerosis, cerebral palsy, multiple sclerosis, and Parkinson. Some groups fund research, and if you have a good idea for a small research project, it might be worthwhile to contact the relevant association.

Augumentative and Alternative Commuication

Among the many support groups for individuals who use augmentative and alternative communication (AAC) devices, SLPs often have to teach parents to be advocates for their children who use AAC devices (Seligman-Wine, 2007). Product developers, such as the Rehabilitation Engineering Research Center (RERC; rerc-aac.psu.edu.), have the goal of enabling individuals with complex communication needs to maximize their participation in education, employment, health, and community activities. Dissemination projects to reach AAC stakeholders include the RERC AAC website; webcasts and YouTube channel; e-blasts; conference presentations, proceedings, and journal publications; consumer newsletters, blogs, and technical assistance; and free e-prints.

Aphasia

Founded in 1987, the National Aphasia Association (NAA; https://www.aphasia.org/) is the first national organization dedicated to advocating for persons with aphasia and their families. It has the following goal: to provide access to research, education, rehabilitation, and therapeutic and advocacy services to individuals with aphasia and their caregivers. The NAA serves as a clearinghouse for resources, and offers a community of support for individuals with aphasia and their caregivers.

Autism

According to its mission statement, the goals of Autism Speaks (https://www.autismspeaks.org) are to promote solutions, across the spectrum and throughout the life span, for the needs of individuals with autism and their families through advocacy and support; to increase understanding and acceptance of people with autism spectrum disorder; and to advance research into causes and better interventions for autism spectrum disorder and related conditions. The organization supports research through grants and fellowships to evaluate new interventions and support services.

Childhood Apraxia of Speech

The Childhood Apraxia of Speech Association of North America (CASANA) (http://www.apraxia-kids.org) is the only national nonprofit organization representing the needs of children with apraxia and their families (NIDCD, 2017). The goals are to provide information, education, and some financial support for speech therapy; provide support for a national conference and regional training institutes; and provide research support that connects families to researchers, funds research projects, and hosts research symposia.

Cleft Lip and Palate

There are many support groups for individuals with cleft lip and palate and their families. For example, the mission of cleftAdvocate (http://www.cleftadvocate.org) is to provide educational opportunities, on- and off-line support networks, and social interaction and advocacy guidelines. Operation Smile (https://www.operationsmile.org/), founded in 1982, is a volunteer and fundraising organization that provides surgery to repair cleft lips and palates for children around the world, while Smile Train (https://www.smiletrain.org/), founded in 1999, supports local doctors in 87 countries who perform surgical repairs. The Cleft Lip and Palate Association (CLAPA; https://www.clapa.com), organized in 1979, is based in the United Kingdom and serves as a partnership between people affected by cleft and health professionals. CLAPA helps members understand research in cleft palate and helps health professionals, patients, and their families get involved either as a participant or as part of a research team.

Cochlear Implants

The goals of the American Cochlear Implant Alliance (https://www.acialliance.org/blogpost/1334356/248481/Adult-CI-Support-Groups) are to encourage and support research on candidacy, criteria, and the broad impacts of cochlear implants for children and adults; advance awareness of best practices related to cochlear implants among patients and their families, clinicians (including primary care doctors and other health professionals), early interventionists, educators, policy-makers, payers, and the general public; and educate and encourage policy-makers and payers to take steps that expand access to cochlear implants.

Dysphagia

The National Foundation of Swallowing Disorders (http://swallowingdisorderfoundation.com) has the mission of improving quality of life for individuals with dysphagia. By enhancing direct patient support, education, and research, as well as raising public, professional, and governmental awareness, their goals are to advance the prevention and treatment of swallowing disorders. Some support organizations in the United Kingdom focus on disorders that include dysphagia among its symptoms, such as stroke (http://www.stroke.org.uk) and patients on intravenous and naso-gastric nutrition treatment (PINNT; https://pinnt.com).

Hearing Loss

Founded in 1979, the mission of the Hearing Loss Association of America (HLAA; https://www.hearingloss.org/) is to open the world of communication to people with hearing loss by providing information, education, support, and advocacy. HLAA seeks to reduce the stigma associated with hearing loss, to advocate at grassroots and national levels for communication access such as assistive devices in public spaces, and to use educational programs to protect hearing. The association offers hearing help such as finding a professional, learning about technology, and joining a community.

Laryngectomy

The Web Whispers (http://www.webwhispers.org) support group was started in 1996 for those who had questions about larynx cancer treatments, surgery, recovery, and what life is like after laryngectomy surgery. Its mission is education, rehabilitation, and support, and its membership is composed of patients, caregivers, medical professionals, and suppliers of the special products that individuals need after laryngectomy. The National Association of Laryngectomee Clubs (http://www.laryngectomy.org.uk/) in the United Kingdom includes the Lost Chord Club (http://www.lostchordstoke.org.uk) whose mission is similar to Web Whispers.

Stuttering

According to its mission statement, the National Stuttering Association (NSA) (https://westutter.org/) is a nonprofit organization empowering children and adults who stutter, their families, and professionals through support, education, advocacy, and research. NSA provides support through local chapters and programs for advocacy, families, and education, and hopes to be a catalyst for research on efficacy of research as well as the cause and cure of stuttering. According to its mission statement, the Stuttering Foundation (https://stutteringhelp.org/), established in 1947, provides free online resources, services, and support to individuals who stutter and their families, as well as support for research into the causes of stuttering. The Foundation also offers training programs and materials on stuttering and cluttering (books, DVDs) for professionals. I have received funding from the Stuttering Foundation for a symposium on ethics and research in stuttering, as well as financial support for a PhD student's dissertation research on stuttering. Since 2001, the Stuttering Association for the Young (SAY; http://www.say.org/) has been a nonprofit organization offering programs that address the physical, social, and emotional impacts of stuttering. Programs aimed at more effective communication include Camp SAY, speech therapy, the Confident Voices after-school and weekend program, and Storytellers for teens. Early in their existence, when SAY was called Our Time,

I received funding from the Stuttering Foundation for the Our Time teen theatre company to perform at the CUNY Graduate Center.

ADVOCATING FOR THE PROFESSIONS

Advocacy involves building relationships. In *grassroots advocacy*, people work together to support a cause or a position. Student activities (for example, through the National Student Speech-Language-Hearing Association [NSSLHA]) may involve such grassroots activities as university hearing screenings, bake sales to support the Speech and Hearing Center, or posters representing best practices in speech, language, and hearing interventions displayed on your university's Research Day. In *legislative advocacy*, professionals and student leaders may visit the federal, state, and local governments that are responsible for creating and passing laws as well as monitoring existing legislation. In *regulatory advocacy*, professionals and student representatives may visit the federal, state, and local agencies that are responsible for interpreting and implementing the legislation passed by governmental bodies. At all stages of advocacy, a command of research support in human communication and its disorders strengthens arguments to promote and advance the interests of CSD.

Some examples of advocacy in our professions involve older debates, such as the whole-language philosophy (Shapiro, 1992) and points of view regarding auditory integration training for autism (Monville & Nelson, 1994; Nelson, 1994); and more recent discussions, such as the use of implementation science as a model for cognitive-communication screenings of adults with acute stroke (Hinckley, 2014); and current practices for evaluating speech-language outcomes for preschoolers with communication disorders using the International Classification of Functioning-CY Body Functions and Activities components (Cunningham et al., 2017, pp. 459–460).

A major topic for advocacy in CSD is the concept of highest-qualified provider. Many states in the United States that license individuals as speech-language pathologists and audiologists follow guidelines set by ASHA, including the master's degree for SLPs and the AuD for audiologists as the minimum degree for best practices. Some states, especially ones where graduate-trained CSD professionals are in short supply, allow licensing of audiologist assistants and SLP assistants. Physicians and hearing-aid dealers are exempt from the requirement to have audiology licensure. A proposal to add a third category of audiology technician or assistant who would not need an audiology license resulted in a flurry of articles, proposed position statements, and letters to the editor of the *American Journal of Audiology* in the mid-1990s when requirements for the AuD were established. Many professionals with CCC-A abandoned ASHA at that time for AAA, an organization that they thought did a better job of advocating for their best interests. In its chapter on speech-language pathology and audiology regulations, ASHA (2016) proposed model regulations for state licensure that allows recognition of audiology assistants who have only a high school diploma and SLPs who have only an associate's degree.

Advocating for highest-qualified provider means that, at least in some states, individuals (especially schoolchildren) may not receive the CSD services they need. On the other hand, allowing technicians or assistants to do the job under the supervision of professionals may result in inadequate service or convince heads of schools or medical offices that they can save money by paying lower-qualified people less while still complying minimally with some state and federal regulations. In the debate about highest-quality provider, knowing the research on both sides of the topic is essential for both legislative and regulatory advocacy.

IN THE NEWS

University News

Most colleges and universities have an office for university news. The office will usually include a media kit to help researchers prepare a press release for local or even national newspapers. There should also be a section for a speakers' bureau that will list areas of research specialization in such categories as health and education where CSD members can be listed as media experts. A profile section lists accomplishments of students, faculty, and alumni that include recent research projects. Use Box 15–3 for practice in filling out a news release form.

Association Publications

The *ASHA Leader* has guidelines for members to submit articles or blogs that can reach the roughly 200,000 ASHA members. Find the writing guidelines for the *Leader* at https://leader.pubs.asha.org/SS/Writers_Guidelines_for_The_ASHA_Leader.aspx and remember that you are writing for a newsmagazine, not a scholarly journal. Find the blogger application form for the *Leader Live* at https://blog.asha.org/blogger-application-form/ and fill out the Guest Contributor Application Form. A sample of some newsworthy items includes a report from SIG 9 on hearing disorders in children (Blaiser, 2017), an online conference on autism spectrum disorders (Faustino & Longden, 2016), and data snapshots of ASHA researchers (ASHA Researchers, 2010).

New research is often presented in the context of continuing education at local and state levels. For example, proposals to the New York State Speech, Hearing, and Language Association (NYSSHLA) should be sent to http://www.nysslha.org/continuing-education/, where the editors of the NYSSHLA *Communicator* will determine whether or not to list the event in the association newsletter. Other state associations have similar mechanisms for dissemination of new research findings. All ASHA members must earn at least 30 hours of continuing education every 3 years, whether you are a new member, an established member, or even a life member. Many members opt to complete the Award for Continuing Education (ACE) that requires at least 70 hours of continuing education in the same 3-year period. ASHA sends an ACE certificate to these members and a letter to their employers. Lifelong learning is a good way to stay on top of the latest research and to keep your own research skills sharp.

Box 15–3. Sample News Release Form

Share Your News or Story with Us

Our communications and marketing team is eager to get the word out about your research. We welcome content ideas for our various channels, which include the following:

- University website
- School and program newsletters (print and electronic)
- Weekly e-mail sent campus-wide on Mondays
- University social media channels
- University Magazine for alumni
- Magazine on faculty scholarship
- Media relations

Below is a form to help you share news and information. We review and consider all submissions, and will update you with thoughts and plans for covering your suggested news. To request an event post, please use the "Event Listing Request" form instead.

Name: ________________ First ________________ Last

University Email: __________ Enter Email __________ Confirm Email

Department/Organization: ____________________________

Please share the category/categories of your news:

☐ Student Achievements
☐ Faculty Research
☐ Alumni Accomplishments and Contributions
☐ Campus Events
☐ Other Initiatives

Please share your primary audiences:
Check all that apply

☐ University faculty
☐ University staff
☐ University graduate student
☐ University undergraduate student
☐ Alumna/Alumnus
☐ Prospective students and families
☐ Parents of current students
☐ The media
☐ The public
☐ Other

Please let us know about any specific goals, such as event attendance or participation, raising awareness, supporting a strategic initiative, and so forth.

Please tell us about your news in as much detail as possible, including dates and locations, contact information, and assets you already have (photos, background information, flyer, website, etc.).

Do you need a photo taken for this news?

☐ Yes ☐ No

Please allow at least two weeks lead time for content.

CONCLUSION

In closing this chapter as well as the book, it is important to acknowledge that some new researchers are concerned that they will not have important questions to test as hypotheses or that they will run out of questions. While new researchers certainly need mentors to hone their thinking about research—understanding what is achievable as a project in comparison to a program of research—it is more likely that you will run out of time before you run out of questions. Some techniques of counseling that are associated with dissemination are also helpful as exercises to help the clinical researcher formulate experimental ideas. Counseling skills are crucial if we are to communicate effectively as clinicians and as researchers to each other and to other stakeholders in our mutual quest to help individuals with speech, language, and hearing disabilities. There are quiet and loud techniques (Holland, 2012). Quiet techniques focus on listening in terms of clarifying, disclosing, and affirming, as well as practice with listening to help clients and families understand the process of change. Loud techniques include informing, explaining, teaching, and advising. Helping others to change is the goal, and it is often necessary for the clinician to enlist the client, who may also act as a student clinician's mentor (see Chapter 9); the families and caregivers, who are frequently unofficial SLP assistants; and the researcher, who needs to know what helps in order to refine protocols and hypotheses. These quiet and loud techniques, that Holland (2012) offers clear and entertaining ways to practice, contribute to your success as a clinician or a researcher. If you can identify as both, that is, as a clinician–researcher, then you have the best job in the world.

ADVANCED STUDY

The author proposes that skills in nontraditional dissemination of research are necessary for an individual to be granted power of professor. With new generations of scholars and researchers needed every 10 years, professors and master clinicians have an obligation to prepare individuals with adequate knowledge and skills to undertake the tasks of scholarship and research, and nontraditional dissemination of research is a key component. For evidence of the requisite skills in understanding nontraditional dissemination of research, complete the following and have your instructor, academic adviser, mentor, or CSD department chair review that you have completed the requirements and sign and date where indicated.

Student's Name: ______________________________

1. List three links in the marketing chain for dissemination that are broken, and suggest ways to strengthen the chain.
2. Describe and give an example of a difference between Web 1.0 and Web 2.0 technologies.
3. What do you think Rosenbek means by "active ingredients" in a validated therapy protocol?
4. Do an Internet search of a CSD support group in an area of your interest. Describe it and copy and paste the URL.
5. What are the three ways to advocate? Give one example for each way.
6. How would you submit a blog item to the online version of the *ASHA Leader*?

Date of Completion: ______________________________

Faculty/Supervisor Signature: ______________________________

REFERENCES

American Speech-Language-Hearing Association. (2016). *Model regulations for state licensure of audiologists, speech-language pathologists, and audiology and speech-language pathology assistants*. Retrieved from https://www.asha.org/uploadedFiles/State-Licensure-Model-Regulations.pdf

ASHA Researchers: Data Snapshots. (2010). *The ASHA Leader, 15*(12), 20–22. doi:10.1044/leader.AN2.15122010.20

Baylow, H., Goldfarb, R., & Steinberg, R. (2014). Swallowing effect and suspected neuromuscular fatigue in adults with acute stroke: A videofluorographic analysis. *Journal of Medical Speech-Language Pathology, 21*, 333–342.

Bernhardt, J. M., Mays, D., & Kreuter, M. W. (2011). Dissemination 2.0: Closing the gap between knowledge and practice with new media and marketing. *Journal of Health Communication, 16*(Suppl. 1), 32–44.

Bik, H. M., & Goldstein, M. C. (2013). An introduction to social media for scientists. *PLoS Biology, 11*, e1001535.

Blaiser, K. (2017). Special interest group 9, hearing and hearing disorders in childhood. *The ASHA Leader, 29*(3), 8–29. doi:10.1044/leader.SIGS.22032017.np

Cunningham, B. J., Washington, K. N., Binns, A., Rolfe, K., Robertson, B., & Rosenbaum, P. (2017). Current methods of evaluating speech-language outcomes for preschoolers with communication disorders: A scoping review using the ICF-CY. *Journal of Speech, Language, and Hearing Research, 60*, 447–464.

Devitt, P. (2016). How to use social media to disseminate research findings. *Nursing Children and Young People, 28*, 20.

Faustino, P., & Longden, D. (2016). ASD: On its best behavior. *The ASHA Leader, 21*(2). doi:10.1044/leader.OV.21022016.np

Feuerstein, J. L., Olswang, L. B., Greenslade, K. J., Dowden, P., Pinder, G. L., & Madden, J. (2018). Implementation research: Embracing practitioners' views. *Journal of Speech, Language, and Hearing Research, 61*, 645–657.

Hapner, E. R. (2012). Community- and office-based oral, head, and neck cancer screening and education. In R. Goldfarb (Ed.), *Translational speech-language pathology and audiology* (pp. 69–74). San Diego, CA: Plural Publishing.

Hapner, E. R., & Wise, J. C. (2011). Results of large scale head and neck cancer screenings of NASCAR fans. *Journal of Voice, 25*, 480–483.

Hinckley, J. J. (2014). A case for the implementation of cognitive-communication screenings in acute stroke. *American Journal of Speech-Language Pathology, 23*, 4–14.

Hinckley, J. J., & Douglas, N. F. (2013). Treatment fidelity: Its importance and reported frequency in aphasia treatment studies. *American Journal of Speech-Language Pathology, 22*, S279–S284.

Holland, A. L. (2012). Counseling around the edges of traditional treatment. In R. Goldfarb (Ed.), *Translational speech-language pathology and audiology* (pp. 343–352). San Diego, CA: Plural Publishing.

Kreuter, M. W., & Bernhardt, J. M. (2009). Reframing the dissemination challenge: A marketing and distribution perspective. *American Journal of Public Health, 99*, 2123–2127.

Lanyon, L. E., Rose, M. L., & Worrall, L. (2013). The efficacy of outpatient and community-based aphasia group interventions: A systematic review. *International Journal of Speech-Language Pathology, 15*, 359–374.

Mastergeorge, A. M. (2007). Maternal belief systems: The discourse of cultural practice as evidence. *Topics in Language Disorders, 27*, 62–73.

Monville, D. K., & Nelson, N. W. (1994). Parental viewpoints on change following auditory integration training for autism. *American Journal of Speech-Language Pathology, 2*, 41–53.

National Institute on Deafness and other Communication Disorders. (2017). *Childhood Apraxia of Speech Association of North America (CASANA)*. Retrieved from https://www.nidcd.nih.gov/directory/childhood-apraxia-speech-association-north-america-casana

Nelson, L. K. (2012). Promoting resilience in young children: A role in prevention of communication disorders. In R. Goldfarb (Ed.), *Translational speech-language pathology and audiology* (pp. 43–49). San Diego, CA: Plural.

Nelson, N. W. (1994). Clinical research, the placebo effect, responsibility to families, and other concerns stimulated by auditory integration training. *American Journal of Speech-Language Pathology, 2*, 106–111.

Rosenbek, J. C. (2012). The science of dissemination. In R. Goldfarb (Ed.), *Translational speech-language pathology and audiology* (pp. 37–42). San Diego, CA: Plural Publishing.

Searcy, K. L., Stahmer, A., & Brookman-Frazee, L. (2012). SoCal BRIDGE collaborative across treatment disciplines. In R. Goldfarb (Ed.), *Translational speech-language pathology and audiology* (pp. 59–66). San Diego, CA: Plural Publishing.

Seligman-Wine, J. (2007). Supporting families of children who use AAC. *The ASHA Leader, 12*(10), 17–19. doi:10.1044/leader.FTR1.12102007.17

Serpanos, Y. C., & Berg, A. L. (2012). Noise exposure and the potential impact on hearing in the pediatric population. In R. Goldfarb (Ed.), *Translational speech-language pathology and audiology* (pp. 107–112). San Diego, CA: Plural Publishing.

Shapiro, H. R. (1992). Debatable issues underlying whole-language philosophy: A speech-language pathologist's perspective. *Language, Speech, and Hearing Services in Schools, 23,* 308–311.

United States Environmental Protection Agency Noise Control Act, 42 U.S.C. §4901 (1972).

Yoshinaga-Itano, C. (2004). Levels of evidence: Universal newborn hearing screening (UNHS) and early hearing detection and intervention systems (EHDI). *Journal of Communication Disorders, 37,* 451–465.

INDEX

E

F

G

H

I

J

L

M

N

O

P

Q

R

S

T

U

V